Index of Prescription Drugs 1998

Index of Prescription Drugs 1998

Frederick H. Meyers, MD
Professor of Pharmacology
University of California, San Francisco
San Francisco, California

Constantine J. Gean, MD, F.A.C.P.M.
Associate Clinical Professor
Division of Occupational and Environmental Medicine
Department of Medicine
University of California, Irvine
Irvine, California

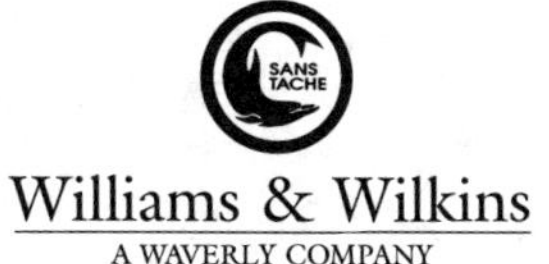

Williams & Wilkins
A WAVERLY COMPANY
BALTIMORE • PHILADELPHIA • LONDON • PARIS • BANGKOK
BUENOS AIRES • HONG KONG • MUNICH • SYDNEY • TOKYO • WROCLAW

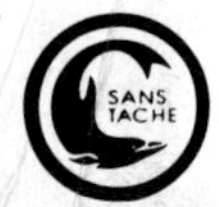

Editor: Donna Balado
Managing Editor: Jennifer Schmidt
Marketing Manager: Tara Williams
Cover Designer: Shepherd, Inc.
Typesetter: Maryland Composition Co., Inc.
Printer and Binder: Vicks Lithograph & Printing

351 West Camden Street
Baltimore, Maryland 21201-2436 USA

Rose Tree Corporate Center
1400 North Providence Road
Building II, Suite 5025
Media, Pennsylvania 19063-2043 USA

Accurate indications, adverse reactions and dosage schedules for drugs are provided in this book, but it is possible that they may change. The reader is urged to review the package information data of the manufacturers of the medications mentioned.

Printed in the United States of America

ISBN 0-683-03463-4

The publishers have made every effort to trace the copyright holders for borrowed material. If they have inadvertently overlooked any, they will be pleased to make the necessary arrangements at the first opportunity.

To purchase additional copies of this book, call our customer service department at **(800) 638-0672** or fax orders to **(800) 447-8438.** For other book services, including chapter reprints and large quantity sales, ask for the Special Sales department.

Canadian customers should call **(800) 665-1148,** or fax **(800) 665-0103.** For all other calls originating outside of the United States, please call **(410) 528-4223** or fax us at **(410) 528-8550.**

Visit Williams & Wilkins on the Internet: http://www.wwilkins.com or contact our customer service department at **custserv@wwilkins.com.** Williams & Wilkins customer service representatives are available from 8:30 am to 6:00 pm, EST, Monday through Friday, for telephone access.

98 99 00 01 02
1 2 3 4 5 6 7 8 9 10

Preface

No book of this size can pretend to be an adequate guide to drug therapy. It can, however, be an aid to your memory and a guide to placing a new or unfamiliar drug in a familiar category and making your previous training and experience relevant. The alphabetical listing includes many of the euphonious trade names that contrast with the awkward generic names, allowing identification of the generic version, if available, and the flood of less than essential imitative compounds. If the drug introduces a pharmacologic class or effect new to you or to most everyone, the alphabetical listing will refer to a note in Part I that will provide a brief definition.

Nowadays, with the changes in the organization of medical practice and the participation of third parties in the choice of drugs, "providers" must be able to react knowingly to drugs and drug names prescribed by many different physicians and suggested by many agents, including the patient. The information in this book should allow the identification of a drug and the propriety of a dose or indication, which is to say that inclusion does not imply our approval or recommendation. Students, house staff, nurses, and pharmacists should find the book especially useful.

The almost dictionary approach of this book promises convenience and speed. Should you need further help in concisely and conveniently organizing drugs into clinical categories, a more comprehensive companion volume to this book is available: Pocket Drug Guide—Third Edition.

Acknowledgments

Williams & Wilkins has lent essential support in the persons of Timothy S. Satterfield, editor and publisher, and in the skilled work of Jennifer L. Schmidt.

Joan M. Meyers provided immeasurable help with the manuscript.

Contents

Guide to Part I, Definitions of Drug Classes

PART I

DEFINITIONS OF DRUG CLASSES

How can health professionals organize their information about the overwhelming number of drugs on the market today? With the confusion of names and the aggressive (and skilled) advertising, it is easy to accept each product as unique and probably superior without considering that it may be merely an imitative compound marketed to gain a share of an established market. Much more productive is an effort to place drugs in defined categories so that information and experience previously acquired becomes applicable to the "new" drug. The number of such categories is daunting but manageable. From time to time a genuinely new category appears, but there has been no difficulty in recognizing the startling advances as they have occurred.

The following classification is deliberately inconsistent in that it begins with a classification based purely on mechanism of action but then, for your convenience, and with some duplication, considers also drugs and special preparations used in particular organ systems.

CENTRAL NERVOUS SYSTEM AGENTS

Sedative-Hypnotics

This very large group of drugs and environmental agents vary widely in chemical structure but have pharmacologic effects that are similar if not identical. Included are not only the familiar drugs listed below, but also the gases and volatile liquids selected for use as general anesthetics and abused drugs, such as PCP and inhalants such as the toluene in glue and other inhalants. **Pharmacologic Effects:** Given in increasing doses, all of these drugs cause a diffuse depression of the central nervous system that ascends from the sacral cord and descends from the cortex, taking the subject through the stages of anesthesia. The effects, approximately in a dose-related order, include relief of anxiety, impaired psychomotor performance, impaired judgment, drowsiness, induction of normal sleep, reduced REM sleep, disinhibition with excitement, ataxia, nystagmus, slurred speech, euphoria, aphasia for the drugged period, anticonvulsant, loss of consciousness (surgical anesthesia with loss of swallowing and cough reflexes), voluntary muscle weakness (loss of polysynaptic cord reflexes), and respiratory depression. **With Continued Administration:** anticonvulsant, habituation, and withdrawal. Withdrawal is manifested by CNS stimulation with anxiety, sleep disturbances, hyperactivity, tremor, elevated BP, mania, and convulsions. It is common with shorter-acting hypnotics including alcohol; rare after the administration of phenobarbital or chlordiazepoxide. Behavioral and metabolic tolerance develop to a very limited extent. **Side Effects:** Adverse reactions are predicted from the above listing. Overdose toxicity is most dangerous with the shorter-acting drugs and when alcohol or other drugs are present. **Contraindications and Cautions:** Use with reduced dose and careful observation in combination with opiates. Dosages of coumarin anticoagulants must be adjusted if barbiturate type of sedative is initiated or discontinued. Patient should be warned about driving under the influence, and refills should be limited to the amounts required by a patient who is compliant with the doctor's instructions.

The further differentiation of the available compounds is based entirely on their speed of onset and duration of action. The chemical classification is not important; that is, the benzodiazepines are not safer than the barbiturates if a comparison is made between drugs with similar durations of action given in comparable doses.

Ultrashort Acting Hypnotics

The recent introduction of five benzodiazepines (clonazepam, lorazepam, temazepam, triazolam, and zolpidem) with properties entirely similar to those of alcohol requires the use of this category previously reserved for injectable induction agents. All are very rapidly acting but very brief acting hypnotics. Taken at bedtime, these drugs provide the first part of the cycle (euphoria and a brief period of sleep) but, when the patient awakens only an hour or two later, he or she is tempted, like the drinker, to repeat or increase the dose. Thereafter, when he or she awakens, the difficulty in going to sleep is intensified by the anxiety and stimulation of early withdrawal. Habituation causes even more problems when the drug is used during the day. The labeling is for bedtime use for a brief period, and their use for daytime sedation is not justified by postmarketing experience.

Other Injectable Induction Agents

Thiopental and propofol are examples of rapidly acting, short acting hypnotics used only for brief procedures or to permit intubation.

Short Acting Hypnotics

Drugs of this class, exemplified by flurazepam, should not be replaced by the ultra-short agents as the most commonly used bedtime medications. The period of sleep latency is shortened, and the action is terminated long before time for awakening. Minimal signs of withdrawal appear even with therapeutic doses. Patients receiving bedtime hypnotics regularly may, if they do not take their accustomed dose, feel the anxiety and sleep disturbances of minor withdrawal, which they misinterpret as establishing a continued need for the drug ("sleeping pill habit").

Intermediate-Acting Sedative-Hypnotics

The period of sleep latency is roughly double that after use of the short acting hypnotics, but the duration of the effect comes closer to matching the total duration of the desired sleep. Indeed, hangover may occur. These drugs, for example diazepam, are widely used for continuous, daytime sedation, but with a greater hazard of habituation and misuse than with the long-acting sedatives next described.

Long-Acting Sedatives

The most common indication for the use of sedatives, however it may be described, is for the symptomatic relief of anxiety. The long-acting sedatives carry minimal dangers of habituation or impaired motor function and judgment. Acute toxicity (as in suicidal attempts) is negligible. These agents must be given cumulatively. When the dosage is changed, the change in effect cannot be evaluated for several days.

Narcotic Analgesics

Narcotic analgesics act on the CNS to alter the perception of pain and other unpleasant stimuli so that, although still present, they are less troubling. These analgesics are derived from opium or chemically related synthetics ("opioids"). Seen with continued administration is the development of tolerance (almost but not quite absolute), a withdrawal state (hyperexcitability), and habituation. A compulsive drive to use (addiction) is a major problem with IV use of the strong narcotics, but not a major problem in the care of patients with pain because the addicting rush is not felt. "Oral habits" are not difficult to manage. Do not undertreat patients in pain. Adverse reactions include dysphoria, constipation, postural hypotension, nausea, sedation or stimulation, bradycardia, meiosis, coma, and respiratory depression.

The analgetic agents (agonists) are classified not by absolute (mg) potency but by the intensity of the pain that they can relieve. They also differ in their suitability for oral administration.

Narcotic Analgesics of Greatest Potency

Morphine, methadone, or hydromorphone can comfort a patient with even the most severe traumatic or cardiac ischemic pain. The latter two are far superior to morphine given by mouth for severe pain.

Narcotic Analgesics of Intermediate Potency

Between the categories of greatest and lowest potency are meperidine and oxycodone.

Narcotic Analgesics of Lowest Potency

Codeine and hydrocodone are useful against mild pain, e.g., post extraction, minor trauma, and most bursitis. They are also selectively more active against diarrhea. Stimulation often is prominent.

How does one select from the above groups? Sometimes, prior information is the determinant, e.g., renal colic or a myocardial infarct will require the strongest. Often, the optimal agent is determined by beginning with a non-narcotic and moving up the scale until relief is adequate.

Narcotic Antagonists

Minor chemical changes on the above drugs confer the ability to combine with opiate receptors but not to further activate the process. Depressant (but not stimulant) effects of the narcotics are reversed or prevented by such antagonists. Withdrawal will be precipitated in a dependent individual. Prior administration will deny addicts their pharmacologic reward and naltrexone is one treatment for heroin abuse.

Mixed Agonist-Antagonists

Some derivatives are at the same time both agonists and antagonists, the net or manifest effect depending upon the dose and the state of the patient

In small doses, they may be used as analgetics. With larger doses, unpleasant confusion and distorted perception occur. In the tolerant patient, withdrawal occurs.

Opioids With Purely Stimulant Effects

The depressant effects of opioids (analgesia, sedation, respiratory depression) are antagonized by the above antagonists

Remaining are the stimulant effects ranging from euphoria to convulsions. These effects are found in pure form in an old opiate, thebaine, and in propoxyphene, which has never been shown to be an analgetic but is habituating (pleasant to take) and, in large single doses, lethal (V. fibrillation).

Muscle Relaxants

Sedative-Hypnotics

The search for agents that would selectively block the reflexes underlying muscles that are spastic or in painful spasms has been unsuccessful. The complication is that the sedative hypnotics have the desired effect but only in anesthetic doses. However, the sedative (anxiety relieving) action does reduce the pain caused by muscle tension. Thus, the drugs commonly used are either acknowledged or unacknowledged sedatives, for example, diazepam or carisoprodol.

Other, Negligible, Compounds

Two atropine-like drugs are of negligible importance. If baclofen is useful, it is with the dangerous intrathecal use.

Miscellaneous

Dantrolene is active but toxic, and its use is limited to malignant hyperthermia. Unlike the previous drugs, it acts on muscle rather than on the CNS.

Anticonvulsants

Anticonvulsants suppress or limit conduction from an epileptogenic focus. As an approximation for the present purpose, epileptic states can be classed as major motor (grand mal) or partial [absences (petit mal) and psychomotor].

Sedative-Hypnotics

All sedative-hypnotics are anticonvulsant, but withdrawal or fluctuations in effect may precipitate convulsions. For chronic administration, therefore, a sedative with a long duration of action is used, i.e., phenobarbital, generally in combination with a nonsedating anticonvulsant. Short-acting hypnotics available in injectable form (diazepam) have an immediate effect and are useful in acutely terminating a convulsant state.

Hydantoins and Equivalent

Phenytoin is the type compound and is also generally the drug first used major motor convulsions; it often is supplemented by phenobarbital or one of the miscellaneous drugs listed below. Cerebellar signs (ataxia, nystagmus, diplopia) are frequent. Dosage often is controlled with blood levels.

Carbamazepine is similar to phenytoin. The sedation that it causes is similar to that of the TCAs rather than the usual sedatives. Treatment of trigeminal neuralgia is usually initiated with phenytoin or carbamazepine.

Succinimides

Drugs of choice, ethosuximide most often, for absences

Miscellaneous Anticonvulsants

Valproic acid is an important example of a drug used supplementary to the above

Antipsychotics

Typical Antipsychotics

The antipsychotic or neuroleptic drugs are of great importance because of their ability to control manic behavior and to less regularly modify schizophrenic behavior and ideation, especially paranoia.

Side effects invariably occur; indeed the dose often is that just below one causing intolerable or disabling side effects. In contrast to the sedatives, the neuroleptics cause dysesthetic sedation, a subjectively unpleasant feeling of lassitude and depression. Patients are aroused easily from their indifferent state and retain all protective reflexes. These feelings, together with the extrapyramidal symptoms, account for the poor compliance of patients on these drugs and the consequent use of the injectable depot preparations. Sleep does not reach the deeper levels, REM sleep is increased, and patients remember their dreams and complain of nightmares. Paradoxically, the neuroleptics may cause excitement and increased violence on occasion. **Autonomic:** Atropine-like. The bradycardia, peripheral vasodilation with postural hypotension, and failure of ejaculation is explained by beta-adrenergic and central sympatholytic effects. Shivering is suppressed. **Endocrine:** Hypothalamic depression reduces gonadotropin and growth hormone elaboration and increases lactogenic hormone with amenorrhea and nonpuerperal lactation (in the male also, usually with a painful lump of breast tissue). Presumably, the weight gain caused by some phenothiazines is related. **Extrapyramidal:** Reversible: Parkinson equivalent. Dystonias, usually static and involving the shoulder and jaws but sometimes violently athetoid and with oculogyric movements. Akathisia. Irreversible: Tardive dyskinesia is intensified when the causal antipsychotic is withdrawn. Recovery is limited and requires months or years. **Ventricular dysrhythmias:** Quinidine-like effects on the ECG (QT and QRS prolongation) are easily demonstrable. Ventricular fibrillation occurs unpredictably and without a clear dose-effect relation. **Others:** Convulsant threshold is lowered. Neuroleptic malignant syndrome. Unrecognized as such, these drug-induced states may be treated as intercurrent diseases.

Interactions: See conscious sedation. Sedatives further depress during the day but at bedtime help correct the "can't stay awake all day, can't sleep all night" feeling.

Not all of the antipsychotics are phenothiazine derivatives, but all are similar in effect. One, promethazine causes unusually prominent sedation. Some are said to cause less sedation and more prominent extrapyramidal effects.

Atypical Antipsychotics

Clozapine, risperidone and olanzapine have none of the extrapyramidal effects but are otherwise equivalent to the phenothiazine types mentioned above. All are so expensive that they are being used only in selected patients.

Antimanic Agents

See lithium in addition to the antipsychotics.

Tricyclic Antidepressants (TCAs)

The introduction and heavy promotion of new stimulants more or less similar to the amphetamines (fluoxetine, bupropion and others) is leading to a long overdue review of the treatment of "depression" and of the pharmacology of the TCAs.

The TCAs are in every respect similar to the antipsychotics except that they are used with a ceiling on the dose so that the extrapyramidal effects (except for akathisia) are seen only rarely. Their effectiveness in controlling psychotic behavior has been demonstrated.

The adverse effects that should be emphasized first and foremost include the dysesthetic sedation or lassitude. These antidepressants do not elevate mood, on the contrary, patients may become suicidal.

Also, like the antipsychotics, the TCAs are quinidine-like (cause ventricular arrhythmias) and have led to significant numbers of accidental and suicidal deaths. Other adverse reactions are as listed for antipsychotics. There is a dangerous serotonergic-sympathomimetic interaction when they are used in combination with fluoxetine or with MAO inhibitors.

TCAs were shown to be as effective as electroconvulsant therapy in terminating a major, psychotic depression. However, that small market was expanded by blurring the distinction between the disease entity *depression,* and *depression,* the symptom of anxiety or agitated depression, as it was called until the profession was taught to call it "mixed anxiety and depression."

Stimulants

Note that the mild euphoriants propoxyphene, caffeine, and nicotine are listed or discussed elsewhere. Adding the people using those drugs to those using the stimulants now to be discussed, we conclude that, given free availability, people may choose alcohol or marijuana as a social drug, but for chronic, everyday use, they would prefer a stimulant.

Monoamine Oxidase (MAO) Inhibitors

Inhibitors of MAO A block the oxidative deamination of norepinephrine and serotonin within the CNS. The accumulation of the amines in the adrenergic neurone leads to a sequence of excited behaviors described under sympathomimetic stimulants immediately below. Dangerous, hypertensive reactions may occur when MAO inhibitors are used in combination with other sympathomimetics, meperidine, dextromethorphan, possibly other narcotics, and fluoxetine.

The metabolism of tyramine ingested with fermented foods is also blocked and rare reactions occur. A CNS MAO B inhibitor of dopamine metabolism (selegiline) is listed in the section on Parkinsonism.

Sympathomimetic Stimulants

A number of amines related to ephedrine exert their action through peripheral and CNS norepinephrine, epinephrine and probably dopamine. Peripherally, a mixture of alpha and beta agonist effects is seen. Behaviorly, there is euphoria, tremulousness, anxiety, excitement, distorted perception, and paranoia. Appetite is suppressed, but on a fixed dose, body weight begins to return toward base line after 2–3 weeks. Habituation is very common. Only a small minority of doctors used these agents as antidepressants until the aminergic agents below were introduced. The several drugs were first classified according to their addiction liability, that is, the strongest agents were placed in schedule 2 (See Appendix B), the other diet pills in 3 or 4.

Atypical Diet Pills

At least one of the scheduled diet pills (fenfluramine) was different from the others in that stimulation and habituation were not often reported and that sedation did appear. Dexfenfluramine, briefly available, was an effective anorexic, but sedation is so prominent that a stimulant was invariably prescribed with it, and it has neuro- and cardiotoxicity.

Unscheduled Aminergic Agents

The four amines cross referenced to this category (amantadine, bupropion, sertraline, and rimantadine) appear similar to an amphetamine or diet pill. Which CNS amines are involved and to what extent is not clear.

Specific Serotonin Reuptake Inhibitors (SSRI)

The two SSRIs (fluoxetine and paroxetine) are more clearly related to serotonin. Descriptively, their effect is similar to the previously mentioned aminergic amines.

Antiparkinson Agents

Rigidity and tremor appear because dopaminergic neurones are lost. Treatment aims to restore a dopaminergic influence on the remaining, postlesional neurone.

Dopamine Precursors

Dopamine itself cannot reach the neurones, but a precursor, levodopa, can, and it can be converted to dopamine at the proper site. It can also be metabolized peripherally and, to increase the amount that reaches the CNS, a peripheral inhibitor of decarboxylase, carbidopa, is given in combination with DOPA.

Agonists

Pergolide, bromocriptine and cabergoline act on dopamine receptors.

Inhibitor of MAO, Type B

Selegiline, given with levodopa, retards the metabolism of dopamine and prolongs the effect of levodopa.

Parasympatholytics

Denervation supersensitivity of the cholinergic neurone next in the sequence further mediates the extrapyramidal signs. Cholinolytics that reach the CNS (tertiary amines) have limited use and usefulness in symptomatic management.

ACTING ON AUTONOMIC NERVES OR TISSUES

Cholinergic Agents (Parasympathomimetics)

Acetylcholine is the mediator or transmitter of nerve activity across: (1) the junction of preganglionic, parasympathetic nerve and the intrinsic nerves of the effector (smooth muscle or gland) or on the effector directly; (2) between the pre- and post-ganglionic fibers of sympathetic ganglia; (3) between the preganglionic fibers and the secretory cells of the adrenal medulla, which cells are analogous to sympathetic ganglion cells; and (4) the voluntary nerve-muscle junction. Agents that mimic the effects of acetylcholine (choline esters or equivalent alkaloids) or prevent its destruction (cholinesterase inhibitors) will, therefore, be expected to have a combination of effects: cholinergic (often called muscarinic after the alkaloid); sympathomimetic (ganglionic or nicotinic); and voluntary neuromuscular.

Choline Esters and Equivalent Alkaloids

Pilocarpine is still the cholinergic agent most commonly used.

Smooth muscle of the gut, bladder, bronchioles, and pupillary constrictor is stimulated. Exocrine secretions are increased; the increased respiratory tract fluid is most dangerous. The eye is accommodated for near vision. Blood pressure is affected unpredictably because of the opposing muscarinic and nicotinic influences. Principal use is in the treatment of glaucoma with some application in urinary retention and postoperative ileus. Nicotine is an alkaloid with prominent nicotinic effects and appreciable CNS stimulation.

Cholinesterase Inhibitors, Reversible

Acetylcholine is destroyed rapidly following liberation. When a cholinesterase inhibitor occupies or chemically inactivates the postsynaptic cholinesterase, the mediator accumulates and cholinergic effects intensify. Inhibitors of the reversible type are hydrolyzed by the enzyme or otherwise metabolized and act for only a few hours. In addition to the effects listed for the choline esters, large doses of cholinesterase inhibitors initially stimulate (cyclic depolarization) voluntary muscle with fasciculation and occasional gross movement. Ultimately, the accumulation of acetylcholine causes failure to repolarize and paralysis.

In addition to the treatment of glaucoma and the stimulation of smooth muscle, a drug of this class is used to terminate the effect of curariform drugs and to treat myasthenia gravis. A tertiary amine (physostigmine) has been used to reverse CNS anticholinergic toxicity from a TCA.

Cholinesterase Inhibitors, Irreversible

These agents act by phosphorylating the enzyme and irreversibly terminating activity until new enzyme is synthesized. The organophosphates have minor therapeutic importance but are widely used as insecticides in intensively cultivated regions. Treatment of intoxication requires atropine and prompt protopam.

Cholinesterase Inhibitor, Central

Among their several effects, tacrine and donepezil inhibit CNS cholinesterase. They have very limited usefulness in Alzheimer's disease.

Parasympatholytics

The parasympatholytics are competitive antagonists to acetyl choline, but only at the parasympathetic neuro-effector junction. The intrinsic and parasympathetically stimulated contractions of gastrointestinal, ciliary, pupillary, and biliary muscle are inhibited, as are exocrine secretions (salivation, sweating). The drying of bronchial secretions may be deleterious, but inhaled belladonna alkaloids are useful bronchodilators, especially in nocturnal asthma.

Even therapeutic doses may cause constipation, tachycardia, ileus, postural hypotension, dizziness, urinary retention, blurred near vision, dry mouth and skin. The danger from the drugs is not great except in children when temperature regulation is disturbed. Contraindications include glaucoma and prostatism.

Tertiary Amines

Atropine and others are tertiary amines that reach and act on the CNS. Comparable to the antipsychotics, antihistamines and TCAs, the tertiary parasympatholytics cause subjectively unpleasant (dysesthetic) sedation, excitement, altered perception, convulsions, and coma.

Quaternary Amines

The synthetic substitutes for belladonna (propantheline) that are esters of quaternary aminoalcohols lack the sedative and other CNS effects of atropine.

Sympathomimetics

The terminations of the postganglionic sympathetic nerves release norepinephrine to act on the receptors. Secretory cells of the adrenal medulla are homologous with postganglionic cells but contain an additional enzyme that methylates norepinephrine and releases epinephrine into the circulation. The two natural mediators (in contrast to some of the synthetics named) act on both of the adrenergic receptor types but with a different balance and different net results. Some of the synthetics act purely on one receptor type only. ALPHA receptor activity or alpha adrenergic effect is vasoconstriction in all beds. BETA receptor or beta adrenergic effects are: vasodilation of all beds, increased cardiac rate (direct not reflex), increased force of cardiac contraction, smooth muscle relaxed, glycogenolysis (elevated blood sugar), subjective anxiety, and tremor. The sympathomimetic drugs differ in the fractionation between alpha and beta and in their duration or action, i.e., their suitability for chronic, oral use.

With Mixed Alpha and Beta Agonist Effects

Epinephrine, predominantly a beta agonist, constricts vessels in the skin and splanchnic area but is a vasodilator in muscle beds for "fight or flight." It is in its net effect a vasodilator, i.e., it lowers total peripheral resistance, and its effect of cardiac stimulation can become manifest as a rise in systolic and pulse pressure (unless reflex tachycardia narrows the pulse pressure).

Dopamine is, in small ("renal") doses, a pure vasodilator; with increasing doses vasoconstriction appears and its effects eventually equal those of norepinephrine.

Ephedrine is a mixed alpha and beta agonist acting indirectly, that is, through the sympathetic mediators present. It and its analogues are phenylisopropylamines, slowly metabolized, and it may be given by mouth for an effect of some hours. These analogues have prominent CNS stimulant properties discussed above under the sympathomimetic stimulants or amphetamines.

Predominantly Alpha Agonists

Norepinephrine elevates both systolic and diastolic pressures and appears at first glance to be a pure alpha agonist. Actually, it has cardiac stimulating effects, but cardiac output is not increased in the face of the increased resistance to ejection. Tissue perfusion is decreased.

For many years, even in the face of recognition of the utility of vasodilators in the treatment of shock, norepinephrine and congeners were used because they maintained BP until the patient recovered independent of treatment or expired because of it.

Unselective Beta 1 and 2 Effects

Drugs that are analogues of the direct and indirect acting amines but with a bulky substituent on the amine N act as beta agonists.

Some (e.g., isoproterenol) act on the heart (increased rate and force of contraction) and blood vessels (vasodilation) as well as bronchiolar and uterine smooth muscle. They are used by infusion in shock as an alternative to dopamine and by inhalation in asthma; some are active after oral administration.

Hydralazine, studied before beta adrenergic receptor blockers were available, is generally called a direct vasodilator. Re-examination of the literature shows it to be a beta agonist.

Beta 2 Selective Effects

Some "beta 2 selective" agonists act on bronchiolar or uterine smooth muscle with minimal cardiovascular side effects. The differential effect disappears as the dose is increased.

Sympathomimetics, Incomplete

Used only in nose drops or sprays, these drugs cause vasoconstriction (decongestion) but no other sympathomimetic effects.

Sympathoplegics or Sympatholytics

The following five drug groups are those that reduce the amount of sympathetic nerve activity exerted on the blood vessels (meaning, primarily, veins) when used on hypertensive patients. Some of their properties can be understood by reference to the level at which they act. The centrally acting adrenergic inhibitors—reserpine, methyldopa, clonidine, and others—act on the hypothalamus, above the level integrating the reflexes controlling blood pressure. Used alone, they have a minimal effect on blood pressure, and the fall in BP will not be postural because their effect is minimized by reflex adjustment. When the drugs act at the level of the ganglia, the adrenergic neurone, or the receptors, the efferent reflex flow cannot reach the blood vessels and the hypotension is postural because of venous pooling and can be as intense as is desired. Agents used in the treatment of hypertension that act on blood vessels without significant effects (except reflex to decreased BP) on the heart are listed as vasodilators in the section on cardiovascular drugs.

Alpha Adrenergic Receptor Blockers

These drugs (e.g., prazosin) block the effect of norepinephrine on the postsynaptic (alpha 1) receptors on vascular smooth muscle. As capacitance vessels are dilated and as effective plasma volume and venous return fall, cardiac output and, therefore, blood pressure, decrease. The decrease in blood pressure is postural or orthostatic, i.e., the effectiveness of the drug is increased to the extent that gravity intensifies the pooling. The effect of sympathetic blockade is also manifested on the outflow tract of the bladder by partial relief of the symptoms of prostatism. The male orgasm may be delayed, but erectile difficulties are not intensified; in fact, useful degree of turgor may be induced. As the drug effect appears, a limited degree of tolerance develops as plasma volume is expanded. Adjustment of the dosage will be minimal if the plasma expansion is minimized by the concurrent administration of a thiazide or other diuretic.

The hypotension, which is reversed rapidly by the supine position, is perceived as the important adverse reaction. The possibility is intensified by stillstanding, heat, the vasodilation that persists after exercise, alcohol, and other hypotensive drugs, e.g., the opiates, antidepressants, antihistamines, and others.

Ganglionic Blockers

These drugs block transmission across both sympathetic and parasympathetic ganglia. Hypotension as profound as is desired can be produced; however, at times a change in the pulse rate, constipation, ileus, urinary retention, pupillary dilation, paralysis of accommodation, dry mouth, and erectile and ejaculatory failure also can be produced. These drugs have been replaced almost completely by agents that act selectively on the sympathetic nervous system; mecamylamine remains.

Adrenergic Neuron (Postganglionic) Blockers

Guanethidine, the type compound of this group, replaces norepinephrine in the sympathetic nerve. The mediator no longer being released, both alpha and beta effects are lost. Postural hypertension is induced but so also is bradycardia, decreased force of cardiac contraction with CHF, and diarrhea. The drug has largely been abandoned.

Centrally-Acting Adrenergic Inhibitors

Reflex control of BP in the face of postural and other change is initiated by afferents that enter the CNS below the hypothalamic site at which these drugs act. Sympathetic outflow is reduced, but because lower integrative centers are not influenced, the hypotension induced is limited in degree and is not postural. In addition, behavioral effects comparable to those of the antipsychotic agents are induced. Indications: Hypertension: Adequate for mild or moderate elevations if combined with diuretic. Prophylactic for migraine attacks. Off label use for symptomatic relief of narcotic withdrawal symptoms, but mecamylamine is probably better. Adverse: See below for individual agents, but all have the following effects: dysesthetic sedation (subjectively unpleasant lassitude but easy arousal); depressed mood; light sleep with much REM activity; bradycardia; and rebound hypertension with abrupt cessation.

Beta Adrenergic Receptor Blockers

Beta blockers may be unselective (blocking Beta 1 and 2) or cardioselective (blocking largely Beta 1). These remarkable drugs have multiple mechanisms of action and multiple applications.

Effects Related to Beta Blocking Activity

Beta 1 blockade leads to decreased cardiac output and cardiac work, CHF, bradycardia, rapid AV nodal conduction, and AV block. Beta 2 blockade leads to peripheral vasoconstriction, bronchiolar constriction, increased uterine contractility at term, and possibly impaired glucose tolerance.

Effects Related to Central Sympathoplegic Effect

Daytime dysesthetic sedation, increased REM sleep, prophylactic effect against migraine comparable to clonidine, nonpostural BP lowering limited in degree. Consensus holds that BP lowering is peripheral; however, that position is not well supported.

Effects Related to Membrane Stabilizing Action

Comparable to quinidine or lidocaine. Antiarrhythmic effect is not present in all compounds.

Effects Related to Inherent Beta Agonist Effect

Not present in all compounds.

Indications

Hypertension (with diuretic); relief of angina by reducing cardiac work; convert atrial arrhythmias; slow ventricular rate in presence of rapid atrial rate in lieu of digitalis; after mild cardiac infarct to defer dysrhythmias and reduce work; normalize signs and symptoms in hyperthyroidism; glaucoma; prophylaxis of migraine; familial tremor; neuropathic pain and stage fright or other overt anxiety. The difference between cardioselective and nonselective blockers is relative and disappears at higher doses.

Alpha and Beta Receptor Blocker

Marketed but awaiting evaluation (Labetalol).

Xanthines

Xanthines are phosphodiesterase inhibitors and act on many autonomic tissues and on the CNS. Bronchiolar smooth muscle relaxation is the only effect applied therapeutically with theophylline and congeners. Two similar inhibitors are suggested for use as inotropic agents. The CNS effect, of course, accounts for the popularity of caffeinated beverages.

CARDIOVASCULAR AGENTS

Vasodilators

Post-Arteriolar (Antianginal and Related Agents)

Drugs of this class act directly on vascular smooth muscle but not on the heart nor on or through the autonomic or central nervous system. Except for coronary artery spasm, there are no examples of drugs dilating large, named arteries, especially those made inelastic by atherosclerosis. The "coronary vasodilators" and "peripheral vascular" agents do act on veins. The result is venous pooling, decreased venous return, and a decrease in cardiac output and resistance to ejection. The resulting decrease in cardiac work relieves the pain of angina, but the decrease in perfusion pressure may even intensify claudication. This formulation is based on studies in diseased humans not in normals or dogs with arterioles still elastic.

Nitroglycerine is the important nitric oxide donor used to abort or prevent angina. Nitroglycerin remains effective with continued use except under special circumstances that include the simultaneous administration of "long acting" nitrates to which absolute tolerance develops within a few days of use.

Angiotensin Converting Enzyme (ACE) Inhibitors

Hypertensinogen is converted by renin to angiotensin I. The conversion of angiotensin I to angiotensin II is blocked by an angiotensin converting enzyme (ACE) inhibitor. The vasoconstricting and aldosterone elaborating effect of angiotensin II does not appear. There are weaknesses in the formulation, but a useful degree of arteriolar dilation with a mild, nonpostural fall in BP occurs, and it can be intensified by a thiazide.

ACE inhibitors are used in hypertension, congestive heart failure, and in protection against the development of diabetic nephropathy (other nephropathy is a contraindication, as is pregnancy).

Side effects include cough, headache, diminished or unpleasant taste, dizziness, gastritis, fatigue, rash, and proteinuria.

Two drugs, losartan and moexipril, are actually angiotensin II receptor blockers, but so far need not be distinguished from ACE inhibitors. They do not cause the cough.

Calcium Channel Blockers

The action current of excitable tissues begins with the rapid entry of sodium (0) and is followed by a plateau (2) as calcium more slowly enters the cell. The calcium entry blockers act on this phase to slow the electrical activity and to decrease the amount of calcium that reaches the contractile proteins. Vascular smooth muscle is relaxed, myocardial contractility is reduced, and AV nodal conduction is slowed and its refractory period prolonged. This diffuse effect on excitable tissues suggests multiple uses and multiple adverse effects, including a sudden reflex tachycardia with short acting compounds or preparations.

The ten agents are allowed to claim effectiveness in the treatment of hypertension and/or angina, but a serious problem in evaluation of the many drugs already marketed exists. For example, the value of beta blocker-diuretic treatment having already been established in randomized studies using death as an end point, the use of untreated controls presents an ethical problem. Such randomized studies as are available suggest that the use of Ca blockers in hypertensive patients or those with coronary artery disease is associated with an excess of deaths.

The drug group is not homogenous and sustained action products or inherently long-acting drugs such as amlodipine should be safe, but the available data for these ten drugs is inadequate. The conservative consensus would not start untreated patients with hypertension, CHF, angina or a recent MI on calcium-channel blockers, long or short acting. Patients already on drugs of this group can be continued if the extended release forms are used.

Other adverse reactions are worsening angina or TIAs, headache, dizziness, ankle edema independent of CHF, and CHF.

Miscellaneous Vasodilators

Diazoxide is a congener of the thiazides with no diuretic action but with the arteriolar dilating effect intense enough to be useful in hypertensive crisis. Minoxidil is not used much in hypertension but is marketed (OTC) as a scalp lotion for the treatment of baldness. Hydralazine is discussed under beta agonists. Alprostadil, PGE_1: See alphabetical listing.

Vasoconstrictors and Oxytocics

These drugs constrict arteries (not arterioles) and initiate or stimulate contractions of the ripe uterus. They are used for the following:
Migraine (Ergot alkaloids and derivatives and sumatriptan)
Postpartum bleeding (Ergot alkaloids, oxytocin, carboprost)
Induction of labor (oxytocin)
Abortion (carboprost, dinoprostone)

Antiarrhythmic Agents

In the conventional classification, quinidine and similar common agents are called *Class 1*. The beta adrenergic blockers are called *Class II*. *Class III* contains bretylium, a sympathoplegic whose usefulness is questioned. The calcium channel blockers, which promise usefulness against supraventricular tachycardias, are put in *Class IV.* Digitalis (unclassified) still has usefulness in these problems.

Group I Antiarrhythmic Agents

Drugs of this group are sodium channel blockers with local anesthetic activity. As a result, the rhythmicity of myocardial tissue is depressed and the rate of firing of the ectopic focus slows until it is less than that of the normal pacemaker. AV and intraventricular conduction times are prolonged with QT and QRS prolongation, leading to ventricular ectopic activity including ventricular tachycardia and fibrillation. This kind of misadventure is seen also with parasympatholytics, antihistamines, antidepressants, and antipsychotics, which are, in turn, antiarrhythmics. A sudden increase in ventricular rate in the presence of a rapid atrial rate caused by decreased refractory period of AV node can be prevented by pretreatment with digitalis or propranolol. Do not use with any degree of AV block.

Drugs of this group are used to convert supraventricular dysrhythmias to NSR and to prevent recurrences. They also are used after myocardial infarctions to suppress ectopic ventricular activity premonitory of V fibrillation. It appears that, to date, efforts in coronary care units have precipitated about the same number of episodes as they have prevented.

Miscellaneous Antiarrhythmic Agents

Amiodarone (Cordarone) is a very effective Type I antiarrhythmic but has multiple other effects (is sometimes said to be Class I, II, III and IV). It has a half life of three or more weeks, and a loading dose may have to be continued for that long to saturate body depots before the effectiveness can be evaluated. Toxic reactions are common and subjectively distressing and persist for weeks. It probably does benefit angina and CHF but should be reserved for desperate problems. Decrease digitalis before beginning its use.

Cardiotonic Glycosides

Cardiac glycosides or "digitalis" (digoxin, digitoxin) affect all areas of the heart. They increase the force (velocity) of ventricular contraction; slow AV conduction and prolong the refractory period; decrease normal sinus rate; increase ectopic impulse formation in the atria, ventricles, and conducting tissue; and alter the order of repolarization with ST sagging, shorter QT, and nonreciprocal T lowering or inversion.

In congestive failure, they restore the ability of the pump to increase its output in response to increased activity with resultant diuresis, decreased venous pressure, decrease in heart size (more complete emptying), and decrease in the tachycardia of CHF. The addition of vasodilators (ACE inhibitors) or diuretics does not conflict except when the thiazides deplete potassium. In supraventricular tachycardias, including fibrillation and flutter, ventricular rate is decreased by digitalis, NSR often is restored, and recurrences generally are prevented.

Adverse reactions include all degrees of heart block, bradycardia, and any supraventricular or ventricular arrhythmia—from extrasystoles to V fibrillation—without premonitory warning. Intermittent anorexia and nausea is said to be the earliest sign. Treat overdose by stopping digitalis, replete potassium if depleted, and use propranolol for arrhythmias unless second or third degree block is present. Do not use if DC countershock is contemplated (use propranolol instead to slow V rate). Do not give IV calcium to a digitalized patient. The dose of digitalis (digoxin) must be decreased before amiodarone is started.

RENAL AGENTS

Sodium Diuretics

Thiazide Diuretics and Related Agents

The thiazides have two primary effects. They dilate arterioles and, by themselves, have a minor effect on BP. Combined with hypotensive drugs, they often control mild to moderate hypertension. They reduce renal reabsorption of sodium by an action on the *cortical* portion of the loop. Excess extracellular fluid is lost but plasma volume decreases only transiently. However, the increase in plasma volume that accompanies the use of BP-lowering drugs is prevented and the amount of agent needed is kept from increasing.

In addition to treating essential hypertension, thiazides are used to treat the following: CHF; other fluid retention states; acute pulmonary edema (benefit appears before diuretic effect); and diabetes insipidus.

Thiazides also cause potassium loss as the amount of sodium presented to ion exchange site increases. K depletion is most likely with great loss of edema fluid or dietary restriction. Other adverse effects include impaired CHO tolerance, elevated uric acid with manifest gout in predisposed patients, intensified erectile difficulties and allergic reactions as with other sulfonamides. Combination therapy for hypertension probably causes an excess of myocardial infarcts.

Potent ("Loop") Diuretics

The loop diuretics, such as furosemide, act on the medullary portion of the loop of Henle and can, in large enough doses, destroy the countercurrent mechanism and the concentrating power of the kidney, leading to dehydration with shock or deafness. Their effectiveness in hypertension is less than that of hydrochlorothiazide, but they are preferable for use in renal insuffiencey. Except for ethacrynic acid, they are "sulfas."

Potassium-Sparing Diuretics

Spironolactone, an aldosterone antagonist, is a weak sodium diuretic that causes potassium retention. It is combined with a thiazide whenever possible. The relation to physiologic steroids may lead to gynecomastia, decreased libido, menstrual irregularities, and postmenopausal bleeding.

The other two (triamterene, amiloride) potassium-sparing diuretics are very weak, and the usual combinations with a thiazide offer no advantage over a thiazide alone.

Osmotic Diuretics

Osmotic diuretics are water diuretics rather than sodium diuretics. They are not resorbed from the kidney tubules, nor do they cross other membranes. They are used to maintain urine volume or to extract water and lower intraocular or intracranial pressure.

Antiinflammatory Steroids

Systemic Effects

Exemplified by prednisolone, the corticosteroids provide the following: (1) suppression of inflammation from any cause whether traumatic, infectious or allergic, and whether the inflammation is destructive or protective. Lymphoid tissue atrophy. Eosinopenia. Immunologic reactions inhibited at a stage earlier than manifest inflammation; (2) adrenal suppression and atrophy. Abrupt cessation of treatment or increase in demand by illness or injury can result in relative or complete Addisonian state; (3) protein catabolic effect with osteoporosis following atrophy of the protein matrix. Also muscle wasting and thinning of skin with scarring (striae); (4) other metabolic effects: round facies, fat accumulation in upper back and trunk but with wasting otherwise. Insulin requirement increased; and (5) CNS stimulation with euphoria and wakefulness progressing with large doses in a few patients to excitement and distorted perception. **Adverse Reactions:** Most are predicted from the above. Increased susceptibility to infections, scar formation defective with large, chronic dosage. Adrenal insufficiency upon withdrawal, a Cushingoid state (lacking hirsutism, acne and plethora). **Contraindications:** Glaucoma, diabetes, osteoporosis, post menopausal state, psychosis, bacterial infections that cannot be controlled by antibiotics, ophthalmic herpes, peptic ulcer. **Cautions:** Use every second day (early morning) dosing to minimize adrenal atrophy. Use local applications to get high local concentrations without significant systemic levels. Of the steroids developed subsequent to hydrocortisone, none offer any advantage over prednisone.

Intra-articular Use

Very slowly soluble salts of many cortisones are available for injection into joint spaces, inflamed bursae, etc. A high local concentration is maintained but systemic levels are negligible.

Topical Use

See under topical agents.

Deep Inhalation (Pulmonary)

Solutions can be administered by inhalation with aerosol particles small enough to be carried deeply into the lung parenchyma exerting bronchodilating and antiinflammatory effect.

Inhalation (Nasal)

Solutions administered by spray form particles so large that they are deposited in the upper respiratory tract.

Intraocular Use

The corticosteroids can precipitate or intensify glaucoma and can spread herpetic infection disastrously, especially when given by intraocular drops. However, by suppressing inflammation with scar formation, the drops can preserve vision.

Mineralocorticoids

Fludrocortisone is a pharmacologic analogue of aldosterone and acts to control (increase) renal reabsorption of sodium and the coupled loss of potassium. Adrenal insufficiency is treated with fludrocortisone supplemented by hydrocortisone.

Inhibitors of Glucocorticoid Synthesis

These drugs (aminoglutethimide for one) reduce corticosteroid elaboration by several mechanisms. They are used in treatment of Cushing's disease and to test hypothalamic-pituitary responsiveness.

Androgenic/Anabolic Steroids

The androgens initiate and maintain the secondary male characteristics, including the behavioral; they accelerate linear growth but also close epiphyses. They are protein anabolic to muscle, bone, hair, and skin; they also inhibit LH and FSH and cause sodium retention. Those listed other than testosterone are alleged, without good basis, to be selectively more active as anabolic agents. In the male, side effects include acne, edema, elevated BP, increased libido, aggressiveness, and testicular atrophy; in women, side effects include virilization. When used as replacement therapy in men, the slowly absorbed, oily solutions of sparingly soluble esters are still preferred, although more acceptable transdermal products are imminent. Widespread use exists in athletes to increase body bulk and explosive strength but not endurance. Some use to stop ovulation in the presence of endometriosis.

Testosterone Antagonists

A diverse group. One is useless (finasteride), one is toxic (cyproterone), and one (flutamide) is useful in combination with LHRH antagonist in cancer of the prostate.

Estrogens

In addition to the cyclic effect on the epithelia of the female reproductive tract and breast, the estrogens have anabolic and sodium retaining effects and inhibit the hypothalamic-pituitary axis. Therefore, they are used in the initial phase of the menopause to lower FSH and relieve vasomotor and emotional instability; throughout the postmenopausal years to prevent osteoporosis and other catabolic changes; in the pill; and in large doses as an antiandrogen and inhibitor of the hypothalamic-pituitary axis in palliation of cancer of the prostate.

Progestins

Progestins transform an estrogen-prepared endometrium from the proliferative to the secretory stage and are essential to maintain a pregnancy. They inhibit LH and FSH secretion and prevent ovulation. They are components of the oral contraceptives and are used by themselves as contraceptives. During hormone replacement therapy, they are added to the estrogen to reduce toxicity of estrogens on uterus.

Antiestrogens

Tamoxifen, for example, competes for estrogen receptors and is active against some breast cancers.

Antiprogestins

Mifepristone is a progestin and corticoid receptor antagonist on trophoblastic and endometrial tissue and is about to become an important abortifacient.

Oral Contraceptives

Combinations of an estrogen and a semisynthetic (orally active) progestin, oral contraceptives prevent implantation or inhibit ovulation.

All of the preparations available today are low potency compared with more toxic OCs of past years. **Monophasic** brands contain the same amounts of estrogen and progestin in 21 tablets with or without seven dummy tablets for the withdrawal period. **Biphasic** and **triphasic** preparations contain increased amounts of progestin in the tablets to be taken the second 10 days or the second and third weeks of administration. No advantage is apparent.

Hypothalamic Releasing Factor Antagonists

These analogues are polypeptides that differ only slightly from endogenous Luteinizing Hormone Releasing Factor or hormone (LHRH). After initial stimulation of LH release, the analogues block their receptors, and LH and FSH levels and corresponding (estrogen and) testosterone levels fall to castrate levels. Given with an antiandrogen, they are useful against cancer of the prostate.

Anterior Pituitary Hormones

A diverse group of bioengineered growth hormone, recombinant FSH, chorionic gonadotropin (FSH) and ACTH. Clomiphene, a small molecule, is cross-indexed to this group because it induces ovulation somehow through FSH.

Posterior Pituitary Hormones

See pitressin and oxytocin in the alphabetical listing.

Insulins

The manifest function of insulin as a drug is the same as the resultant of its several physiological functions: to maintain the level of blood glucose within limits in the face of the postprandial and overnight rise. Those patients who are not controlled by diet and the oral antidiabetic agents vary in the amounts (units) that they require and in the pattern of their changing needs over the 24 hours. To meet the need for insulins of varying durations of action, the solubility, i.e., the rate of absorption, of crystalline insulin has been altered in several ways. These preparations are gathered at one place in the alphabetic listing under *insulin.* Bioengineered human insulin does differ slightly from beef or pork insulin and may have slightly more rapid onset of action and of decay.

Oral Antidiabetic Agents

Non-insulin-dependent diabetes mellitus (NIDDM) is associated with the release of enough residual insulin to prevent ketosis but not enough to maintain blood glucose at the properly low level. In addition, tissue sensitivity to insulin is reduced.

The first type of orally active agent, the sulfonylureas (such as tolbutamide), modify both defects and are used when diet inadequately controls hyperglycemia. "Second generation" sulfonylureas, e.g., glyburide, carry more danger of hypoglycemic reactions.

One study associated an excess of deaths from cardiovascular disease with tolbutamide treatment, but the resultant warning is generally ignored.

The biguanides (metformin) reduce blood sugar even in insulin-dependent diabetes by increasing the release (not synthesis) of insulin. They do not lower fasting blood sugar but do lower the postprandial rise. The first biguanide marketed had to be withdrawn because of episodes of lactic acidosis, but the present drugs appear to be much safer. Because lactate accumulation is increased by any degree of tissue hypoxia, these drugs should not be used in patients with CHF or COPD.

Thyroid Replacements

Partially purified preparations of the desiccated gland have largely been replaced by T_4 (levothyroxine) and, to a much lesser extent, T_3. Triiodothyronine (liothyronine has a half-life of 1 day compared with 4 days for T_4). The signs of overdose are those of hyperthyroidism, an intense beta agonist surge. Only in patients with profound myxedema may absorption be so slowed that a parenteral preparation is needed.

Thyroid Stimulating Hormones

Protirelin is the tripeptide, hypothalamic thyrotropin releasing factor (TRH). Its infusion provides a sensitive method for the diagnosis of borderline hyper- or hypothyroid function.

Thyrotropin or TSH is the thyroid stimulating hormone of the anterior pituitary. Its use in diagnosis has been replaced by assays of the hormone itself.

Antithyroid Agents

The two antithyroid agents, methimazole and propylthiouracil, are thioamides that block organification, the oxidation of iodide to iodine, and its incorporation into tyrosine residues. Over several weeks, as the store of hormone is depleted, a eu- or hypothyroid state is reached. As the sole treatment, it implies long treatment and frequent relapses after withdrawal. Relapse is least frequent when levothyroxine is given concurrently to inhibit TSH.

Iodine also blocks organification and inhibits TSH release. If treatment with an antithyroid drug or ^{131}Iodine is anticipated, it should not be used until after treatment is underway. Iodine reduces the size and vascularity of the thioamide treated gland in preparation for surgery.

The beta blockers (propranolol) provide rapid symptomatic relief of hyperthyroidism.

METABOLIC AGENTS

Lipid Lowering Drugs

Combined with dietary treatment and the control of other risk factors, the lipid lowering drugs defer myocardial infarcts and may even allow regression of atherosclerotic deposits.

HMG-COA Reductase Inhibitors

The "statins" inhibit the enzyme (hydroxymethylglutaryl-CoA reductase) that governs the rate limiting step in the synthesis of cholesterol. Cholesterol is depleted, and the uptake of LDL from plasma is promoted. The lowering is dose-related and may reach 30–40% if a second drug is used.

Bile Acid Binding Resins

Bile acids combine with the insoluble, nonabsorbable polymer in the intestine and are excreted rather than reentering the enterohepatic cycle. Cholesterol is depleted because it is then used for the synthesis of replacement bile acids.

Other Lipid Lowering Agents

Gemfibrozil is used in hypertriglyceridemia but has no effect on cholesterol. Probucol is less effective than the statins in lowering cholesterol, yet trials show regression of lesions, possibly because it is an antioxidant. Niacin is inexpensive and was the first to have an effect on longevity demonstrated.

Regulators of Calcium Kinetics

D Vitamins and Related

The naming of the D vitamins is based on D3 or cholecalciferol, which is monohydroxylated. With the addition of another hydroxyl, 25(OH)-D3 or calcifediol is formed. Finally, a third hydroxyl is added in the kidney and calcitriol, the ultimate "D vitamin," is formed. It should be considered a gene-acting steroid hormone released by the kidney. The D vitamins are used in infants as nutritional supplements and, instead of parathyroid hormone, in hypothyroidism. Excessive doses can cause metastatic calcification.

Other Calcium Regulators

The diphosphonates, especially IV pamidronate (and, to a much lesser degree, calcitonin) decrease osteoclastic activity to an impressive degree. They are useful in Paget's disease and in recalcifying osteoporosis. Estrogens have only a feeble effect on an established osteoporotic process but, of course, prevent early bone loss and also have an anabolic effect on skin and muscle and relieve the symptoms of the early menopause.

Anticoagulants and Coagulants

Heparin and Related Agents

Prevention and treatment of deep vein thrombosis. Low molecular weight heparin (dalteparin, enoxaparin) can be given subcutaneously (home care) in a fixed dose, has a longer duration of action and is less expensive. Note protamine as the antagonist to heparin.

Inhibitors of Prothrombin Synthesis

The final step in the synthesis of prothrombin (and also Factors VII, IX, and X) is the Vitamin K dependent carboxylation of glutamic acid residues. The coumarins (warfarin) are noncompetitive antagonists to vitamin K; functional prothrombin is not produced and levels fall as preformed prothrombin is exhausted. Initial large doses shorten the latent period, which is covered by heparin. Dosage must be adjusted, first daily, then at longer intervals. Coumarin effects are altered by inducers of hepatic microsomal enzymes, such as phenytoin and phenobarbital.

Antiplatelet Agents

The platelet aggregation phase of clotting results in a platelet plug around which fibrin is deposited. *Aspirin* (but not other NSAIDs) is the prototype, and it is of established value in deferring MIs in males with risk factors, including simply age. It is also used in TIAs. It blocks the synthesis of thromboxanes and stops the self-accelerating process of aggregation. Bleeding time (the test) is prolonged, but blood loss is not increased.

Ticlopidine is a less active aspirin equivalent. Dipyridamole has the same effect but with a different mechanism as aspirin and is used to maintain patency of bypass grafts and after valve replacements.

Thrombolytic Agents

The thrombolytic agents, given soon after the thrombosis IV or by close intra-arterial infusion, lyse the fresh clot dramatically. They also have a generalized fibrinolytic (hemorrhagic) effect. See alteplase, streptokinase, or anistreplase.

Clotting Factors

See antihemophilic factor VIII and coagulant factor IX.

Other Hemostatic Agents

Aminocaproic acid and tranexamic acid are fibrinolytic (inhibitors of plasminogen activators). The first is labeled for use in bleeding in general, the second for control of bleeding in hemophiliacs during dental procedures. Aprotinin is a protease inhibitor that favors the accumulation of fibrin and is used during bypass procedures.

Specific Ions

See under each ion.

Agents Used in the Treatment of Gout

Treatment of gout involves aborting the acute attacks and preventing further damage by lowering the blood levels and depleting the tissues of urate. Colchicine reduces leukocyte mobility and phagocytosis of urate crystals and is the prototype of the mitotic spindle inhibitors listed under cancer chemotherapy. It is rapidly effective against acute attacks and prevents the recurrent attacks that often occur early in chronic treatment. Its administration requires care, and diarrhea often cannot be prevented. Indomethacin or prednisone often is used instead. The other NSAIDs can be used only if the dose is increased until the anti-inflammatory effect becomes manifest.

Chronic treatment involves either probenecid or sulfinpyrazone to increase uric acid excretion or allopurinol to reduce its production. The latter is preferred with high blood levels or tophaceous gout.

Vitamins

See cyanocobalamin, folic acid and folinic acid, and phytonadione in the alphabetical listing.

Enzymes

For enzymes not mentioned in other categories, see alglucerase, lactase, and galactosidase in the alphabetical listing.

INFLAMMATION, ALLERGY, IMMUNOMODULATION

Non-Narcotic Analgesics

Aspirin and Related NSAIDs

Aspirin, acetaminophen, and relatives are often discussed in relation to the centrally acting narcotic analgesics.

However, they act peripherally through prostaglandins and other mediators of pain and inflammation. All of these drugs relieve minor or moderate pain less intense than that requiring codeine or other opioid for its control. In large, chronic doses, they are anti-inflammatory.

Aspirin

A small amount of ASA is absorbed before the acetyl group is hydrolyzed, accounting for the effect on platelet function and its use in deferring thrombotic episodes. Bleeding time (the test) is prolonged; however, increased blood loss postoperatively has not been shown. Aspirin is, however, usually discontinued before surgery.

Other Salicylates

These drugs are obsolete except possibly for diflunisal.

Acetic and Propionic Acid Derivatives (NSAIDs)

NSAID is an industrial term exploiting the physician's fear of the anti-inflammatory steroids. Given in doses that cause equivalent side effects, aspirin and the NSAIDs are essentially similar. Indomethacin is an exception in that it is a more potent anti-inflammatory agent if also more toxic. In addition to the familiar GI upsets and bleeding, the aspirin-like drugs have caused chronic renal toxicity, interstitial nephritis, and subtle CNS effects. They are characterized chemically here to separate them from the categories below.

Other NSAIDs

Of the other analgesics that do not fit in the previous categories, only piroxicam need be mentioned. It can be given once daily.

Other Non-narcotic Analgesics

The important drug in this category is acetaminophen, which is a useful analgesic and antipyretic that is free of GI and other side effects. It is not anti-inflammatory with any dose. Large single doses may cause hepatic necrosis.

Phenylbutazone and oxyphenbutazone are impressively more potent analgesics than any of the above, but, in most opinions, are prohibitively toxic.

Antihistamines (H_1 Antagonists)

Histamine acting on H_1 receptors is the principal mediator of Type 1 allergic reactions (hay fever, allergic rhinitis, urticaria, and anaphylaxis). Dilation of blood vessels, constriction of nonvascular smooth muscle (especially bronchiolar), and hives or laryngeal edema if caused by histamine liberation, are antagonized by H_1 antihistamines. However, their action is too slow to be useful in acute anaphylaxis, in which case epinephrine should be used. Gastric acid secretion is the only function mediated by H2 receptors.

Thus, the only established indication for these drugs is the hay fever type of allergic reaction.

Several older antihistamines, especially diphenhydramine (Benadryl), produce dysesthetic sedation as defined for the antipsychotics. Some patients experience stimulation and tremulousness which, in young children, has progressed to convulsions. Atropine-like and quinidine-like side effects also occur.

The quinidine-like effects are intensified dangerously when loratadine or terfenadine are given together with macrolide antibiotics or imidazole antifungals.

Newer antihistamines from chlorpheniramine cause minimal sedation or other side effects with the usual doses.

Motion Sickness Prevention

Motion sickness can be ameliorated or prevented by cholinergic-blocking agents (scopolamine) or by selected antihistamines. Of the drugs available, dimenhydrinate, a different salt of Benadryl, gives far more frequent side effects.

Antihistamines, Miscellaneous

Cyproheptadine is used for improved appetite and weight gain in children.

Eicosanoid (Prostaglandin) Related

Eicosanoids are metabolites of arachidonic acid such as the prostaglandins (listed in Part II), the leukotrienes and prostacyclin. They have been used for their vasodilating and uterine stimulating effects. Now inhibitors of leukotriene formation (zileuton) and leukotriene receptor blockers (zafirlukast) are used in chronic asthma.

Adjuncts to Cancer (and Other) Therapy

Cytokines are a large group of widely differing proteins, including the colony stimulating factors, the interferons, the interleukins, and other mediators of inflammation. Their original source was cultured human cells: macrophages, T lymphocytes, endothelial cells, and, to stretch the classification to include epoetin, kidney cells. The controlling genes were cloned for the production of useable amounts of the proteins.

Hemopoietic Colony-Stimulating Factors

The colony-stimulating factors (CSF), acting on progenitor or stem cells in the marrow, hasten recovery of the myeloid elements after chemotherapy or bone marrow transplantation. Filgrastim (G-CSF) acts on neutrophiles; sargramostim (GM-CSF) acts on granulocyte and macrophage precursor cells.

Immunomodulators

Aldesleukin, the interferons, BCG, cyclosporin, tacrolimus, and antilymphocyte globulin act through the immune system. Indications are listed under each agent in Part II.

Cytotoxic Immunosuppressants

Often called *slow acting antirheumatic drugs,* these drugs are held or hoped to halt progression of rheumatoid arthritis and related autoimmune states by causal therapy rather than the symptomatic relief provided by NSAIDs or corticosteroids. Two such drugs, the folate analogue methotrexate and azathioprine, have established efficacy and tolerable toxicity.

Other Antirheumatics

Hydroxychloroquine, the gold salts, and penicillamine are of uncertain usefulness and cause frequent side and toxic effects.

CANCER CHEMOTHERAPY

Cancer chemotherapy is dramatically useful against a few neoplasms but palliative or ineffective against the common dangerous, solid tumors. The early occurrence of distant micrometastases, most often before the neoplasm is clinically detectable, presents an insurmountable problem for surgical and radiation therapy, which cannot focus on the microscopic implants. Chemotherapy reaches the invisible spread and is the only treatment that promises any great progress in the future.

Treatment usually involves multiple agents and relatively complex scheduling. The treatment is generally protocol driven and constantly changing to achieve small additional gains.

A generalization about the toxicity of cytotoxic agents is possible because they do not act selectively on malignant tissue but on all rapidly growing and dividing cells as well. The less differentiated cells of the bone marrow, crypts of the enteric glands, and hair follicles are affected; thrombocytopenia, granulocytopenia, anemia, mucositis, enteritis, and alopecia are common. Nausea and vomiting may be intolerable for some patients after, for example, platinum, and are prominent after most of the drugs listed below. In addition, specific agents have specific organ toxicity. Patients who survive for a long period may develop second primaries. These drugs must be handled like other carcinogens. Drug resistance may develop in metastases or locally recurring tumors that were originally sensitive.

Cytotoxic agents that find application in general medicine (immunosuppressants) were mentioned immediately above.

Alkylating Agents

Polyfunctional alkylating agents transfer methyl groups to guanine and other bases. When two or more reactive groups are affected, crosslinking occurs. Abnormal base pairing results in abnormal RNA and defective protein synthesis.

Chelates of Platinum: These very useful drugs (cisplatin is an example) are classified tentatively with the alkylating agents.
Nitrogen Mustards: Cyclophosphamide is an example of this most frequently used group.

Nitrosoureas: Prodrugs such as carmustine are transformed into lipid soluble metabolites that are used against brain tumors.
Other Alkylating Agents: See busulfan and dacarbazine.

Mitotic Spindle Inhibitors

Promote Tubulin Depolymerization: Microtubular assembly is terminated, leading to metaphase arrest.
Promote Tubulin Polymerization: See paclitaxel (Taxol).

Antimetabolites

Antimetabolites are similar enough to the physiologically important substance to replace them in a reaction chain, but different enough that the reaction cannot continue or the product is not functional and cell proliferation is retarded.
Folate Analogue: See methotrexate, the one member of this class.
Pyrimidine Analogues: Block methylation of deoxyuridylic acid to thymidylate and, therefore, the synthesis of DNA.
Purine Analogues: Analogues of guanine and hypoxanthine, they are incorporated in DNA, and RNA synthesis is altered.

React with DNA

A number of antibiotics (doxorubicin, bleomycin) or synthetics suggested by the structure of the antibiotics react with or are intercalated into DNA.

ANTI-INFECTIOUS CHEMOTHERAPY

The initial choice of an antibacterial (antibiotic or synthetic) is made on the basis of recorded experience with the clinical state, that is, without certain knowledge of the infectious agent (culture) and certainly without sensitivity testing. The large number of agents from which this "best guess" must be chosen, nevertheless, can be organized into a few classes based on their "spectrum of activity."

Here is one oversimplified spectrum. Beginning at the top, two lines could be drawn for each class: one that begins where predicted usefulness appears and ends where other agents are clearly preferable. For example, the line for *Benzyl Penicillins and Equivalent Cephalosporins* would begin with the spirochetes and extend into the enteric gram negative rods with a gap at *Lactamase Producing Staph.* Another type of representation showing actual bacterial sensitivity for the aminoglycosides would extend virtually from top to bottom. However, because of toxicity, the aminoglycosides are not used except for Gram negative rods and acid fast organisms or in combination when no other choice promises effectiveness.

Idealized Spectrum of Antibacterial Activity
Category

Spirochetes
Gram Positive Bacilli
Gram Positive Cocci
Lactamase Producing
Staphylococci
E. fecalis (Gp D Strep.)
Gram Negative Cocci
Gram Negative Bacilli, Enteric
Gram Negative Bacilli, Other
Acid Fast Rods
Chlamydiae
Mycoplasma
Rickettsiae

Lactam Antibiotics—Penicillins and Cephalosporins

The lactam antibiotics, penicillins and cephalosporins, interfere with the synthesis of the bacterial cell wall, a rigid structure outside of the plasma membrane and not found in animal cells.

The penicillins are, therefore, remarkably free of adverse effects. Allergic reactions are rare but anaphylaxis does occur; fungal or bacterial overgrowth may occur, and those lactams that are not absorbed completely may cause some cramps or diarrhea. The cephalosporins also cause anaphylaxis, skin rashes, nephritis, granulocytopenia, and hemolytic anemia. Cross-sensitization is low, but cephalosporin should not be used in patients with a history of Type I reactions to penicillin.

The native penicillins and, to a lesser extent, the cephalosporins are destroyed by bacterial, especially staphylococcal, beta-lactamase. To overcome this limitation and to extend the spectrum in the gram negative direction, many semisynthetic derivatives have been made. Seemingly endless substitutions have been made on the core penicilloic and cephalosporanic acids.

Benzyl Penicillins and Equivalent Cephalosporins

Penicillins G and V both derive from fermentation. Pen G is less stable in the stomach but more active after absorption or parenteral administration (all penicillins should be given at other than mealtimes).

The "first generation" cephalosporins (for example, cephalexin and cefazolin) are more resistant to Staph lactamase than the benzyl penicillins.

Penicillins Resistant to Staphylococcal Lactamase, Somewhat Less Active versus Gram Positives

Cloxacillin and others make up one group of semisynthetics that are active against lactamase-producing streptococci.

Formulations (Penicillin) Containing a Lactamase Inhibitor

Clavulanic acid and sulbactam are potent inhibitors of bacterial beta-lactamase. Given in combination with amoxicillin or ticarcillin, they maintain the concentration of the antibiotic at the site of bacterial growth.

Others (Non-Lactam) Resistant to Staphylococcal Lactamase

Vancomycin acts on cell wall synthesis but is not a lactam. It is reserved generally for use in resistant staphylococcal infections.

Penicillins with Wider Gram Negative Coverage, Less Active Against Gram Positives, Inactivated by Staph Lactamase Comparable Cephalosporins

Amoxicillin is used in mixed infections of the respiratory tract, in UTI with coliforms, in combination for Helicobacter, and is an alternate treatment for typhoid-paratyphoid. It has been replaced by ceftriaxone for treatment of H. influenzae meningitis. Second generation cephalosporins have about the same spectrum but are resistant to Staph lactamase.

Wider Gram Negative Coverage; Activity versus Gram Positives Retained, Enter CNS

The third generation cephalosporins can be summarized at the extreme of their indications:

Effective in meningitis and some activity versus P. aeruginosa: cefoperazone, cefotaxime, ceftriaxone, cefuroxime.

Uncertain effectiveness in meningitis and some activity versus P. aeruginosa: ceftazidime, cefsulodin, ceftizoxime.

Piperacillin, carbenicillin, mezlocillin, and ticarcillin have sometimes been placed in this category on the basis of their wider spectrum that extends perhaps to P. aeruginosa. They may be more properly placed above with amoxicillin because they are inactivated by lactamase and require concomitant aminoglycoside administration in serious Pseudomonas infections. They are not equivalent in meningitis.

Other Beta-Lactams

The beta-lactamase inhibitors (e.g., clavulanic acid) incorporated in the preparations above are very weak antibacterials. Two related simple beta-lactams are marketed. A monobactam, aztreonam, is active against gram negative rods. A carbapenem, imipenem, has a wide spectrum of activity. It has appreciable toxicity. It is combined with cilastin, an inhibitor of renal dihydropeptidase, to prevent its rapid inactivation.

Macrolide Antibiotics

Macrolides (e.g., erythromycin) are important because of their special indications: diphtheria, chlamydial infections, and pneumonias possibly caused by Mycoplasma or Legionella. They also have activity against gram positives comparable to penicillin but are not destroyed by lactamase. Erythromycin must be given with an enteric coating to prevent its destruction in the stomach. The newer azithromycin, clarithromycin and dirithromycin are absorbed better and have a slightly longer chemical half-life. Dosage of the erythromycins cannot be increased without pronounced nausea.

Lincomycin and clindamycin are not macrolides in structure but are similar to erythromycin pharmacologically. They are used occasionally against anaerobic infections.

Aminoglycosides

The aminoglycosides (e.g., streptomycin, gentamycin, neomycin) are bactericidal over much of the spectrum introduced above, from spirochetes through acid fast organisms. However, problems of toxicity, resistance, and absorption make them less than the perfect antibiotic.

Resistance develops invariably and quickly. It is plasmid controlled, i.e., transmissible, and is a public health problem with tuberculosis. They are ototoxic (cochlear and vestibular), nephrotoxic, and skin sensitizing with prolonged use or contact.

Aminoglycosides are, therefore, used only against gram negative enteric bacilli, when sepsis is present or suspected and against an enterococcal or gram negative endocarditis. Penicillin given concurrently may facilitate entry into the bacterial cell. With renal insufficiency, the drug may accumulate and cause additional toxicity. Dose and interval should be adjusted on the basis of creatinine and drug blood levels.

Streptomycin is now used in tuberculosis only with disseminated or progressing disease. Neomycin and kanamycin are used topically and by mouth to sterilize the gut.

Tetracyclines

The tetracyclines are bacteriostatic over practically the entire spectrum. If they are somewhat less potent than alternative drugs in general, their action against Mycoplasma, Chlamydiae, and Legionella make them useful in, for example, a pneumonia when the causative agent may be uncertain.

Resistance against the common bacteria is a problem in hospital practice and, to a minor extent, in the community even though it has been used widely in medicine and agriculture for fifty years.

Absorption is incomplete (calcium in food or medication further delays it) and the modification of flora leads to nausea, cramps, and diarrhea, or at least soft stools. Candida may overgrow in the mouth, vagina, or gut. If any of the seven tetracyclines is taken late in pregnancy or in children under the age of 8 years, the yellow drug may be deposited in the enamel with permanent staining. Deformation from enamel hypoplasia may occur rarely.

Perhaps the most common uses are in UTI, chronic respiratory tract infections, and acne. It is not invariably successful as a substitute for a lactam. Other uses are suggested by its spectrum discussed previously. The seven tetracyclines differ from one another in their duration of action.

Quinolones

It is the fluoroquinolones (ciprofloxacin and norfloxacin are examples) that are exciting many people. Six of these synthetics are marketed, but their evaluation is still incomplete. They are also too expensive for chronic use in the presence of so many alternate drugs.

Quinolones are bactericidal by inhibiting DNA gyrase and blocking DNA synthesis. They are not active against spirochetes but cover the balance of the orienting spectrum presented in the introduction above, through Legionella, Mycoplasma, Chlamydiae, and at least one mycobacterium. The limits to their usefulness cannot be defined at this time, nor can the problems with resistance be predicted.

Common adverse reactions include nausea, vomiting, headache, abnormal LFTs, skin rash, tendinitis, and insomnia. The insomnia has progressed to excitement, psychotic behavior, and convulsions. The effects (probably the blood levels) of caffeine and theophylline are increased by concomitant use. Photosensitivity, anaphylactic-like reactions, and colitis have been reported.

Nalidixic Acid and Cinoxacin must now be regarded as obsolete.

Sulfonamides

The first important antibacterial was sulfanilamide, which was followed by many other sulfonamide competitive antagonists to para-amino-benzoic acid (PABA). They are almost obsolete today except as a component of the important mixture defined next. Their spectrum extends from the gram positives into the enteric gram negative rods.

The modern soluble variants (sulfamethoxazole or trisulfapyrimidines) may still be used for uncomplicated UTIs. Sulfacetamide is still used topically in the eye. Some sulfasalazine is still used for inflammatory bowel disease; the ingested drug is split in the colon into a sulfa and the active component, 5-ASA.

Toxicity includes serious allergic reactions: arthritis, hepatitis, Stevens-Johnson syndrome, and others.

Sulfonamide-Trimethoprim Mixture

The sulfonamides, competitive antagonist to PABA, prevent the synthesis of the endogenous folate required by many pathogens. Trimethoprim, unrelated to the sulfonamides, inhibits dihydrofolate reductase, so that such folate as is formed is not converted to the tetrahydro, active form. These two reactions, acting sequentially, give a far more powerful bacteriostatic effect than the sulfas alone.

The combination (trimethoxazole, TMP-SMZ) is used in UTIs, prostatitis, and in Pneumocystis carinii pneumonia.

In addition to the adverse reactions associated in small numbers with the sulfas, the combination can cause a folate deficiency in the host with megaloblastosis. Concurrent administration of folic acid is preventive.

Non-Sulfonamide Urinary Tract Agents

Three unimportant obsolete drugs are included for identification only.

Antituberculous and Related Agents

This section purports only to define or identify the drugs mentioned in the alphabetical listing. To establish a treatment regimen for tuberculosis, the recommendations of the CDC or other comprehensive source is required. Treatment always uses at least two agents so that emerging resistant strains are suppressed by the second or third agent.

Agents of First Choice

Isoniazid (INH), rifampin, and ethambutol are the primary agents. Under some circumstances, pyrazinamide and streptomycin would also qualify. Treatment commonly begins with the first two of these three agents, preferably INH and rifampin. If resistance to INH is established by sensitivity testing or if resistance is suspected on the basis of area of origin, ethambutol should be added.

Second Line Agents

In case of a failure to respond or a relapse, and guided by sensitivity studies, a regimen that may include streptomycin or capreomycin is derived.

Agents for Atypical Mycobacteria

See the listings for dapsone and rifabutin.

Miscellaneous Antibacterials

CHLOROMYCETIN is a small molecule that was originally a fermentation product but is now synthetic. It has a broad spectrum of activity including many anaerobes and the rickettsiae, but it also caused aplastic anemia in a prohibitive number of cases. Also, excessive doses in newborns led to the "gray baby syndrome." It is still considered for use in brain abscess, serious H. influenzae, or typhoid infections, and as an alternative to tetracycline in rickettsial disease.

POLYMYXINS are surface active polypeptides once used systemically. They are prohibitively nephrotoxic and now, as Polymyxin B, are used topically.

SPECTINOMYCIN is related to the aminoglycosides. It is marketed only for IM use in treating gonorrhea when the patient is sensitive to lactams or is infected with a resistant strain.

METRONIDAZOLE, in addition to being a useful parasiticide, is bactericidal to anaerobes.

Systemic Antiviral Agents

General Class	Site of Inhibitory Effect *Drug Name*	Indication
Uncoating of Virus	**In Susceptible Cells** *Amantadine* *Rimantidine*	 **Influenza A** **Influenza A**
Purine and Pyrimidine Analogues	**DNA Polymerase** *Acyclovir* *Cidofovir* *Famciclovir* *Foscarnet* *Ganciclovir* *Valacyclovir* *Vidarabine* **DNA Synthesis** *Ribavirin*	**Herpes** **CMV** **Herpes zoster** **CMV** **retinitis** **CMV** **Herpes** **Herpex** **Respiratory syncytial**
Nucleoside Analogues (dideoxy-nucleo-sides)	**Reverse Transcriptase** *Delavirdine* *(Rescriptor)* *Didanosine* *(Videx, ddI)* *Lamivudine* *(Epivir)* *Nevirapine* *(Viramune)* *Stavudine* *(Zerit)* *Zalcitabine* *(Hivid)* *Zidovudine* *(Retrovir, AZT)*	 **All HIV**

General Class	Site of Inhibitory Effect *Drug Name*	Indication
Protease Inhibitor	**Viral protein**	
	Indinavir (Crixivan)	**HIV**
	Nelfinavir (Viracept)	**HIV**
	Ritonavir (Norvir)	**HIV**
	Saquinavir (Invirase)	**HIV**

Systemic Antifungal Agents

The section on dermatologic agents list a number of effective and safe drugs, imidazole and others, for the control of the dermatophytoses and candidiasis. Systemic drugs for the systemic mycoses are less satisfactory.

Amphotericin B is an antibiotic that is active against all of the fungi pathogenic for humans but also nephro- and hepatotoxic, and the long treatment is unpleasant. *Flucytosine* (converted to fluorouracil) can be used against Candida and Cryptococcus but in combination with amphotericin to prevent the invariable emergence of resistors. The *imidazoles* are being used for Candida (esophageal or systemic) and dermatophytosis. *Griseofulvin* by mouth accumulates in the keratin of the diseased skin or nails and in time is effective.

Antiparasitic Agents

The listing contains most of the drugs of this class easily available in the United States but only a sampling of the total. Indications can be sought under the listing for key drugs.

Malaria: Chloroquine, primaquine, Fansidar
Amoebae: Metronidazole, quinacrine
Pneumocystis: Pentamidine, trimethoprim-sulfamethoxazole

Worms: Pyrantel, mebendazole, thiabendazole
Scabies: Lindane, pyrantel

GASTROINTESTINAL AGENTS

Inhibitors of Gastric Acid Secretion (H2 Antagonists, Proton Pump Inhibitors)

All stimulants to gastric acid secretion except gastrin act through a final common pathway involving histamine acting on a subgroup (H2) of histamine receptors. The H2 antagonists (cimetidine is the only one to consider) reduce basal and food-stimulated acid secretion. Omeprazole and lansoprazole block hydrogen ion secretion even more effectively by an effect on the ATPase of the parietal cells. Indications include the following: treatment of signs of hyperchlorhydria; promote healing and prevent recurrence of duodenal esophageal or benign gastric ulcers; and prevent stress ulcers in post-op, burn, and other vulnerable patients. The advantage in the pump inhibitors is insuffient to justify not using the inexpensive cimetidine.

Antacids

Effects: The hydrated oxides of aluminum, magnesium, and, to a lesser extent, calcium carbonate are nonabsorbable. They neutralize and form salts with HCl in the stomach, but, in the alkaline intestine, their original state is restored. Thus, they cannot cause alkalosis or other systemic effects. Sodium is absorbed from sodium bicarbonate, and a systemic effect is invariable. Aluminum and magnesium gels are able to absorb other drugs (e.g., tetracycline) and slow absorption. All antacids may alter dissolution and absorption.

Antiemetics

Motion sickness

Motion sickness is a problem different from the other emetogenic states and is much easier to treat. The relevant drugs, antihistamines and scopolamine are mentioned in discussion of antihistamines above.

Antiemetics (Serotonin Antagonists)

Blockers of serotonin type three receptors (ondansetron, for example) are the only antiemetics dependably effective against the nausea and vomiting from cisplatin and other cytotoxic agents.

Antiemetics (Minor)

See listings for metoclopropamide and phenothiazines such as promethazine.

Laxatives and Bowel Cleansers

Isosmotic or Hypertonic Solutions

Isotonic solution (4L) of polyethylene glycol and electrolytes (e.g., NuLYTELY) is taken by mouth over a 2.5-hour period to prepare the bowel for surgery or imaging.

Irritant Laxatives

Irritant laxatives act on the wall of the intestine to stimulate activity with no effect on the possibly inspissated material therein. Examples include cascara and castor oil.

Bulk and Saline Laxatives

Milk of magnesia or psyllium gel hold water in the lumen and stimulate activity by distending the bowel.

Fecal Softener Laxatives

Mineral oil forms an emulsion with the contents of the colon and is dependably active. The detergents are probably less effective as emulsifying agents but may have some irritant effect.

Anti-Diarrheal Agents

Relatively benign diarrheas that do not require fluid replacement or specific chemotherapy may be controlled most dependably with small, frequent doses of a weak narcotic such as codeine or small doses of paregoric or diphenoxylate. OTC mixtures of a very weak narcotic are available (loperamide).

Miscellaneous GI Agents

Lactulose is a disaccharide metabolized in the colon to low MW acids that trap ammonia. It is used in hepatic failure. It also becomes osmotically active.

Mesalamine and olsalazine taken by mouth liberate 5-ASA in the colon for the treatment of inflammatory bowel disease.

DERMATOLOGIC AGENTS AND PREPARATIONS

Only two drug groups beyond those already defined are introduced in this section. However, there are indications and dose forms distinctive to the organ system, and this outline may be useful.

The vehicle used to apply the drug may have therapeutic properties of its own and the preparation must be chosen to match the acuteness or chronicity of the process. Wet preparations and powders dry acute lesions; ointments macerate (hydrate) the underlying skin.

Antiinflammatory Steroids, Topical

Some steroids available topically are more potent than others; however, because the concentration is adjusted, the differences are not important. Possibly the fluorinated derivatives are an exception. Absorption from an ointment is greater than from a cream, and absorption from both is increased by the use of an occlusive dressing of plastic film. Repeated use builds up a reservoir in the skin and once daily application is sufficient.

The catabolic effect is shown by atrophy of the skin after large amounts for extended periods. Observe the limits suggested with each preparation. See earlier text for contraindications and systemic effects.

Topical Anti-infectious Agents

For those occasions when topical application of antibacterials is indicated, the requisite preparations are listed under the specific agent. Mixtures containing bacitracin, polymyxin B, or neomycin are in common use. In treating acne erythromycin, clindamycin, tetracycline, and metronidazole are available in topical preparations.

Topical Fungicides

Nystatin and amphotericin B can be used against candidiasis but not against dermatophytes. The imidazoles are active against both.

(Ecto) Parasiticidal Agents

Permethrin (OTC), a synthetic analogue of pyrethrin, has the highest cure rate after a single application.

Keratolytic and Keratoplastic Agents

The keratoplastic effect is a consequence of the keratolytic process. Acne, the common indication, requires OTC abrasives and benzoyl peroxide, topical or systemic antibiotics, tretinoin, and, if necessary, isotretinoin by mouth.

Antipsoriatic Agents

Inflammation and plaque formation is controlled by topical steroids, the retinols (tretinoin, isotretinoin, and etretinate) and calcipotriene.

Miscellaneous

Hydroquinone (reversibly) and monobenzone (irreversibly) reduce hyperpigmentation.

OPHTHALMIC AGENTS AND PREPARATIONS

Only two drug groups beyond those already defined are introduced in this chapter. However, the indications and dose forms are distinctive to the organ system, and this outline may be useful.

Agents Used in the Treatment of Glaucoma

Drops instilled in the treatment of glaucoma (e.g., pilocarpine) usually constrict the pupil, and the contraction of the ciliary muscle increases outflow of aqueous humor from the angle. The same and other drugs reduce the rate of secretion. The properties of drug groups already described should be recalled because absorption after transport through the naso-lacrimal duct can lead to side effects.

Beta-Adrenergic Receptor Blockers

Alpha-Adrenergic Blocking Agent

Dapiprazole is listed here because it reverses the mydriasis and lowers IOP after local anesthesia or phenylephrine.

Sympathomimetic

Parasympathomimetic (Miotics)

Choline Esters and Related

Pilocarpine and the beta blockers are the most frequently used.

Cholinesterase Inhibitors

Prostaglandin

See latanoprost for this dramatic new drug.

Carbonic Anhydrase (CA) Inhibitors

Acetazolamide and two others reduce aqueous secretion by reducing the availability of bicarbonate. They are useful in chronic (open angle) and preoperatively in acute glaucoma. These are sodium diuretics for only a few days of administration, but the effect on the eye (and urinary excretion of bicarbonate) persists. CA inhibitors also are used to prevent and treat acute mountain sickness.

Osmotic Agents

Hypertonic solutions of substances that do not enter the cells (urea, glycerol, mannitol) can be used to extract fluid and rapidly lower pressure.

Mydriatics, Non-Cycloplegic

Sympathomimetics dilate the pupil for examination without paralyzing accommodation.

Mydriatics, Cycloplegic (Cholinergics, Parasympathomimetics)

Used preparatory to refraction or to maintain mydriasis with infection.

Anti-inflammatory Steroids

See under Endocrine Agents.

Anti-inflammatory, Non-steroidal

Four NSAIDs are available as ophthalmic drops to prevent miosis during surgery or to treat inflammation after surgery.

Mast Cell Stabilizer

Lodoxamide is comparable to cromolyn, which is no longer available in ophthalmic dose form. It is used for hay fever.

Antihistamine

See levocabastine (combination of two antihistamines).

Local Anesthetics

Two are available for use on the conjunctiva in addition to the usual injectables.

Anti-infective Agents

See individual agents in alphabetical listing.

Adjuncts to Surgery

For chymotrypsin, hyaluronate, and botulinum toxin, see under alphabetical listing.

RESPIRATORY AGENTS

The most widely used drugs in this category have already been defined mechanistically as autonomic and endocrine agents. However, the indications and dose forms are distinctive to the organ system, and this outline may be useful.

Lung Surfactant

Neonatal respiratory distress syndrome (RDS) is associated with a deficiency of surfactant acting on the alveolar membrane. Some benefit follows the intratracheal provision of DPPC (dipalmitoylphosphatidylcholine) together with spreading agents essential for its action. Colfosceril and beractant are synthetic and natural (bovine) sources of the combination.

Mucolytics

Acetylcysteine acts on disulfide bonds and dornase fragments DNA. Both liquefy the viscid secretions of cystic fibrosis. Acetylcysteine also increases glutathione synthesis and protects against hepatic necrosis after acetaminophen overdose.

Expectorants

See part III.

Antiallergic Agents, Non-Steroidal

Cromolyn and congener are thought with some basis to act by preventing the release of histamine from mast cells. They must be given as fine powders or aerosolized suspensions for prophylaxis of asthma or for prevention or treatment of allergic rhinitis.

Antitussives

The most dependable antitussives are small doses of codeine or a stronger narcotic depending upon the need. See Part III

Anti-inflammatory (Cortico-) Steroids

These are used for systemic effect, for deep (pulmonary) inhalation, and for nasal inhalation.

Parasympatholytic for Deep Inhalation

Sympathomimetics (Beta Agonists)

Used in asthmatics by injection, by mouth, and by deep inhalation.

Sympathomimetics for Nasal Decongestion

Refer to alpha and mixed agonists but especially to topical use of incomplete sympathomimetics.

GENERAL AND LOCAL ANESTHESIA AND CONSCIOUS SEDATION

General Anesthetics and Adjuncts

Typical "balanced anesthesia" begins with premedication as described below; induction and intubation with a short acting, injected agent; maintenance with nitrous oxide or a Freon; and exposure and deepened anesthesia with a curariform drug and a narcotic.

Complete Anesthetics

The pharmacology of the general anesthetics is exactly the same as that of the sedative-hypnotics except that gases or volatile liquids are selected for use. These drugs can be given by inhalation with breath-by-breath control of dose and rapid reversal of effect. The fluorohalohydrocarbons are used because they are not explosive and cause minimal postoperative vomiting. They require assisted respiration and careful induction as with all halogenated hydrocarbons. Examples are enflurane (Ethrane), isoflurane (Forane), desflurane (Suprane) and sevoflurane (Ultane).

Agents for Induction

These agents are discussed with ultra-short acting hypnotics.

Neuromuscular Blocking Agents

With one exception (weakening electroshock convulsions), these drugs are used to permit intubation and secure exposure at surgery.

Depolarizing Agent: Succinylcholine acts like an excess of acetylcholine at the voluntary nerve muscle junction. After a brief period of stimulation with fasciculation, the muscles remain depolarized and paralyzed. The effect is brief.

Non-Depolarizing (Competitive) Agents: The longer acting curare alkaloids, for example, pancuronium (Pavulon) or atracurium (Tracrium), are competitive antagonists to acetylcholine at this one site. Their effect can be terminated by a cholinesterase inhibitor that allows acetylcholine to accumulate.

Preprocedural Agents (Conscious Sedation)

If a relatively minor but anxiety producing procedure is to be performed, it is desirable to have the patient deeply sedated but not to cross the line between deep sedation and general anesthesia when the protective reflexes are lost and danger is increased greatly.

Sedatives

For procedures that are not painful, it is possible to give a sedative such as diazepam or midazolam by vein, fractionally, and get relief of anxiety and amnesia without approaching the border. Even so, one person should observe the patient without the distraction of other functions; indeed, such caution is required by statute in some states. Analgesia is poor, and a narcotic analgetic may be added in small doses.

Incomplete Anesthetics

Two sedatives, nitrous oxide and ketamine, are peculiar in that they cannot take the patient into general anesthesia regardless of dose. Injected ketamine is long acting and excitement during recovery is common.

Antipsychotic-Opiate Combination

When an antipsychotic is injected with a narcotic, the sedation is increased significantly but the respiratory depression is not increased. If allowance is made for the commonly occurring postural hypotension, the mixture is safe. With the patient in a semierect position or with other hypotensive drugs, it can cause trouble. Mixtures of promethazine-meperidine, fentanyl-droperidol, and atropine-morphine are used.

Local Anesthetics

Some local anesthetics are **injectable only,** that is, are active if deposited around a nerve or sensory ending but, except in prohibitively alkaline solution, do not penetrate and anesthetize mucous membranes. Others, like lidocaine, have favorable pK and are **injectable or topical.**

Two (OTC) are insoluble and are **topical (mucosal) only.** None will act on the intact skin.

ANTIDOTES AND AGENTS USED IN MANAGEMENT OF POISONINGS

The following treatments may be useful in managing intoxications with the (toxic agents) listed. Dosage and preparations can be found in the alphabetical listing:

Acetylcysteine	(Acetaminophen)
Amyl Nitrite	(Cyanide)
Apomorphine	(Induce emesis)
Atropine	(Organophosphates)
Bicarbonate	(Methanol)
Charcoal, activated	(Adsorb ingested agent)
Deferoxamine	(Iron)
Digoxin Immune FAB	(Digoxin)
Dimercaprol	(BAL) (Mercury)
Edetate Ca Na_2	(Lead)
Flumazenil	(Benzodiazepine sedation)
Ipecac, syrup of	(Induce emesis)
Methylene Blue	(Methemoglobinemia)
Na Nitrite	(Cyanide)
Na Thiosulfate	(Cyanide, Bleach)
Neostigmine	(Curariform)
Opiates	(Naloxone)
Oxygen	(Carbon monoxide)
Penicillamine	(Cu, Hg, Pb, As)
Pralidoxime	(Organophosphates)
Protamine	(Heparin)
Phytonadione	(Warfarin)
Trienitine	(Cu alternate)

PART II

INDEX OF PRESCRIPTION DRUGS

GENERIC NAME Trade Name	INDICATIONS AND DOSAGES	DOSE FORMS	GROUP (G)/SUBGROUP (SG) Relative Cost within Group
8-Arginine Vasopressin	See VASOPRESSIN		Antidiuretic Hormone
8-Lysine Vasopressin	See LYPRESSIN		Antidiuretic Hormone
15-methyl PGF2a	See CARBOPROST		Oxytocic
25-Hydroxychole calciferol	See CALCIFEDIOL		D Vitamin Prodrug
25[OH]-D3	See CALCIFEDIOL		D Vitamin Prodrug
5 FC	See FLUCYTOSINE		Antifungal, systemic
8-MOP	See METHOXSALEN		Pigmenting Agent
A-Hydrocort	See HYDROCORTISONE		Corticosteroid
A-poxide	See CHLORDIAZEPOXIDE		Sedative, Long Acting
A-Spaz	See DICYCLOMINE		Parasympatholytic
AB	See AMPHOTERICIN B		Antifungal, systemic
Abbokinase	See UROKINASE		Thrombolytic
ABCIXIMAB ReoPro Centocor	**Inhibit Thrombogenesis After Angioplasty**		METABOLIC AGENTS (G) Coagulant-Anticoagulant (SG) Inhibit Platelet Aggregation SSG)
ACARBOSE Precose	**Diabetes (NIDDM):** PO: Initially 25 mg tid at start of each meal then adjust at monthly intervals to 50–100 mg tid	**Tablets:** 50, 100 mg	ENDOCRINE AGENTS (G) Oral Antidiabetic Agents (SG) Delays absorption of glucose (SSG)
Accolate	**See ZAFIRLUKAST**		**Leukotriene Antagonist (Asthma)**
Accupril	**See QUINAPRIL**		**ACE Inhibitor (SG)**
Accurbron	**See THEOPHYLLINE**		**Xanthine Bronchodilator**
Accutane	**See ISOTRETINOIN**		**Keratolytic**

GENERIC NAME Trade Name	INDICATIONS AND DOSAGES	DOSE FORMS	GROUP (G)/SUBGROUP (SG) Relative Cost within Group
ACEBUTOLOL Sectral	**Hypertension:** PO: 400 mg/d initially as 1 or 2 doses; 200–1200 mg/d maintenance, given in 2 doses. **Ventricular Arrhythmias:** PO: 200 mg bid initially; 600–1200 mg/d maintenance, given in 2 doses. When discontinuing, taper dose over two or more weeks.	**Tablet:** 200, 400 mg	AUTONOMIC NS AGENTS (G) Sympathoplegics (SG) Beta Adrenergic Receptor Blockers (SSG) Cardioselective (Beta 1) (SSG) **Cost:** Medium
ACETAMIN-OPHEN OTC, Generic, Tylenol, APAP, Feverall	**Pain, Fever:** PO: 325–650 mg q4–6h; max. dose 4.0 gm/d. Pediatric (6–12 yrs) PO: 325 mg q4h–6h; max.dose 2.6 gm/d. Pediatric (3–6 yrs) PO: 120 mg q4–6h; max. dose 720 mg/d.	**Capsule:** 80, 160, 500 mg **Tablet:** 160, 325, 500, 650 mg **Tablet:** (Chewable) 80 mg **Granules:** 80 mg **Liquid:** 160 mg/ 5 ml, 500 mg/ 15 ml **Suppository:** 80,120, 125, 300, 325, 650 mg **Elixir:** 80,120,130, 160,325 mg/5 ml **Solution:** 120 mg/ 2.5 ml,100 mg/ml **Suspension:** 160 mg/ 5 ml, 80 mg/ 0.8 ml	ANTI-INFLAMMATORY ETC. AGENTS (G) Non-Narcotic Analgesics (SG) **Cost:** Low
ACETAZOL-AMIDE Generic, Diamox	**Chronic Open-Angle Glaucoma:** PO: 250–1000 mg/d in 3–4 doses. **Acute Glaucoma (short-term use):** PO: 500 mg to start, then 125–250 q4h. IV, IM: 500 mg bolus, then 125–250 mg q2–4h. **Acute Mountain Sickness:** PO: 500–1000 mg/day in divided doses (start therapy 1–2 days prior to ascent). **Epilepsy:** PO: 8–30 mg/kg/day given in divided doses; maintenance 375–1000 mg/ day.	**Tablet:** 125, 250 mg **Capsule:** (Ext'd release) 500 mg	OPHTHALMIC AGENTS (G) Used In Glaucoma (SG) Carbonic Anhydrase Inhibitors (SG) **Cost:** Low
ACETOHEX-AMIDE Generic, Dy-melor	**NIDD Diabetes:** PO: 250–1500 mg/d in 1–2 doses).	**Tablet:** 250, 500 mg	ENDOCRINE AGENTS (G) Oral Antidiabetic Agents (SG) Sulfonylurea (SSG) **Cost:** Medium

GENERIC NAME Trade Name	INDICATIONS AND DOSAGES	DOSE FORMS	GROUP (G)/SUBGROUP (SG) Relative Cost within Group
ACETOPHEN-AZINE Tindal	**Psychotic Disorders:** PO: 20 mg tid to start; maintenance 40–80 mg/d (max. dose 400–600 mg/d, in hospitalized patients)	**Tablet:** 20 mg	CNS AGENTS (G) Antipsychotics (SG) Agents Causing Prominent Extrapyramidal Side Effects (SG) **Cost:** Medium
ACETYL-CYSTEINE Generic, Mucosil	**Mucolytic:** Nebulization (face mask, mouth piece, tracheostomy): 1–10 ml of the 20% solution or 2–20 ml of the 10% solution every 2 to 6 hours. RESPIRATORY AGENTS (G) Expectorants and Mucolytic Agents (SG) **Acetaminophen Overdose:** PO, via NGT, or duodenal intubation: 140 mg/kg loading dose, then 70 mg/kg 4 h later and q4h for up to 17 total doses or until acetaminophen assay indicates only nontoxic levels remain.	**Solution:** 10%, 20% (as sodium).	ANTIDOTES (G)
Acetylsalicylic acid	See ASPIRIN		Non-Narcotic Analgesia
Achromycin	See TETRACYCLINE		Tetracycline Antibiotic
Actibine	See YOHIMBINE		Vasodilator
Aclovate	See ALCLOMETASONE		Corticosteroid, Topical
ACTH	See CORTICOTROPIN		Adrenocorticotropin
Acthar	See CORTICOTROPIN		Adrenocorticotropin
Actidil	See TRIPROLIDINE		Antihistamine
Actigall	See URSODIOL		Dissolve Gall Stones
Actimmune	See INTERFERON GAMMA-1B		Cytokine
Actinomycin D	See DACTINOMYCIN		Cancer Chemotherapy
Activase	See ALTEPLASE		Thrombolytic
Accupril	See QUINAPRIL		ACE Inhibitor
Acycloguanosine	See ACYCLOVIR		Antiviral

GENERIC NAME Trade Name	INDICATIONS AND DOSAGES	DOSE FORMS	GROUP (G)/SUBGROUP (SG) Relative Cost within Group
ACYCLOVIR Zovirax, Acyclo-guanosine	**Herpes Simplex Infections (Immunocompromised Patients):** IV: 5 mg/kg (infuse over 1 hour) q8h for 7 days. **Herpes Simplex Encephalitis (Immunocompromised Patients):** IV: 10 mg/kg (infuse over 1 hour) q8h for 10 days. **Varicella-Zoster (Immunocompromised Patients):** IV: 5–10 mg/kg (infuse over 1 hour) q8h for 7 days **Initial Genital Herpes:** PO: 200 mg q4h (5 times per day) for 10 days; max. dose 1 g/d. **Chronic Suppressive Therapy for Recurrent Herpes:** PO: 200 mg bid for 6 months. **Intermittent Therapy:** PO: 200 mg q4h (5 times per day) for 5 days; reinitiate at first sign of recurrence. **Herpes Zoster (acute):** PO: 800 mg q4h 5 times per day for 7–10 days. **Chickenpox:** PO: 20 mg/kg QID for 5 days (max. single dose 800 mg/dose). **Herpes Genitalis; Mucocutaneous Herpes (Immunocompromised Patients):** Topical: Apply 0.5 inch ribbon/4 sq. inch area q3h six times per day for 7 days. IV: 6.2 mg/kg IV, q8h for 7d	**Capsule:** 200 mg **Injection:** (powder) 500 mg/vial, 1000 mg/vial **Tablet:** 400, 800 mg **Ointment:** 5% **Suspension:** 200 mg/ 5ml	ANTI-INFECTIOUS AGENTS (G) Antiviral Agents (SG)
Adalat	See NIFEDIPINE		Ca Channel Blocker
ADAPALENE Differin	**Acne:** Topical: Apply once each evening **Gel:** 0.1%		DERMATOLOGIC AGENTS (G) Keratolytic and Keratoplastic Agents (SG) Acne and Psoriasis (SSG) **Cost:** Moderate
Adapin	See DOXEPIN		TCA, Antidepressant
Adenocard	See ADENOSINE		Antiarrhythmic
ADENOSINE Adenocard Adenoscan	**Supraventricular Tachyarrhythmias (including WPW):** IV: (Rapid bolus), initial dose 6 mg (over 1–2 second period), if not effective, give second dose of 12 mg 1–2 minutes after first dose as rapid IV bolus; repeat 12 mg dose one additional time if needed (max. dose per injection 12 mg). **Substitute for exercise in thallium-201 scintigraphy:** IV: (Continuous infusion), 140 mcg 1 kg/min for 6 min.	**Injection:** 6 mg/ 2ml; 3 mg/ml, 30 ml vial	CARDIOVASCULAR AGENTS (G) Antiarrhythmic Agents (SG) Miscellaneous Antiarrhythmic Agents (SG) **Cost:** Low
Adrenalin	See EPINEPHRINE		Sympathomimetic
Adrenocortico-tropic Hormone	See CORTICOTROPIN		ACTH

GENERIC NAME Trade Name	INDICATIONS AND DOSAGES	DOSE FORMS	GROUP (G)/SUBGROUP (SG) Relative Cost within Group
Adenoscan	See ADENOSINE		Vasodilator
Adriamycin	See DOXORUBICIN		Cancer Chemotherapy
Adrucil	See FLUOROURACIL		Cancer Chemotherapy
Advil	See IBUPROFEN		Non-Narcotic Analgetic
AeroBid	See FLUNISOLIDE		Corticosteroid
Afrin	See OXYMETAZOLINE		Nasal Decongestant
Aftate	See TOLNAFTATE		Antifungal, Topical
Agoral	PO: 7.5–15cc hs.	**Liquid Emulsion** (per 15 cc)**:** mineral oil (4.2 g), phenolphthalein (200 mg).	GI AGENTS (G) Laxatives (SG)
AK-Homatropine	See HOMATROPINE		Parasympatholytic
AK-Taine	See PROPARACAINE		Local Anesthetic
Akineton	See BIPERIDEN		Parasympatholytic, Parkinsonism
Akne-mycin	See ERYTHROMYCIN		Macrolide Antibiotic
Albamycin	See NOVOBIOCIN		Lactamase Resistant Antibiotic
ALBUTEROL Generic, Proventil, Ventolin, Salbutamol	**Bronchospasm:** PO: 2–4 mg tid-QID initially; gradually increase to max. dose 32 mg/d. Geriatric PO: 2 mg tid-QID initially. Pediatric (6–14 yrs) PO: 2 mg tid-QID initially; gradually increase to max. dose 24 mg/d in divided doses. Inhalation: 1–2 sprays q4–6 h Nebulization: 2.5 mg tid or QID.	**Tablet:** 2, 4 mg **Tablet:** (Ext'd release) 8 mg **Syrup:** 2mg/5ml **Inhaler:** 90 mg/ spray (200 sprays)	AUTONOMIC NS AGENTS (G) Sympathomimetics (SG) Unselective Beta 1 and 2 Agonists (SG) **Cost:** Medium
Alcaine	See PROPARACAINE		Local Anesthetic
ALCLOMETA-SONE Aclovate	Apply to affected area 2–3 times per day. Medium Potency	**Ointment:** 0.05% **Cream:** 0.05%	DERMATOLOGIC AGENTS (G) Anti-Inflammatory Steroids, Topical (SG) **Cost:** Medium
Aldactazide	See SPIRONOLACTONE/HCTZ COMBINATION		K Sparing Diuretic
Aldactone Diuretic	See SPIRONOLACTONE		Potassium Sparing
ALDESLEUKIN Interleukin-2, Proleukin	**Metastatic Renal Cell Carcinoma:** IV: 600,000 IU/kg q8h (give IV over 15 min.; give a total of 14 doses with initial course, rest 9 days, then give another 14 doses)	**Powder:** for injection/ reconstitution: 22 million IU/ vial.	ANTI-INFLAMMATORY, ETC AGENTS (G) Immunomodulators (SG)
Aldoclor	See METHYLDOPA-DIURETIC COMBINATION		Hypotensive-Diuretic Combination
Aldomet	See METHYLDOPA		Hypotensive (Central Sympathoplegic)

GENERIC NAME Trade Name	INDICATIONS AND DOSAGES	DOSE FORMS	GROUP (G)/SUBGROUP (SG) Relative Cost within Group
Aldoril	See METHYLDOPA-DIURETIC COMBINATION		Hypotensive-Diuretic Combination
ALENDRONATE Fosamax	**Established Postmenopausal Osteoporosis:** PO: 10 mg/d in the AM before anything by mouth (even coffee) give with plain water. Eat no food and maintain erect position for 30 min. **Paget's disease:** PO: 40 mg/d for 6 months. Retreatment guided by alkaline phosphatase. See also Pamidronate.	**Tablet:** 10 mg	METABOLIC AGENTS (G) Calcium Kinetics Regulators (SG) Other Calcium Regulators (SG) **Cost:** High
ALESSE	**Oral Contraception:** PO: Levonorgestrel 0.1 mg and ethinyl estradiol 20 mcg. 21 such tabs in 28 day pack.		
Aleve	See NAPROXEN		Non-Narcotic Analgetic
Alfenta	See ALFENTANIL		Narcotic Analgetic
ALFENTANIL Alfenta	**Narcotic Analgesic, Adjunct to Anesthesia:** IV: 8–20 mcg/kg induction; then 0.5–1 mcg/kg/min maintenance.	**Injection:** 500 mcg/ml	CNS AGENTS (G) Narcotic Analgesics And Related Agents (SG) Narcotic Analgesics of Intermediate Potency (SG) **Cost:** High
Alferon N	See INTERFERON ALFA-3		Cytokine
ALG	See ANTI-THYMOCYTE GLOBULIN		Immunomodulator
ALGLUCERASE Glucocerebrosidase-B-glucosidase, Ceredase	**Gaucher's Disease:** IV: 60 U/kg (infused SLOWLY over 1 to 2 hours) initial dose; then repeat dose qod to q 4 weeks, depending on severity. Taper dose to minimal effective dose with downward adjustments q 3–6 months.	**Injection:** 10, 80 U/ml	METABOLIC AGENTS (G) Enzymes (SG) **Cost:** Medium
Alka-Mints	See CALCIUM CARBONATE		Antacid
Alkeran	See MELPHALAN		Cancer Chemotherapy
Allegra	See FEXOFENADINE		Antihistamine
ALLOPURINOL Generic, Zyloprim, Lopurin	**Gout, Prophylaxis:** PO: Initially 100 mg/d, then increase weekly by 100 mg/d; maintenance = 200–300 mg/d in mild cases and 400–600 mg/d in severe cases (max. dose 800 mg/d). **Control of Gouty Attacks:** PO: 200–600 mg/d (max single dose 300 mg; max daily dose 800 mg) **Uric Acid Nephropathy, Prevention During Chemotherapy:** PO: 600–800 mg/d for 2–3 days (also vigorously hydrate). **Recurrent Calcium Oxalate Stones:** PO: 200–300 mg/day.	**Tablets:** 100,300 mg **Suspension:** 5 mg/ml	METABOLIC AGENTS (G) Agents Used In The Treatment Of Gout (G) **Cost:** Low
Alomide	See LODOXAMIDE		Mast Cell Stabilizer
Alpha Nine SD	See COAGULANT FACTOR IX		Hemophilia B

GENERIC NAME Trade Name	INDICATIONS AND DOSAGES	DOSE FORMS	GROUP (G)/SUBGROUP (SG) Relative Cost within Group
ALPHA-D GALACTOSIDASE OTC, Alpha-D-Galactosidase, Beano	PO: 3–8 qtt per average-sized meal.	**Liquid:** 175 galactose units per 5 drop dosage	METABOLIC AGENTS (G) Enzymes (SG)
Alphagan	See BRIMONIDINE		Glaucoma (Central Sympatholytic)
Alphamul	See CASTOR OIL		Irritant Laxative
ALPRAZOLAM Generic, Xanax	**Sedation:** PO: 0.25–0.5 mg tid (max. dose 4 mg/d).	**Tablet:** 0.25, 0.5, 1, 2 mg **Liquid:** 0.5 mg/5ml, 1 mg/ml	CNS AGENTS (G) Sedative-Hypnotics (G) Intermediate-Acting Sedative Hypnotics (SG) **Cost:** High
ALPROSTADIL Caverject Muse Prostin VR Pediatric, Prostaglandin E1 PGE1	**Temporary Maintenance of Ductus Arteriosus Patency:** Begin infusion with 0.1 mcg/kg/minute. Maintain at the lowest effective dosage, e.g., between 0.01 and 0.1 mcg/kg/minute (max dose: 0.4 mcg/kg/minute) **Erectile Dysfunction:** Intracavernous Injection: 2.5 mcg initial injection (dorso-lateral proximal third of penis); Subsequent injections of 5 mcg and more (increase in 5 mcg increments) to endpoint of erection lasting not > 1h (max. single dose = 60 mcg, Do not use > once/d), and not more often than 3 times a week.	**Injection:** 500 mcg/ml **Muse Urethral Suppository:** 125, 250, 500, 1000 mcg pellets in hollow applicator. Insert prn. Successful in more than half of attempts. Cost: Minimum of $20/insertion. **Injection:** 500 mcg/ml	CV AGENTS (G) Vasodilators (SG) Arteriolar Dilators and Miscellaneous Agents (SSG) **Cost:** High
Altace	See RAMIPRIL		ACE Inhibitor
ALTEPLASE Activase, TPA	**Acute Myocardial Infarction:** IV: initially 15 mg bolus then 50 mg infusion over 30 min then 30 mg infusion over 60 min **Pulmonary Embolism:** IV: 100 mg (given over 2h).	**Injection:** (powder) 20 mg (11.6 million IU) per vial, 50 mg (29 million IU) per vial	METABOLIC AGENTS (G) Anticoagulants and Coagulants (SG) Thrombolytic Agents (SSG) **Cost:** Very High
Alternagel	See ALUMINUM HYDROXIDE GEL		Antacid
ALTRETAMINE Hexamethylmelamine Hexalen	CANCER CHEMOTHERAPY (G) React With DNA (SG) Other Miscellaneous (SSG)		
Alu-Cap	See ALUMINUM HYDROXIDE GEL		Antacid
ALUMINUM CARBONATE Basaljel	**Hyperphosphatemia:** PO: 2 caps or tabs or 10 ml of suspension q2h as often as 12 times a day. Capsule, Tablet, Suspension (Tablets and capsules contain equivalent of 500 mg of aluminum hydroxide, suspension 400 mg/ml.)		GASTROINTESTINAL AGENTS (G) Antacids (SG) Acid Neutralizing (SG) **Cost:** Low

GENERIC NAME Trade Name	INDICATIONS AND DOSAGES	DOSE FORMS	GROUP (G)/SUBGROUP (SG) Relative Cost within Group
ALUMINUM HYDROXIDE GEL Generic, OTC, Amphojel, Gelumina, Alternagel, Alu-Cap	**Gastric Hyperacidity:** PO: 500–1500 mg (or 5–30 ml suspension) 3–6 times/d (between meals and hs). **Capsule:** 400, 500 mg	**Tablet:** 300, 500, 600 mg **Suspension:** 320, 450 ,600, 675 mg/ 5ml	GASTROINTESTINAL AGENTS (G) Antacids (SG) Acid Neutralizing (SG) **Cost:** Low
ALUMINUM HYDROXIDE with **MAGNESIUM HYDROXIDE** Generic, OTC, Maalox, Mylanta, Magnox, etc.	**Gastric Hyperacidity:** PO: 5–10 ml QID. PO: 1–2 tabs QID.	**Maalox:** **Tablet:** 225 mg Al hydroxide; 200 mg hydroxide. **Mylanta:** with 20 mg Simethicone.	GASTROINTESTINAL AGENTS (G) Antacids (SG) Acid Neutralizing (SG) **Cost:** Low
ALUMINUM HYDROXIDE with **MAGNESIUM TRISILICATE** Generic, OTC, Gelusil	**Gastric Hyperacidity:** PO: 1–2 tsp. PO: 2 tabs.	**Tablets:** chewable	GASTROINTESTINAL AGENTS (G) Antacids (SG) Acid Neutralizing (SG) **Cost:** Low
Alupent	See METAPROTERENOL		Beta Adrenergic Agonist
AMANTADINE Generic Symmetrel Symadine	**Influenza A:** PO: 100 mg bid Pediatric PO: 2.2–4.4 mg/kg bid **Parkinson's:** PO. 100 mg bid	**Capsule:** 100 mg **Syrup:** 50 mg/ml	ANTI-INFECTIOUS AGENT (G) Antiviral, Systemic (SG) Also CNS AGENT (G) Stimulant (SG) Aminergic Agent (SG)
Amaryl	See GLIMEPIRIDE		Oral Antidiabetic
AMBENYL	See PART III		
Ambien	See ZOLPIDEM		Hypnotic, Ultra Short
AMCINONIDE Cyclocort	Topical: Apply to affected area 2 to 3 times a day.	**High Potency:** **Ointment:** 0.1%. **Medium Potency:** **Cream:** 0.1%. **Lotion:** 0.1%.	DERMATOLOGIC AGENTS (G) Anti-Inflammatory Steroids, Topical (SG) **Cost:** High
Amen	See MEDROXYPROGESTERONE		Progestin
Amethopterin	See METHOTREXATE		Folate Antagonist
Amicar	See AMINOCAPROIC ACID		Hemostatic
Amidate	See ETOMIDATE		Induction of Anesthesia
AMIFOSTINE Ethyol	CANCER CHEMOTHERAPY (G) Reduce Toxicity of Cisplatin		

GENERIC NAME Trade Name	INDICATIONS AND DOSAGES	DOSE FORMS	GROUP (G)/SUBGROUP (SG) Relative Cost within Group
AMIKACIN Generic, Amikin, Amikacin	**Serious Infection:** IM, IV: 15 mg/kg/d given in 2–3 divided doses, may start with an initial loading dose of 10 mg/kg followed by lower maintenance doses, e.g., 7.5 mg/kg q12h (max. dose 1.5 g/d; desirable peak serum levels 15–30 mcg/ml, trough levels should not exceed 10 mcg/ml; usual duration of treatment 7–10 days). **Uncomplicated UTI:** IM, IV: 250 mg q12h (response should be noted in 24–48 hours, discontinue if no response in 3–5 days).	**Injection:** 250 mg/ml **Injection:** (pediatric) 50 mg/ml	ANTI-INFECTIOUS AGENTS (G) Aminoglycosides & Related Agents (SG) **Cost:** Very High
Amikin	See AMIKACIN		Aminoglycoside Antibiotic
AMILORIDE Midamor, Moduretic (Amiloride a component)	**Diuretic:** PO: 5 mg/d to start; 5–20 mg qd maintenance.	**Tablet:** 5 mg	RENAL AGENTS (G) Sodium Diuretics (SG) Potassium-Sparing Diuretics (SG) **COST:** Low
AMINOCAPROIC ACID Amicar	**Bleeding:** PO, IV: 5g initially, then 1 to 1.25 g qh, (should yield plasma levels of 0.13 mg/ml; max. dose 30 gm/d); usually continue for 8 hours or until bleeding is controlled. IV given slowly, i.e., 4 to 5 g in 250 ml of diluent during the first hour.	**Tablet:** 500 mg **Syrup:** 250 mg/ml **Injection:** 250 mg/ml	METABOLIC AGENTS (G) Anticoagulants And Coagulants (SG) Other Hemostatic Agents (SSG)
Aminodur	See AMINOPHYLLINE		Xanthine Bronchodilator
AMINOGLUTETHIMIDE Cytadren	**Cushing's Syndrome:** 250 mg at 6-hour intervals. The dosage may be increased in increments of 250 mg daily at intervals of 1–2 weeks to a total daily dose of 2g.	**Tablet:** 250 mg	ENDOCRINE AGENTS (G) Inhibitor of Corticosteroid Synthesis (SG)

GENERIC NAME Trade Name	INDICATIONS AND DOSAGES	DOSE FORMS	GROUP (G)/SUBGROUP (SG) Relative Cost within Group
AMINOPHYLLINE Generic, Aminodur, Aminophyllin	Note: 1.2 mg aminophylline anhydrous = 1.0 mg theophylline anhydrous = 1.3 mg aminophylline dihydrate. Theophylline solubilized with ethylenediamine. **Bronchospasm (rapid attainment of therapeutic levels)** (therapeutic serum concentration is 10–20 mcg/ml). PO: 5.8 mg/kg initial dose, then maintenance as follows: 3.5 mg/kg q8h (nonsmokers); 2.3 mg/kg q8h (>60 yrs., cor pulmonale); 1.2–2.3 mg/kg q12h (CHF) NOTE: Give all IV doses slowly (less than 25 mg/min). Use in conjunction with serum levels measured as theophylline. **IV (Healthy nonsmokers):** 6.0 mg/kg loading dose, then 0.7 mg/kg/hour for 12 hours; thereafter 0.5 mg/kg/hour. **IV (Healthy smokers):** 6.0 mg/kg loading dose, then 1.0 mg/kg/hour for 12 hours; thereafter 0.8 mg/kg/hour. **IV (>60 yrs, cor pulmonale):** 6.0 mg/kg loading dose, then 0.6 mg/kg/hour for 12 hours; thereafter 0.3 mg/kg/hour. **IV (CHF, liver disease):** 6.0 mg/kg loading dose, then 0.5 mg/kg/hour for 12 hours; thereafter 0.1–0.2 mg/kg/hour. **Pediatric IV (9–16 yrs.):** 6.0 mg/kg loading dose, then 1.0 mg/kg/hour for 12 hours; thereafter 0.8 mg/kg/hour. Pediatric IV (1–9 yrs.): 6.0 mg/kg loading dose, then 1.2 mg/kg/hour for 12 hours; thereafter 1.0 mg/kg/hour.	**Tablet:** 100, 200 mg (79, 158 mg anhydrous theophylline) **Tablet:** (Ext'd release) 225 mg (178 mg anhydrous theophylline) **Oral Solution:** 105 mg/5ml (90 mg/5 ml anhydrous theophylline) **Injection:** 250 mg/ml (197 mg/10ml anhydrous theophylline) **Suppositories:** 250, 500 mg (197.5, 395 mg anhydrous theophylline)	CV AGENTS (G) Xanthines (SG) **Cost:** Low
AMINOSALICYLIC ACID Generic, p-aminosalicylic acid, PAS, Pamisyl, Parasal, Teebacin	**Tuberculosis (given in combination):** PO: Adult: 200 mg/kg/d given in 4 doses q6h (max. dose 12,000 mg/d). Pediatric PO: 150–200 mg/kg/d in 3–4 divided doses (max. dose 12,000 mg/d).	**Tablet:** 0.5 g	ANTI-INFECTIOUS AGENTS (G) Antituberculous and Related Agents (SG) Antituberculous Second Line Agents (SSG) **Cost:** Low

GENERIC NAME Trade Name	INDICATIONS AND DOSAGES	DOSE FORMS	GROUP (G)/SUBGROUP (SG) Relative Cost within Group
AMIODARONE Cordarone	**Life-Threatening Ventricular Arrhythmias:** PO: 800–1600 mg/d for 1–3 wk, reduce to 600–800 mg/d for 1 month, then maintenance of 200–400 mg/d (max. maintenance dose 600 mg/day); give doses greater than 1000 mg/day ac in 3 divided doses. **Note:** Quinidine (Type I) plus alpha- and beta-adrenergic receptor blocking action. May be used against all arrhythmias including those associated with Wolf-Parkinson-White syndrome. Also useful against angina and CHF independent of antiarrhythmic effect. Toxic especially with digoxin. See discussion, Part 1.	**Tablet:** 200 mg IV: 50 mg/ml in 3 ml vial.	CV AGENTS (G) Antiarrhythmic Agents (SG) Miscellaneous Antiarrhythmic Agents (SSG) **Cost:** Very High
Amitone	See CALCIUM CARBONATE		Antacid
Amitril	See AMITRIPTYLINE		Antidepressant (TCA)
AMITRIPTYLINE Generic, Elavil, Amitril, Emitrip	**Endogenous Depression:** PO: 75–100 mg/d to start in 3–4 doses; maintenance 25–150 mg/d. Geriatric/adolescent PO: 10 mg tid plus 20 mg hs. IM: 20–30 mg QID. (Do not give IV.)	**Tablet:** 10, 25, 50, 75, 100, 150 mg **Injection:** 10 mg/ml	CNS AGENTS (G) Tricyclic Antidepressants (SG) **Cost:** Low
AMLODIPINE Norvasc	**Chronic Stable and Vasospastic Angina; Hypertension:** See discussion, Part 1	**Tablet:**	CV AGENTS (G) Vasodilators (SG) Calcium Channel Blockers (SSG) **Cost:** High
AMMONIUM CHLORIDE	**Hypochloremia, Metabolic Alkalosis:** IV: Mix one to two vials (100 to 200 mEq) in 500 or 1000 ml isotonic (0.9%) sodium chloride (do not exceed a concentration of 1% to 2% ammonium chloride or an administration rate of 5 ml/min in adults); follow sequential serum bicarbonate levels to adjust dose.	**Injection:** 26.75% solution (5 mEq/ml)	METABOLIC AGENTS (G) Specific Ions (SG)
AMOBARBITAL Generic, Amytal	**Hypnotic:** IV: 65–200 mg (do not exceed the IV rate of 50 mg/min.). IM: 65–200 mg hs (deep IM injection; do not inject more than 5 ml of solution. Max. dose may go as high as 500 mg).	**Injection:** Powder for injection in 250 mg vials, in 500 mg vials	SEDATIVE-HYPNOTICS (G) Intermediate-Acting Sedative Hypnotics (SG) **Cost:** Medium
AMOXAPINE Generic, Asendin	**Endogenous Depression:** PO (>15 yrs): 150 mg/d to start in 2–3 doses; maintenance 200–300 mg/d (max. dose 400 mg/d). Geriatric PO: 25 mg bid or tid to start; maintenance 100–300 mg/d.	**Tablet:** 25, 50, 100, 150 mg	CNS AGENTS (G) Tricyclic Antidepressants (SG) **Cost:** Medium

GENERIC NAME Trade Name	INDICATIONS AND DOSAGES	DOSE FORMS	GROUP (G)/SUBGROUP (SG) Relative Cost within Group
AMOXICILLIN Amoxil, Larotid, Polymox, Trimox, Wymox, Generic	**General Infections:** PO: 250–500 mg q8h. Pediatric PO: 20–40 mg/kg/d given in 3 divided doses. **Gonorrhea:** PO: 3 g single dose (give with 1 g probenecid and follow by tetracycline 500 mg QID for 7 days). **Bacterial Endocarditis Prophylaxis (dental, respiratory procedures):** PO: 3 g 1 hour prior to procedure then 1.5 g 6 hours after initial dose. Alternate Regimen: 1–2 g amoxicillin IM or IV + 1.5 mg/kg gentamicin IV or IM 1 hour prior to procedure; [(6 hours after initial dose give 1.5 g amoxicillin) OR (8 hours after initial dose repeat parenteral gentamicin)]. Pediatric PO: 50 mg/kg + 2 mg/kg gentamicin IV or IM hour prior to procedure; [(6 hours after initial dose give 25 mg/kg amoxicillin) OR (8 hours after initial dose repeat parenteral gentamicin)].	**Tablet (chewable):** 125, 250 mg **Capsule:** 250, 500 mg **Oral Suspension:** (powder) 50 mg/ml, 125 mg/5 ml, 250 mg/5 ml when reconstituted	ANTI-INFECTIOUS AGENTS (G) Lactam Antibiotics—Penicillins & Cephalosporins (SG) Wider Gram Negative Coverage (SSG) Penicillins (Semi-Synthetic) (SSG) **Cost:** Low
AMOXICILLIN and **CLAVULANIC ACID** Augmentin	**Infections:** PO: one 500 mg tab q12h or one 250 mg tab q8h **Severe Infections and Infections of Respiratory Tract:** PO: one 875 mg tab q12h or one 500 mg tab q8h	**Tablet:** (chewable) 125 mg amoxicillin with 31.25 mg clavulanic acid, 250 mg amoxicillin with 62.5 mg clavulanic acid **Oral Suspension:** (powder) 125 mg amoxicillin and 31.25 mg clavulanic acid per 5 ml, 250 mg amoxicillin and 62.5 mg clavulanic acid per 5 ml	ANTI-INFECTIOUS AGENTS (G) Lactam Antibiotics (SG) Formulations Containing A Lactamase Inhibitor (SSG) **Cost:** Medium
Amoxil	See AMOXICILLIN		Lactam Antibiotic
AMPHETAMINE Generic, racemic amphetamine, Benzedrine, Adoral	**Exogenous Obesity:** PO: 5–30 mg/d in 1–3 doses (given 30 min before meals). PO (Ext'd Release): 10–15 mg qAM. **Attention Deficit:** Pediatric PO (3–5 yrs): 2.5 mg/d to start; increase by 2.5 mg/d q1week PRN; use lowest effective dose. Pediatric PO (>5 yrs): 5 mg q12–24h to start; increase by 5 mg/d q1week; maintenance 10–40 mg/d.	**Tablet:** 5, 10 mg	CNS AGENTS (G) Sympathomimetic Stimulants (SG) Schedule II Agents (SG) **Cost:** Medium

GENERIC NAME Trade Name	INDICATIONS AND DOSAGES	DOSE FORMS	GROUP (G)/SUBGROUP (SG) Relative Cost within Group
Amphojel	See ALUMINUM HYDROXIDE GEL		Antacid
Amphotec	See AMPHOTERICIN		Systemic Antifungal
AMPHOTERICIN B Fungizone Amphotec	**Fungal Infections:** IV: 0.25 mg/kg to start, may increase by 5–10 mg/d; maintenance 0.5–1 mg/kg/d (max. dose 1.5 mg/kg). Infuse over 6 hours. Treatment may require several months. **Candidiasis:** (GI, HIV-related, Azole Refractory): PO: Labeled dose of suspension is 1 ml QID [3–5 ml often used]	**Injection:** (powder) 50 mg per vial **Oral Suspension:** 100 mg/ml	ANTI-INFECTIOUS AGENTS (G) Systemic Antifungal Agents (SG) **Cost:** Low
AMPHOTERICIN TOPICAL Generic, Fungizone	**Cutaneous and Mucocutaneous Candida:** Topical: Apply to lesions 2–4 times/day. Treatment may require 1–4 weeks (longer for interdigital lesions, paronychias and onychomycoses)	**Cream:** 3% **Lotion:** 3% **Ointment:** 3%	DERMATOLOGIC AGENTS (G) Topical Fungicides (SG) **Cost:** Medium
AMPICILLIN Generic, Omnipen, Penbritin, Polycillin, Principen	**General Infections:** PO, IM, IV: 1–12 g daily given in divided doses q4–6h. Pediatric PO, IM, IV: 50–200 mg/kg/d. **Bacterial Meningitis:** IM, IV: 8–14 g/d given in 6–8 divided doses (start initial therapy by IV). Pediatric: IM, IV 100–200 mg/kg/d given in 6–8 divided doses (start initial therapy by IV). **Sepsis:** IM, IV: 150–200 mg/kg/d given in 6–8 divided doses (start initial therapy by IV, give for at least 3 days). **Bacterial Endocarditis Prophylaxis (dental, respiratory procedures):** PO: 1–2 g + 1.5 mg/kg gentamicin (max. gent. dose 80 mg) both given IV or IM hour prior to procedure; [(6 hours after initial dose give 1.5 g amoxicillin) OR (8 hours after initial dose repeat parenteral gentamicin)]. Pediatric PO: 50 mg/kg + 2 mg/kg gentamicin IV or IM hour prior to procedure; [(6 hours after initial dose give 25 mg/kg amoxicillin) OR (8 hours after initial dose repeat parenteral gentamicin)].	**Capsule:** 250, 500 mg **Oral Suspension:** (powder) 100 mg/ml, 125 mg/5 ml, 250 mg/5 ml, 500 mg/5 ml when reconstituted **Powder for Suspension:** 250 mg/100ml when reconstituted **Injection:** (powder) 0.125, 0.25, 0.5, 1, 2, 10 mg **Combination Agents:** Proampacin (3.5 g ampicillin; 1 g probenecid per vial of powder). Polycillin-PRB (3.5 g ampicillin; 1 g probenecid per vial of powder).	ANTI-INFECTIOUS AGENTS (G) Lactam Antibiotics—Penicillins & Cephalosporins (SG) Wider Gram Negative Coverage (SSG) Penicillins (Semi-Synthetic) (SSG) **Cost:** Low
AMPICILLIN and **SULBACTAM** Unasyn	**Infection Due To β-Lactamase Producing Agents:** IM, IV: 1.5 g (1 g ampicillin and 0.5 g sulbactam)—3 g (2 g ampicillin and 1 g sulbactam) q6h (max dose of sulbactam = 4 g/d).	**Powder (for injection):** 1.5 g (1 g ampicillin and 0.5 g sulbactam), 3.0 g (2 g ampicillin and 1 g sulbactam).	ANTI-INFECTIOUS AGENTS (G) Lactam Antibiotics—Penicillins & Cephalosporins (SG) Formulations Containing A Lactamase Inhibitor (SG) **Cost:** Medium

GENERIC NAME Trade Name	INDICATIONS AND DOSAGES	DOSE FORMS	GROUP (G)/SUBGROUP (SG) Relative Cost within Group
AMRINONE Inocor	**Congestive Heart Failure:** IV: 0.75 mg/kg bolus (injected slowly) over 2–3 min initially, then 5–10 mcg/kg/min (max. dose 10 mg/kg/d).	**Injection:** 5 mg/ml	CV AGENT (G) Xanthines (SG) Xanthine Equivalent (SG) **Cost:** Very High
Amvisc	See HYALURONATE		
AMYL NITRITE Generic	**Relief of Angina Pectoris:** Inhalation: One nasal inhalation and may repeat (1 to 6 inhalations per capsule). Cyanide Intoxication: Inhale vapor from crushed ampoule held at nostril. Maintain palpable pulse.	**Frangible Ampoule:** 0.3 ml	CV AGENTS (G) Vasodilators (SG) Post-Arteriolar (Antianginal) (SG) **Cost:** Low
Amytal	See AMOBARBITAL		Sedative-Hypnotic
Anadrol-50	See OXYMETHOLONE		Androgen
Anafranil	See CLOMIPRAMINE		TCA, Antidepressant
ANAGRELIDE Agrelin	**Thrombocytopenia:** PO: Initially 0.5 mg QID, then increase by 0.5/d to 1.5–3 mg/d for platelet count less than 600,000.	**Capsule;** 0.5 mg	METABOLIC AGENTS (G) Coagulants And Anticoagulants (SG) Antiplatelet Agents (SSG)
Anaprox	See NAPROXEN		Non-Narcotic Analgetic
ANASTRAZOLE Arimidex	**Metastatic Ca Of Breast:** PO: 1 mg each day	**Tablet:** 1 mg	ENDOCRINE AGENT (G) Antiestrogen (SG) **Cost:** Moderate
Ancef	See CEFAZOLIN		Lactam Antibiotic
Ancobon	See FLUCYTOSINE		Antifungal, systemic
Androderm	See TESTOSTERONE TRANSDERMAL		Androgen
Andro L.A.	See TESTOSTERONE ENANTHATE		Androgen
Anectine	See SUCCINYLCHOLINE		Curariform
Anestacon	See LIDOCAINE		Local Anesthetic
Angiospan	See NITROGLYCERIN		Vasodilator
ANISOTROPINE Generic, Valpin	**Peptic Ulcer:** PO: 50 mg tid.	**Tablet:** 50 mg	AUTONOMIC NS AGENTS (G) Parasympatholytics (SG) Parasympatholytics, Quaternary Amines (SSG) **Cost:** High
ANISTREPLASE Eminase	Thrombolysis IV: 30 units (give over 2 to 5 minutes).	**Powder:** 30 units	METABOLIC AGENTS (G) Anticoagulants And Coagulants (SG) Thrombolytic Agents (SG)
Ansaid	See FLURBIPROFEN		Non-Narcotic Analgetic
Anspor	See CEPHRADINE		Lactam Antibiotic
ANTHRALIN Generic, Dithranol, Lasan, Drithocreme, Anthro-Derm	**Chronic or Minimal Psoriasis:** Apply minimum amount and strength needed, usually once daily, directly to affected area; rinse and wash skin after treatment.	**Ointment:** 0.1%, 0.25%, 0.4%, 0.5% **Cream:** 0.1%, 0.2%, 0.25%, 0.4%, 0.5%, 1%	DERMATOLOGIC AGENTS (G) Keratolytic And Keratoplastic Agents (SG) Acne and Psoriasis (SSG) **Cost:** High
Anthro-Derm	See ANTHRALIN		Keratolytic (Tar)

GENERIC NAME Trade Name	INDICATIONS AND DOSAGES	DOSE FORMS	GROUP (G)/SUBGROUP (SG) Relative Cost within Group
ANTITHYMO-CYTE GLOBULIN Atgam, Antilymphocyte Globulin, Lymphocyte Immune Globulin, ATG, LIG, ALG	**Renal Transplantation:** IV: 10–30 mg/kg/d (infuse slowly IV over 4 or more hours). **Aplastic Anemia:** IV: 10–20 mg/kg/d (infuse slowly IV over 4 or more hours), give initially for 8–14 days; may give additional alternate day infusions up to a total of 21 doses.	**Injection:** 50 mg/ml.	ANTIINFLAMMATORY, ETC (G) Immunomodulators (SG)
ANTIHEMO-PHILIC FACTOR VIII, NON-RECOMBINANT Hemofil, Koate, Profilate, Humate	See AHF VIII Recombinant.	Koate **Concentrate:** Antihemophilic Factor Profilate HP **Concentrate:** Antihemophilic Factor VIII	METABOLIC AGENTS (G) Anticoagulants And Coagulants (SG) Clotting Factors (SG) **Cost:** Medium
ANTIHEMO-PHILIC FACTOR VIII, RECOMBINANT KoGENate, Recombinate	**Hemorrhage, Mild and Spontaneous (Prophylaxis):** IV: 10 IU/kg initially, observe clinically then repeat if needed with endpoint to raise Factor VIII to 20% of normal. (Note: each 1U of Factor VIII per kg given results in approx. 2% rise in serum Factor VIII). **Hemorrhage, Moderate:** IV: 15–25 IU/kg initially, then 10–15 IU/kg q8–12h with endpoint to raise Factor VIII to 30–50% of normal. **Hemorrhage, Severe:** IV: 50 IU/kg initially, then 20–25 IU/kg q8–12h with endpoint to raise Factor VIII to 80–100% of normal.	**Concentrate:** Antihemophilic Factor VIII	METABOLIC AGENTS (G) Anticoagulants And Coagulants (SG) Clotting Factors (SSG) **Cost:** High
Antilirium	See PHYSOSTIGMINE		Cholinesterase Inhibitor
Antilymphocyte Globulin	See ANTITHYMOCYTE GLOBULIN		Immunomodulator
Antiminth	See PYRANTEL		Antiparasitic
Antivert	See MECLIZINE		Motion Sickness
Anturane	See SULFINPYRAZONE		Increase Urate Excretion
APOMORPHINE Generic	**Induce Vomiting:** Adults 5 mg SC, Children 0.1 mg/kg SC.	**Tablet triturate:** 6 mg	ANTIDOTES AND USED IN POISONINGS (G) Narcotic Analgesics (SG)
APRACLONIDINE Lopidine	**Elevated IOP:** Instill 1 drop into preoperative eye 1 h prior to laser surgery, repeat at the end of surgery. 0.5% solution can be given tid in conjunction with other treatment.	**Solution:** 0.5%, 1.0%	OPHTHALMIC AGENTS (G) Agents used in the treatment of glaucoma (SG) Central Sympatholytic (alpha$_2$-blocker) (SSG) **Cost:** Low

GENERIC NAME Trade Name	INDICATIONS AND DOSAGES	DOSE FORMS	GROUP (G)/SUBGROUP (SG) Relative Cost within Group
APRESAZIDE	See HYDRALAZINE-HCTZ COMBINATION		Hypotensive-Diuretic Combination
Apresoline	See HYDRALAZINE		Hypotensive Agent
APROTININ Trasylol	**Dosage Regimens:** IV: 2 million potassium international units (KIU) loading dose, then 500,000 KIU/hr of surgical procedure as continuous IV infusion. Alternate regimen IV: 1 million KIU IV loading dose, then 250,000 KIU/hr of surgical procedure as continuous IV infusion. (Note: will need full loading dose of KIU placed into the volume needed to operate the pump).	**Injection:** 10,000 KIU/ml	METABOLIC AGENTS (G) Anticoagulants And Coagulants (SG) Other Hemostatic Agents (SG)
Aquamephyton	See PHYTONADIONE (K1)		K Vitamin
Aquaphyllin	See THEOPHYLLINE		Bronchodilator, Xanthine
Aquatensen	See METHYCLOTHIAZIDE		Sodium Diuretic
Aquest	See ESTRONE		Estrogen
ARA-C	See CYTARABINE		Cancer Chemotherapy
Aralen	See CHLOROQUINE		Parasiticide (Malaria)
Aramine	See METARAMINOL		Sympathomimetic
Aredia	See PAMIDRONATE		Inhibit Osteoclasts
Arfonad	See TRIMETHAPHAN		Ganglion Blocker
Aricept	See DONEPEZIL		Central Cholinesterase Inhibitor
Arimidex	See ANASTRAZOLE		Antiestrogen
Aristocort	See TRIAMCINOLONE		Corticosteroid
Arlidin	See NYLIDRIN		Sympathomimetic
Armour Thyroid	See THYROID DESICCATED		Thyroid Replacement
Armour Thyroid	See THYROID DESICCATED		Thyroid Replacement
Artane	See TRIHEXYPHENIDYL		Parasympatholytic
ASA	See ASPIRIN		Non-Narcotic Analgetic
Asacol	See MESALAMINE		Aminosalicylate
Asendin	See AMOXAPINE		TCA, Antidepressant
Asmalix	See THEOPHYLLINE		Bronchodilator, Xanthine
Asminyl	See DYPHYLLINE		Bronchodilator
ASPARAGINASE Elspar Kidrolase	CANCER CHEMOTHERAPY (G) React With DNA (SG) Other Miscellaneous (SSG)		

GENERIC NAME Trade Name	INDICATIONS AND DOSAGES	DOSE FORMS	GROUP (G)/SUBGROUP (SG) Relative Cost within Group
ASPIRIN OTC, Generic, Acetylsalicylic acid, ASA, Ecotrin, ZORprin, Easprin	**Pain, Fever:** PO: 325–650 mg q4–6h (max. dose 4 gm/d). Pediatric PO: 10–15 mg/kg q4–6h (max. dose 60–80 mg/kg/d) If aspirin alone is ineffective, add acetaminophen q4–6h; NO advantage in alternating the two drugs. **Arthritic Conditions:** PO: 2.4–3.6 gm/d in 3 to 4 divided doses to start, increase by 0.325–1.2 gm/d q 1 wk; maintenance 3.6–5.4 gm/d in 4–6 doses. Pediatric PO: 60–110 mg/kg/d in 3 to 4 divided doses; usual maintenance 80–100 mg/kg/d in 4–6 doses. Maintain serum salicylate levels = 150–300 mcg/ml. **Transient Ischemic Attacks, Ischemic Attacks or possible MI (Men):** PO: 650 mg bid; or 325 QID (one study indicates that 300 mg/d may be effective) **MI Prophylaxis:** One tab (150 or 300 mg) qd.	**Tablet:** 325, 500, 650 mg **Tablet:** (chewable) 81 mg **Tablet:** (Enteric) 81, 165, 325, 500, 650, 975 mg **Tablet:** (Ext'd release) 81, 650, 800 mg **Tablet:** (gum) 227.5 mg **Suppository:** 120, 200, 300, 600 mg	ANTI-INFLAMMATORY, ETC AGENTS(G) Nonsteroidal Anti-Inflammatory Agents (SG) **Cost:** Low
Asproject	See SODIUM SALICYLATE		Non-Narcotic Analgetic
Astelin	See AZELASTINE		Antihistamine (H_1)
ASTEMIZOLE Hismanal	**Allergic Reactions (Type I):** PO: (Adults > 11 yrs): 10mg daily.	**Tablet:** 10 mg	ANTI-INFLAMMATORY, ETC AGENTS (G) Antihistamines (H1 Antagonists) (SG) Antihistamines with Mild Sedation (SSG) **Cost:** High
Atabrine	See QUINACRINE		Parasiticide (Malaria)
Atarax	See HYDROXYZINE		Antihistamine
ATENOLOL Generic, Tenormin	**Hypertension:** PO: 50 mg qd initially; 50–100 mg qd maintenance. **Angina:** PO: 50 mg qd initially; 50–100 mg qd maintenance (max. dose: 200 mg qd). **Acute MI:** IV: 5 mg given over 5 minutes, initially; then in 10 minutes give another 5 mg (over 5 min). Oral therapy (50 mg bid) thereafter.	**Tablet:** 25, 50, 100 mg **Injection:** 5 mg/10 ml	CV AGENTS(G) Sympathoplegics (SG) Beta Adrenergic Receptor Blockers (SSG) Cardioselective (Beta 1) (SSG) **Cost:** Low
ATG	See ANTI-THYMOCYTE GLOBULIN		Immunomodulator
Atgam	See ANTI-THYMOCYTE GLOBULIN		Immunomodulator
Ativan	See LORAZEPAM		Hypnotic, Ultra Short

GENERIC NAME Trade Name	INDICATIONS AND DOSAGES	DOSE FORMS	GROUP (G)/SUBGROUP (SG) Relative Cost within Group
ATORVASTATIN Lipitor	**Hypercholesterolemia, hypertriglyceridemia:** PO: 10–80 mg/d	**Tablets:** 10, 20, 40 mg	METABOLIC AGENTS (G) Lipid Lowering Drugs (SG) HMG-CoA Reductase Inhibitors (SSG) **Cost:** Medium but chronic use
ATRACURIUM Tracrium	**Surgery:** IV: 0.4–0.5 mg/kg to start, expect effect in 2–5 min; 0.08–0.1 mg/kg maintenance dose PRN (usually at 15–40 min).	**Injection:** 10 mg/ml	GENERAL ANESTHETICS (G) Neuromuscular Blocking Agents (SG) Non-Depolarizing (Competitive) Agents (SSG) **Cost:** High
Atromid-S	See CLOFIBRATE		Lipid Lowering Agent
ATROPINE Generic	**Antidote to Anticholinesterase Poisoning:** IM, IV: 2–3 mg to start, and repeat until signs of atropine intoxication are seen. **Asystole:** IV: 1.0 mg q 3–5 minutes up to 0.03 to 0.04 mg/kg. **Bradyarrhythmias:** IV: 0.4–1 mg q1–2h PRN (max. dose 2 mg). **Bradyarrhythmias (symptomatic):** IV: 0.5–1.0 mg q 3–5 min up to 0.03 to 0.04 mg/kg. **Preoperative:** SC, IM, IV: 0.4–0.6 mg.	**Injection:** 0.05, 0.1, 0.4, 0.5, 0.8, 1.0 mg/ml. **Tablet:** 0.4 mg	ANS AGENTS (G) Parasympatholytics (SG) Tertiary Amines (SSG) **Cost:** Medium
ATROPINE and **MORPHINE** (combination), Generic	IM,IV,SC: 0.25–2 ml.	**Injection:** Atropine 0.4 mg/ml and Morphine 16 mg/ml combination in 30 ml vials	GENERAL ANESTHETICS AND ADJUNCTS (G) Preprocedural Agents (Conscious Sedation) (SG) Antipsychotic-Opiate Combination (SSG) **Cost:** N/A
ATROPINE-MEPERIDINE Atropine and Demerol, Generic	Varies depending on application and patient.	**Injection:** Atropine 0.4 mg/ml and 50 mg/ml in 2 ml cartridge or Atropine 0.4 mg/ml and Meperidine 75 mg/ml	GENERAL ANESTHETICS AND ADJUNCTS (G) Preprocedural Agents (Conscious Sedation) (SG) Antipsychotic-Opiate Combination (SSG)
Atrovent	See IPRATROPIUM		Cholinolytic (Inhalation)
AUGMENTIN	See AMOXICILLIN and CLAVULANIC ACID		Penicillin and Lactamase Inhibitor
AURALGAN OTIC	**External Otitis:** Instill in ear canal until filled, then insert a cotton pledget moistened with solution into meatus. Repeat q1–2h.		**Otic Solution (per cc):** benzocaine (14 mg = 1.4%), antipyrine (54 mg = 5.4%), glycerin
AURANOFIN Ridaura	**Rheumatoid States:** PO: 6 mg/d in one or two doses. After 6 months may give 3 mg tid (discontinue after 3 months at 9 mg/d if poor response).	**Capsule:** 3 mg	ANTI-INFLAMMATORY ETC (G) Antirheumatic (SG) **Cost:** Medium

GENERIC NAME Trade Name	INDICATIONS AND DOSAGES	DOSE FORMS	GROUP (G)/SUBGROUP (SG) Relative Cost within Group
Aureomycin	See CHLORTETRACYCLINE		Tetracycline
Aurolate	See GOLD SODIUM THIOMALATE		Antirheumatic
AUROTHIO-GLUCOSE Solganal	**Rheumatoid Arthritis:** IM: 10 mg on first week; 25 mg on weeks #2 and #3; then 50 mg/week thereafter until (1) improvement in symptoms, (2) toxicity occurs or (3) until 0.8–1.0 gram total dose is reached. Maintenance dose of 25–50 mg q3–4 weeks may be given if warranted and if toxicity is absent.	**Injection suspension:** 50 mg/ml (in 10 ml vials)	ANTI-INFLAMMATORY ETC (G) Gold Compounds And Antirheumatic (SG) **Cost:** High
Aventyl	See NORTRIPTYLINE		TCA, Antidepressant
Avonex	See INTERFERON BETA 1B		Immunomodulator
Axid	See NIZATIDINE		H2 Antagonist
Azactam	See AZTREONAM (Inj)		Antibacterial
AZATADINE Optimine	**Allergic Reactions (Type I):** PO: 1–2 mg bid.	**Tablet:** 1 mg	ANTI-INFLAMMATORY ETC (G) Antihistamines (H1 Antagonists) (SG) Antihistamines with Mild Sedation (SSG) **Cost:** Medium
AZATHIOPRINE Imuran	**Rheumatoid Arthritis:** PO: 1 mg/kg/d (50–100 mg) given in one dose or in two doses/day; after 2 months may increase q4 wks by 0.5 mg/kg to a maximum dose of 2.5 mg/kg/d (if no clinical response after 12 weeks of treatment, discontinue therapy). **Renal Transplantation:** IV, PO: 3–5 mg/kg/d initially (given on, or 1–3 days before, day of transplantation); maintenance dose 1–3 mg/kg/d (convert to oral when feasible, at same as IV dose).	**Tablets:** 50 mg **Injection:** 100 mg/vial	ANTI-INFLAMMATORY, ETC (G) Cytotoxic Immunosuppressants (Antirheumatic) (SG)
AZELAIC ACID Azelex	**Mild-Moderate Acne:** Topical: Apply bid	**Cream:** 20%	DERMATOLOGIC AGENT (G) Keratolytic Agent (SG) Acne (SSG) **Cost:** Expensive relative to other choices
AZELASTINE Astelin	**Allergic Rhinitis:** nasal spray: two sprays in each nostril bid	**Nasal Spray:**	ANTI-INFLAMMATORY AGENTS, ETC (G) Antihistamine (H_1 antagonist) (SG) **Cost:** Moderately expensive
Azelex	See AZELAIC ACID		Topical for Acne
Azidothymidine	See ZIDOVUDINE		Antiviral
AZITHROMYCIN Zithromax	**Mild to Moderate Infections:** PO (>15 yrs): 500 mg as single dose on the first day followed by 250 mg once daily on days 2–5 for a total dose of 1.5 g. **Chancroid, Chlamydia, Non-gonococcal urethritis:** 1 g as a single dose.	**Capsule:** 250 mg	ANTI-INFECTIOUS AGENTS (G) Macrolide Antibiotics (SG)

GENERIC NAME Trade Name	INDICATIONS AND DOSAGES	DOSE FORMS	GROUP (G)/SUBGROUP (SG) Relative Cost within Group
Azolid	See PHENYLBUTAZONE		Non-Narcotic Analgetic
AZT	See ZIDOVUDINE		Antiviral
AZTREONAM Azactam	**Urinary Tract Infection:** IM, IV: 500 mg or 1g q8–12h. **Systemic Infections:** IM, IV: 1 or 2 g q8–12h (IV recommended if single dose over 1 g or if serious infection). Pediatric IM, IV: 30 mg/kg q6–8h (IV recommended if single dose over 1 g or if serious infection). **Life-threatening Infections:** IV: 2 g q6–8h. Pediatric IV: 50 mg/kg q4–6h.	**Injection:** (powder) 0.5, 1, 2 g	ANTI-INFECTIOUS AGENTS (G) Lactam Antibiotics (SG) Monobactam (SSG) **Cost:** Very High
Azulfidine	See SULFASALAZINE		Prodrug for 5-ASA
B_{12}	See CYANOCOBALAMIN		
BACAMPICILLIN Spectrobid	**Infections:** PO: 400–800 mg q12h. Pediatric PO: 25–50 mg/kg/d given in 2 divided doses. **Gonorrhea:** PO: 1.6 g single dose (give with 1 g probenecid PO and follow by tetracycline 500 mg QID for 7 days).	**Tablet:** 400 mg **Oral Suspension:** (powder) 125 mg/5ml	ANTI-INFECTIOUS AGENTS (G) Lactam Antibiotics(SG) Wider Gram Negative Coverage (SSG) **Cost:** Low
Baciguent	See BACITRACIN		Antibacterial
BACITRACIN Generic, Baciguent	Apply small amount of ointment once or more per day.	**Ointment:** 500 units/gm	OPHTHALMIC AGENTS (G) Antibacterial (SG) **Cost:** Low
BACLOFEN Generic, Lioresal	PO: 40–80 mg/d in 3–4 divided doses.	**Tablet:** 10, 20 mg **Intrathecal:** 10 mg/20 ml, 10 mg/5 ml	CNS AGENTS (G) Muscle Relaxants (SG) Miscellaneous (SSG) **Cost:** Medium
Bactocill	See OXACILLIN		Lactam Antibiotic
BACTRIM IV INFUSION	**Severe Urinary Tract Infections; Shigellosis:** IV: 8–10 mg/kg/d (based on trimethoprim) in 2–4 divided doses, give q6, 8 or 12h by IV infusion for up to 14 days for UTI and 5 days for shigellosis. **P. carinii Pneumonia:** IV: 15–20 mg/kg/d (based on trimethoprim) in 3–4 equally divided doses q6–8h by IV infusion for up to 14 days.		**Injection (per 5 cc):** sulfamethoxazole (400 mg), trimethoprim (80 mg)
Bactrim	See TRIMETHOPRIM SULFAMETHOXAZOLE		Antibacterial
Baking Soda	See SODIUM BICARBONATE		Antacid
BAL	See DIMERCAPROL		Chelating Agent
Balnetar	See TARS AND ANTHRALINS		Kerato-lytic, plastic
Banflex	See ORPHENADRINE		Muscle Relaxant
Banthine	See METHANTHELINE		Parasympatholytic

GENERIC NAME Trade Name	INDICATIONS AND DOSAGES	DOSE FORMS	GROUP (G)/SUBGROUP (SG) Relative Cost within Group
Basaljel	See TPA ALUMINUM CARBONATE		Antacid
BayProgest	See PROGESTERONE		Progestin
BCG, INTRAVESICAL TheraCys BCG, VACCINE Tice BCG	**Primary And Relapsed In Situ Carcinoma Of Bladder:** Use TheraCys or Tice strain **Tuberculosis Vaccination:** Percutaneous (multiple puncture disc), Tice strain only. Freeze dried powder for reconstitution. Both forms are living strains.		ANTI-INFLAMMATORY ETC (G) Immunomodulators (SG)
BCNU	See CARMUSTINE		Cancer Chemotherapy
Beano	See ALPHA-D GALACTOSIDASE		Enzyme
Bebulin	See Coagulation Factor IX		Hemophilia B
BECLOMETH-ASONE Deep (pulmonary): Beclovent, Vanceril Intranasal: Beconase, Vancenase	**Bronchial Asthma:** Inhalation: 2 puffs (84 mcg) tid or QID (max. dose 20 puffs/day [= 420 mcg/day]). Inhalation (children 6 to 12 yrs): 1 or 2 puffs (42–84 mcg) tid or QID (max. dose 10 puffs/day [= 420 mcg]).	**Aerosol:** approx. 42 mcg is delivered by each puff.	RESPIRATORY AGENTS (G) Anti-Inflammatory Steroids (SG) Inhalation and Intranasal (SSG)
Beclovent	See BECLOMETHASONE		Corticosteroid
Bellafoline	See L-ALKALOIDS OF BELLADONNA		Parasympatholytic
BELLADONNA TINCTURE Generic	PO: 0.6–1 ml q6–8h.	**Liquid:** 27–33mg/100 ml	PARASYMPATHOLYTICS (G) Parasympatholytics, Tertiary Amines (SG) **Cost:** Low
Benadryl	See DIPHENHYDRAMINE		Antihistamine
BENAZEPRIL Lotensin	**Hypertension:** PO: initial dose 10mg qd, 20–40 mg/d maintenance in 1 or 2 divided doses.	**Tablet:** 5, 10, 20, 40 mg	CV AGENTS (G) Vasodilators (SG) ACE Inhibitors (SSG) **Cost:** Low
BENDROFLU-METHIAZIDE Naturetin	**Hypertension:** PO: Initially 5–20 mg/d; Maintenance 2.5–15 mg/d. **Edema:** PO: Initially 5–20 mg in 1 or 2 divided doses; Maintenance 2.5–5 mg/d.	**Tablet:** 5, 10 mg	RENAL AGENTS (G) Sodium Diuretics (SG) Thiazide Diuretics and Related Agents (SSG) **Cost:** Medium
Benemid	See PROBENECID		Increase Urate Excretion
Benoquin	See MONOBENZONE		Repigment
Bentyl	See DICYCLOMINE		Anticholinergic
Benzac	See BENZOYL PEROXIDE		Keratolytic (Acne)

GENERIC NAME Trade Name	INDICATIONS AND DOSAGES	DOSE FORMS	GROUP (G)/SUBGROUP (SG) Relative Cost within Group
BENZATHINE PENICILLIN G Generic, Bicillin, Permapen	**Group A Streptococcal Infections:** IM: 1.2 million units (single dose). Pediatric (weight > 27 kg) IM: 900,000 units as a single dose. Pediatric (weight < 27 kg) IM: 300,000–600,000 units as a single dose. **Rheumatic Fever Prophylaxis:** IM: 1.2 million units q4 weeks. **Syphilis (< one year duration):** IM: 2.4 million units in one dose. **Syphilis (> one year duration):** IM: 2.4 million units in one dose qweek for 3 weeks. **Neurosyphilis:** IM: 2.4 million units IM of benzathine pcn once per week for 3 weeks following initial 14-day treatment (which usually consists of 2–4 million units/d IM of Procaine PenG given with probenecid 500 mg PO QID over 10–14 days). **Yaws, Pinta, or Bejel:** IM: 1.2 million units (single dose). **Pneumococcal (Not Meningitis) Infections:**IM : 1,200,000 units (single dose) repeat q2–3 days until patient afebrile for 48 hours. Pediatric IM: 600,000 units (single dose) repeat q2–3 days until patient afebrile for 48 hours.	**Injection:** 300,000 units per ml, 600,000 units per dose, 1,200,000 units per dose, 2,400,000 units per dose	ANTI-INFECTIOUS AGENTS (G) Lactam Antibiotics (SG) Benzyl Penicillins and First Generation Cephalosporins (SSG) **Cost:** High
Benzedrex	See PROPYLHEXEDRINE (INHALER)		Sympathomimetic
Benzedrine	See AMPHETAMINE		Stimulant
BENZOCAINE OTC, Generic, ethyl aminobenzoate	**Topical Anesthesia:** 0.5–20% Apply to the affected area as needed.	**Ointment:** 2% **Cream:** 1, 5, 6% **Gel:** 6, 15, 20% **Liquid:** 20% **Spray:** 20% **Lotion:** 0.5, 2% **Solution:** 2, 3, 5, 9.5, 20% **Lozenges:** 3, 5, 6.25, 10 mg	GENERAL AND LOCAL ANESTHETICS (G) Local Anesthetics (SG) Topical (Mucosal) Only (SSG) **Cost:** Low
BENZONATATE Generic, Tessalon	**Cough:** PO: (Adults and children > 10 yrs): 100 mg tid (max. dose 600 mg/day).	**Capsule:** 100 mg	RESPIRATORY AGENTS (G) Antitussives (SG) **Cost:** Low
BENZOYL PEROXIDE Generic, OTC, Many Proprietaries	**Mild-Moderate Acne:** Topical Preparations: Massage into skin once/d for 3 days; then increase to bid application PRN. Cleansers: wash qd or bid.	**Gel:** 2.5%, 4%, 5%, 10% **Cream:** 5%, 10% **Lotion:** 5%, 5.5%, 10% **Bar:** 5, 10% **Liquid:** 5, 10% **Mask:** 5%	DERMATOLOGIC AGENTS (G) Keratolytic And Keratoplastic Agents (SG) Acne And Psoriasis (SG) **Cost:** Medium
BENZPHETAMINE Didrex	**Exogenous Obesity:** PO: 25–50 mg/d to start; maintenance 25–50 mg/d given 1–3 times daily.	**Tablet:** 25, 50 mg	CNS AGENTS (G) Sympathomimetic Stimulants (SG) Other Schedule 3 or 4 "Diet Pills" (SSG) **Cost:** High

GENERIC NAME Trade Name	INDICATIONS AND DOSAGES	DOSE FORMS	GROUP (G)/SUBGROUP (SG) Relative Cost within Group
BENZQUINAMIDE Emete-con	**Postoperative Nausea, Vomiting:** IM: 50 mg (0.5–1 mg/kg), repeat at 1 hour, then q3–4h PRN (give 15 min before end of anesthesia). IV: 25 mg (0.2–0.4 mg/kg) slowly for one dose, follow with IM maintenance as above.	**Injection:** 50 mg/vial	ANTIEMETICS (G) Antiemetics (Minor) (SG) **Cost:** Very High
BENZTROPINE Generic, Cogentin	**Parkinsonism:** PO: 0.5–1 mg qhs to start; increase 0.5 mg/d q5–6d; maintenance 0.5–6 mg/d. **Drug-Induced Extrapyramidal Disorders:** PO: 1–4 mg qd or bid (re-evaluate need after 1–2 weeks). IM, IV: 1–4 mg bid; follow with 1 to 2 mg PO bid and withdraw when possible (usually 1–2 weeks). **Acute Dystonic Reaction:** IM, IV: 1–2 mg one time followed by 1–2 mg PO bid.	**Tablet:** 0.5, 1, 2 mg **Injection:** 1 mg/ml	ANTIPARKINSONIAN AGENTS (G) Anticholinergics and Related Agents (SG) **Cost:** Low
BEPRIDIL Vascor	**Chronic Stable Angina:** See discussion, Part 1	**Tablet:**	CV AGENTS (G) Vasodilators (SG) Calcium Channel Blockers (SSG) **Cost:** Medium
BERACTANT Survanta	**Prophylactic and Rescue:** Intratracheal: 4 ml/kg. (Many dosing complexities and strategies). **Suspension:** 25 mg phospholipids/ml suspended in 0.9% sodium chloride solution.		RESPIRATORY AGENTS (G) Lung Surfactant (SG)
BETA BLOCKER-DIURETIC COMBINATION Generic, Corzide, Ziac,Timolide, Inderide, Normozide, Lopressor	**Hypertension:** PO: adjust dose within limitation imposed.	**Tablets, Capsules:** Generic combinations in fixed proportion of propranolol/ hydrochlorothiazide: 120/50 LA, 160/50 LA, 80/50, 40/25, and 80/25 mg.	BETA ADRENERGIC RECEPTOR BLOCKER (G) Combined with SODIUM DIURETIC (G)
Betachron	See PROPRANOLOL		Beta Adrenergic Blocker
Betagan	See LEVOBUNOLOL		Beta Adrenergic Blocker
BETAMETHASONE Generic, Celestone Selestoject, Cel-U-Ject	PO: 0.6–7.2 mg/day. IV (Phosphate): 1–9 mg/day. Intraarticular (phosphate-acetate mixture): 0.5–2 ml of the mixture.	**Tablet:** 0.6 mg (not generic) **Syrup:** 0.6 mg/5 ml (not generic) **Phosphate:** 4 mg (3 mg of betamethasone alcohol)/ml (generic) **Phosphate-Acetate Mixture:** 6 mg (3:3)/ml	ENDOCRINE AGENTS (G) Anti-Inflammatory Steroids (SG) **Cost:** Medium

GENERIC NAME Trade Name	INDICATIONS AND DOSAGES	DOSE FORMS	GROUP (G)/SUBGROUP (SG) Relative Cost within Group
BETAMETHASONE BENZOATE Uticort	Apply to affected area 2 to 4 times a day.	**Ointment:** 0.025%. **Gel:** 0.025%. **Cream:** 0.025%. **Lotion:** 0.025%.	DERMATOLOGIC AGENTS (G) Anti-Inflammatory Steroids, Topical (SG) **Cost:** Medium
BETAMETHASONE DIPROPIONATE Generic, Diprolene	Apply 1–2 times a day sparingly to affected area. Maximum 50 grams per week. Highest Potency:	**Ointment:** 0.05%. **Cream:** 0.05%. High Potency: **Lotion:** 0.05%. **Ointment:** 0.05%.	ANTI-INFLAMMATORY STEROIDS, TOPICAL (G) **Cost:** Low
BETAMETHASONE VALERATE Generic, Valisone, Betatrex	Apply to affected area 1–3 times a day. High Potency:	**Ointment:** 0.1%. Medium Potency: **Cream:** 0.01%, 0.1%. **Lotion:** 0.1%. **Cream:** 0.01%	ANTI-INFLAMMATORY STEROIDS, TOPICAL (G) **Cost:** Low
Betapace	See SOTALOL		Beta Adrenergic Blocker
Betaseron	See INTERFERON BETA-1B		Immunomodulator
Betatrex	See BETAMETHASONE VALERATE		Corticosteroid
BETAXOLOL Betoptic, Kerlone	**Hypertension:** PO: 10 mg q/d, maintenance range 10–20 mg/day. PO (Geriatric): Starting dose of 5 mg q/d may be used. When discontinuing, taper dose over two or more weeks.	**Elevated IOP:** 1 drop bid **Tablet:** 10, 20 mg **Ophthalmic Solution:** 0.25, 0.5%	SYMPATHOPLEGICS (G) Beta Adrenergic Receptor Blockers (SG) Cardioselective (Beta 1) (SSG) **Cost:** Low
BETHANECHOL Generic, Urecholine, Duvoid, Vesicholine	**Urinary Retention, Postoperative Ileus:** PO: 10–50 mg tid or QID SC (do not give IM or IV): 2.5–5 mg, repeat q15–30 min. to a maximum of 4 doses. **Tablet:** 5, 10, 25, 50 mg	**Injection:** 5 mg/ml	CHOLINERGIC AGENTS (Parasympathomimetics) (G) Choline Esters and Equivalent (SG) **Cost:** Low
Bethaprim	See TRIMETHOPRIM-SULFAMETHOXAZOLE		Antibacterial
Betoptic	See BETAXOLOL		Beta Adrenergic Blocker
Biaxin	See CLARITHROMYCIN		Macrolide Antibiotic
BICALUTAMIDE Casodex	**Palliation of Prostatic Cancer:** PO: 50 mg daily with LHRH antagonist.	**Tablets:** 50 mg	ENDOCRINE AGENTS (G) Antiandrogen (SG) **Cost:** High
Bicillin	See BENZATHINE PENICILLIN G		Lactam Antibiotic
Bicillin C-R	Benzathine-Penicillin G Procaine Combination		Lactam Antibiotic

GENERIC NAME Trade Name	INDICATIONS AND DOSAGES	DOSE FORMS	GROUP (G)/SUBGROUP (SG) Relative Cost within Group
BICNU	See Carmustine		Cancer Chemotherapy
Biltricide	See PRAZIQUANTEL		Parasiticide
BIPERIDEN Akineton	**Parkinsonism:** PO: 2 mg tid or QID (max. dose 16 mg/d). **Drug-Induced Extrapyramidal Disorders:** PO: 2 mg 1–3 times daily. IV, IV: 2 mg q30 min; max. dose 8 mg/d.	**Tablet:** 2 mg **Injection:** 5 mg/ml	ANTIPARKINSONIAN AGENTS (G) Anticholinergics and Related Agents (SG) **Cost:** Medium
BISACODYL Generic, OTC, Dulcolax	In many OTC mixtures **Laxative:** PO: 10–15 mg (max. dose 30 mg). Pediatric PO (over 6 yrs): 0.3 mg/kg (5–10 mg) at hs, or prior to breakfast. Rectal: 10 mg. Pediatric Rectal (6–12 years): 5 mg.	**Tablet:** (Enteric) 5 mg **Suppository:** 5, 10 mg	GASTROINTESTINAL AGENTS (G) Laxatives And Bowel Cleansers (G) Irritant Laxatives (SG) **Cost:** Medium
BISACODYL TANNEX Clysodrast	**Cleansing Enema:** One packet in 1L warm water or incorporated in barium enema	**Powder:** 1.5 mg bisacodyl and 2.5 g tannic acid	GASTROINTESTINAL AGENTS (G) Laxatives And Bowel Cleansers (G) Irritant Laxatives (SG)
BISMUTH SUBGALLATE Generic, OTC, Pepto-Bismol,	**Indigestion, Diarrhea, Nausea:** PO: 2 tablets (30 ml of regular strength liquid) q30–60 min PRN (max. dose: 8 doses in 1 day). Pediatric PO (9–12 yrs): 1 tablet or 15 ml of regular strength liquid. Pediatric PO (6–9 yrs): 2/3 tablet or 10 ml of regular strength liquid. Pediatric PO (3–6 yrs): 1/3 tablet or 5 ml of regular strength liquid. **Gastric Hyperacidity:** PO: 500–1000 mg QID.	**Tablet:** (chewable) 262 mg **Liquid** (regular Strength): 262 mg/15 ml **Liquid** (extra Strength): 524 mg/15 ml	GASTROINTESTINAL AGENTS (G) Antacids (SG) Surface and Mixed Activity (SSG) **Cost:** Low
BISOPROLOL Zebeta	**Hypertension:** PO: 5 mg qd; maintenance 2.5–20mg/d.	**Tablet:** 5, 10 mg	CARDIOVASCULAR AGENTS Sympathoplegics (SG) Beta Adrenergic Receptor Blockers (SSG) Cardioselective (Beta 1) (SSG)
BITOLTEROL Tornalate	**Bronchospasm:** Inhalation (adults and children > 12 yrs): 2 puffs separated by at least 1–3 minutes, followed by a third puff PRN; to prevent bronchospasm, give 2 puffs q8h (max. dose 12 puffs/day).	**Solution:** (for inhalation) 0.2%. **Aerosol:** 0.8%. Delivers 0.37 mg/puff.	RESPIRATORY AGENTS (G) Sympathomimetics (Beta-Agonists) For Deep Inhalation (SG) **Cost:** Medium
BLEPHAMIDE	**Ophthalmic:** 1 qtt bid to QID. (Apply once or twice at night).		**Ophthalmic Suspension:** sulfacetamide sodium (10%), prednisolone acetate (0.2%) **Ophthalmic Ointment:** sulfacetamide sodium (10%), prednisolone acetate (0.2%)
Blenoxane	See BLEOMYCIN		Cancer Chemotherapy
BLEOMYCIN Blenoxane	CANCER CHEMOTHERAPY (G) React With DNA (SG) Antibiotics (SSG)		
Blocadren	See TIMOLOL		Beta Adrenergic Blocker
Bonine	See MECLIZINE		Motion Sickness

GENERIC NAME Trade Name	INDICATIONS AND DOSAGES	DOSE FORMS	GROUP (G)/SUBGROUP (SG) Relative Cost within Group
Bontril	See PHENDIMETRAZINE		Diet Pill
Botox	See BOTULINUM TOXIN TYPE A		Muscle Paralyzant
BOTULINUM TOXIN, TYPE A Botox	**Strabismus:** Intramuscular (ocular muscles): 1.25 to 5 units, use 2.5 units and lower for strabismus $<$ 20 prism diopters (max. single injected dose = 25 units), assess effect of dose in 1–2 weeks; manufacturer recommends needle electromyography to guide injection placement. **Blepharospasm:** Intramuscular (orbicularis oculi mm.): initial dose =1.25 to 2.5 units (max. single injected dose = 5 units); do not exceed 200 units/month.	**Solution:** 100 units/vial	OPHTHALMOLOGIC AGENTS (G) Adjuncts To Surgery (SG) Acetylcholine block (SSG) **Cost:** High
Brethine	See TERBUTALINE		Sympathomimetic
BRETYLIUM Generic, Bretylol	**Life-Threatening Ventricular Arrhythmias:** IV: 5 mg/kg injection, may give 10 mg/kg in 10 min. PRN (max. total dose 30 mg/kg). IV Maintenance: 1–2 mg/min continuous infusion (or 5–10 mg/kg over $>$8 min q6h). **Other Ventricular Arrhythmias:** IV: 5–10 mg/kg over $>$ 8 min q1–2h until arrhythmia reverses, then IV Maintenance: 1–2 mg/min continuous infusion (or 5–10 mg/kg over $>$8 min q6h). IV: 5–10 mg/kg initial dose, may repeat at q1–2h intervals PRN at varying sites ($<$ 5 ml/site) Maintenance: 5–10 mg/kg q6–8h.	**Injection:** 50 mg/ml	ANTIARRHYTHMIC AGENTS (G) Miscellaneous Antiarrhythmic Agents (SG) **Cost:** Very High
Bretylol	See BRETYLIUM		Antiarrhythmic
Brevibloc	See ESMOLOL		Beta Adrenergic Blocker
Brevital	See METHOHEXITAL		Induction Agent
Bricanyl	See TERBUTALINE		Beta Agonist
BRIMONIDINE Alphagan	**Open angle glaucoma (during trabeculoplasty):** Intraocular: one drop tid	**Ophthalmic Drops:** 0.2%	OPHTHALMIC AGENTS (G) Agents used in the treatment of glaucoma (SG) Central Sympatholytic (alpha$_2$-agonist) (SG)
British Anti-Lewisite	See DIMERCAPROL		Chelating Agent
BROMOCRIPTINE Parlodel	**Parkinsonism:** PO: 1.25 mg bid to start; increase 2.5 mg/d q2–4 week; (max. dose 40 mg/d). Give with meals.	**Tablet:** 2.5 mg **Capsule:** 5 mg	CNS AGENTS (G) Antiparkinsonian Agents (SG) Dopamine Precursors, Agonists and Related Agents (SSG) **Cost:** High

GENERIC NAME Trade Name	INDICATIONS AND DOSAGES	DOSE FORMS	GROUP (G)/SUBGROUP (SG) Relative Cost within Group
BROMPHENIRAMINE OTC, Generic, Dimetane, Veltane	PO: 4 mg q4–6h (max. dose 24 mg/d). PO: (Ext'd Release) 8–12 mg q8–12h (max. dose 24 mg/d). Pediatric (6–12 yrs) PO: 2 mg q4–6h (max. dose 12 mg/d). IV, SC, IV: 5–20mg bid (max. dose 40 mg/day).	**Tablet:** 4, 8, 12 mg **Tablet:** (Ext'd release) 8, 12 mg **Elixir:** 2 mg/5 ml **Injection:** 10 mg/ml	ANTI-INFLAMMATORY, ETC Antihistamines (H1 Antagonists) (SG) Antihistamines with Mild Sedation (SSG) **Cost:** Low
BRONKAID	PO: 1 tablet q4h, up to 5 tabs/d.		**Tablet:** theophylline (100 mg), ephedrine sulfate (24 mg), guaifenesin (100 mg)
Bronkodyl	See THEOPHYLLINE		Xanthine Bronchodilator
BRONKOLIXIR	PO: 10cc q3–4h, up to 4 doses/d.		**Elixir (per 5 cc):** theophylline (15 mg), ephedrine sulfate (12 mg), guaifenesin (50 mg), phenobarbital (4 mg) alcohol (19%)
BRONKOTAB	PO: 1 tablet q3–4h, up to 5 doses/d.		**Tablet:** theophylline (100 mg), ephedrine sulfate (24 mg), guaifenesin (100 mg), phenobarbital (8 mg)
BRONTEX (Schedule III Controlled Drug)	PO: 1 tablet q4h, PRN.		**Tablet:** codeine phosphate (10 mg), guaifenesin (300 mg)
BRONTEX LIQUID (Schedule V Controlled Drug)	PO: 20cc q4h, PRN.		**Liquid (per 20 cc):** codeine phosphate (10 mg), guaifenesin (300 mg)
Bucladin	See BUCLIZINE		Motion Sickness
BUCLIZINE Bucladin	**Motion Sickness:** PO: 50 mg 30 min before embarking and repeat after 4–6 hrs. up to 150 mg/d for extended travel.	**Tablet:** 50 mg	ANTI-INFLAMMATORY, ETC (G) Antihistamines (H1 Antagonists) (G) Motion Sickness Prevention (SG) **Cost:** Medium
BUDESONIDE Deep: Pulmicort, Intranasal: Rhinocort	**Asthma:** Intranasal Spray (adults and children >5 yrs): 256 mcg day initially (give 2 sprays in each nostril bid) (Alt. regimen: 4 sprays in each nostril qAM). **Rhinocort**	**Aerosol:** 32 mcg budesonide per spray.	ANTI-INFLAMMATORY STEROIDS (G) Inhalation and Intranasal (SG) **Cost:** Low
BUMETANIDE Bumex	**Edema:** PO: 0.5–2 mg/d to start; 0.5–10 mg/d maintenance (qod dosing may be best regimen). IV, IM: 0.5–1 mg q2–3h (max. dose 10 mg/d).	**Tablet:** 0.5, 1, 2 mg **Injection:** 0.25 mg/ml	RENAL AGENTS (G) Sodium Diuretics (SG) Potent ("Loop") Diuretics (SG) **Cost:** High
Bumex	See BUMETANIDE		

GENERIC NAME Trade Name	INDICATIONS AND DOSAGES	DOSE FORMS	GROUP (G)/SUBGROUP (SG) Relative Cost within Group
BUPIVACAINE Generic, Marcaine, Sensorcaine	**Infiltration:** 0.25% Peripheral Nerve Block: 0.25–0.5% Dental Alveolar Nerve Block: 0.5%	**Injection:** 0.25, 0.5, 0.75% **Injection:** (with epinephrine) 0.25, 0.5, 0.75%	LOCAL ANESTHETICS (G) Injectable or Topical (Mucosal) (SG) **Cost:** Low
Buprenex	See BUPRENORPHINE		Narcotic Agonist-Antagonist
BUPRENORPHINE Buprenex	**Pain Management:** IM, IV: 0.3 mg q6h PRN (may repeat initial dose once in 30–60 minutes if needed) (max. individual dose 0.6 mg).	**Injection:** 0.324 mg (equivalent to 0.3 mg buprenorphine) per ml	NARCOTIC ANALGESICS AND RELATED AGENTS (G) Mixed Agonist-Antagonist Effects (SG) **Cost:** Medium
BUPROPION Wellbutrin, Zypan	**Stimulant:** PO: Adults initial 100 mg bid, increase to 300 mg/day if necessary, but no sooner than 3 days after beginning tx. (max. dose 150 mg tid). **Smoking Cessation:** 150 mg/d for 3 days then 150 mg/bid 7–12 wks	**Tablet:** 75, 100, 150 mg; **ER tabs:** 100, 150 mg	CNS AGENTS (G) Sympathomimetic Stimulants (SG) Unscheduled Aminergic Stimulant (SSG) **Cost:** Medium
BuSpar	See BUSPIRONE		Nominal Sedative Hypnotic
BUSPIRONE BuSpar	**Sedation:** 15 mg bid	**Tablet:** 5, 10 mg	CNS AGENTS (G) Sedative Hypnotic (SG)
BUSULFAN Myleran	CANCER CHEMOTHERAPY (G) Alkylating Agents (SG) Other Alkylating Agents (SSG)		
BUTABARBITAL Generic, In many proprietary mixtures	**Sedation:** PO: 15–30 mg tid or QID. **Hypnotic:** PO: 50–100 mg hs. **Tablets:** 15, 30, 50, 100 mg	**Elixir:** 30 mg per 5 ml	SEDATIVE-HYPNOTICS (G) Intermediate-Acting Sedative Hypnotics (SG) **Cost:** Low
BUTAMBEN PICRATE OTC, Butesin	**Topical Anesthesia:** Apply PRN	**Ointment: 1**%	LOCAL ANESTHETICS (G) Injectable or Topical (Mucosal) (SG) **Cost:** Medium
Butazolidin	See PHENYLBUTAZONE		Non-Narcotic Analgetic
BUTENAFINE Mentax	**T. pedis, corporis, cruris:** Topical: apply 1% cream qd for 4 wks	**Cream:** 1%	DERMATOLOGIC AGENTS (G) Topical Anti-Infectious (SG) Topical Antifungal (SSG)
Butesin	See BUTAMBEN PICRATE		Local Anesthetic, Topical
BUTOCONAZOLE Femstat	**Vaginal Candidiasis:** Intravaginal: 1 applicator full intravaginally at bedtime for 3–6 days.	**Cream:** 2%.	TOPICAL ANTI-INFECTIOUS AGENTS (G) Topical Fungicides (SG) **Cost:** Medium

GENERIC NAME Trade Name	INDICATIONS AND DOSAGES	DOSE FORMS	GROUP (G)/SUBGROUP (SG) Relative Cost within Group
BUTORPHANOL Stadol	**Pain Management:** IV: 0.5–2 mg q3–4h. IV: 1–4 mg q3–4h.	**Nasal Spray:** 1 spray (1 mg) in one nostril. If additional analgesia is needed, may repeat one spray 60–90 minutes after initial spray. This two dose sequence can be repeated q3–4h PRN (max. dose 2 sprays, one in each nostril, q3–4h). **Nasal Spray:** 10 mg/ ml **Injection:** (1 mg of tartrate salt is equal to 0.68 mg base) 1, 2 mg/ml	NARCOTIC ANALGESICS AND RELATED AGENTS (G) Mixed Agonist-Antagonist Effects (SG) **Cost:** Very High
CABERGOLINE Dostinex	**Hyperprolactinemia:** PO: Initially 0.25 twice weekly then 0.5–1 mg twice weekly after 4 wks. Maximum dose 1 mg twice weekly.	**Tablets:** 0.5 mg (scored)	CNS AGENTS (G) Antiparkinsonian Agents (SG) Dopamine (D_2) Agonist (SSG)
CAFERGOT	**Migraine Headaches:** PO: 2 tabs stat, then 1 tablet q0.5h if needed (max. dose: of 6 tabs per attack). Rectal: Insert 1 stat, then 1 suppository after 1h if needed.	**Tablet:** ergotamine tartrate (1 mg), caffeine (100 mg) **Rectal Suppository:** ergotamine tartrate (2 mg), caffeine (100 mg)	
CAFFEINE OTC, Generic	**Wakefulness Aid:** PO: 100–200 mg q3–4h. **Analeptic:** IM, IV: 250 mg caffeine (max. dose 500 mg caffeine). (Obsolete.)	**Tablet:** 100, 150, 200 mg **Tablet:** (chewable) 100 mg **Tablet:** (Ext'd release) 200 mg **Capsule:** (Ext'd release) 200 mg **Injection:** 250 mg/ml	XANTHINES (G) **Cost:** Low
Calan	See VERAPAMIL		Calcium Channel Blocker
CALCIFEDIOL Generic, 25-Hydroxy-cholecalciferol, 25[OH]-D3, Calderol	**Metabolic Bone Disease, Hypocalcemia (CRF):** PO: 300–350 mcg/week given qd or qod initially, then increase q4 wk until maintenance dose reached (usually 50–100 mcg/d).	**Capsule:** 20, 50 mcg	CALCIUM KINETICS REGULATORS (G) D Vitamins and Related Agents (SG) **Cost:** Very High
Calciferol	See ERGOCALCIFEROL (D2)		D Vitamin Prodrug
Calcijex	See CALCITRIOL		D Vitamin
Calcimar	See CALCITONIN		Calcium-Lowering Hormone

GENERIC NAME Trade Name	INDICATIONS AND DOSAGES	DOSE FORMS	GROUP (G)/SUBGROUP (SG) Relative Cost within Group
CALCIPOTRIENE Dovonex	Topical: Apply twice daily (rub in gently and completely).	**Ointment:** 0.005%	KERATOLYTIC AND KERATOPLASTIC AGENTS (G) Antipsoriatic Agents (SG) **Cost:** High
CALCITONIN-SALMON Calcimar, Miacalcin **CALCITONIN-HUMAN** Cibacalcin	**Hypercalcemia:** IM, SC (Salmon): 4 IU/kg q12h initially; after 2–4 doses, increase to 8 IU/kg q12h PRN; after next 4 doses, increase to a max. dose of 8 IU/kg q6h PRN. **Osteoporosis (postmenopausal):** IM, SC (Salmon): 100 IU/d (give concurrent calcium (1.5 gm/d) and vitamin D (400 units/d)). **Nasal Spray:** 200 IU/d in one nostril. Alternate nostrils. **Paget's Disease:** IM, SC (Salmon): 100 IU/d initially, then maintenance (usually 50 IU qd or qod); monitor with periodic eval. of s/sx, alkaline phos. Note recently introduced phosphonates (pamidronate).	**Calcitonin-Salmon (Calcimar, Miacalcin):** **Injection:** 200 IU/ml (2 ml vials) **Nasal Spray:** Calcitonin-Human (Cibacalcin): **Injection:** 0.5 mg/vials	CALCIUM KINETICS REGULATORS (G) Other Calcium Regulators (SG) **Cost:** High
CALCITRIOL 1,25-Dihydroxy-cholecalciferol, 1,25[OH]2-D3, Rocaltrol, Calcijex	**Hypoparathyroidism:** PO: 0.25 mcg qAM initially, then carefully increase dose every 2–4 wks (monitor serum calcium 2 times/wk during dosage adjustments), maintenance usually 0.5–2.0 mcg/d.	**Capsules:** 0.25, 0.5 mcg. **Injection:** 1 & 2 mcg/ml.	CALCIUM KINETICS REGULATORS (G) D Vitamins and Related Agents (SG) **Cost:** Very High
CALCIUM CARBONATE Generic, OTC, Tums, Alka-Mints, Chooz, Amitone	**Gastric Hyperacidity:** PO: 500–1500 mg PRN	**Tablet:** 500, 600, 650, 1000, 1250 mg **Tablet:** (chewable) 350, 420, 500, 750, 850, 1000 mg **Tablet:** (gum) 500 mg **Suspension:** 1250 mg/5 ml **Lozenges:** 600 mg	ANTACIDS (G) Acid Neutralizing (SG)
Calcium Disodium Versenate	See EDETATE Ca Na_2		Chelating Agent

GENERIC NAME Trade Name	INDICATIONS AND DOSAGES	DOSE FORMS	GROUP (G)/SUBGROUP (SG) Relative Cost within Group
CALCIUM SALTS, ORAL, Generic, OTC, Citracal, PhosLo	PO: 500–2000 mg 1–2 times/d. RDA PO (adults): 0.8–1.5 gm/d (consensus differs, NIH rec. for higher doses to inhibit bone loss associated with age). PO (pregnant/lactating): 1200 mg/d. Pediatric PO (children > 1yr.): 800 mg/d. Pediatric PO (adolescents): 1200 mg/d.	**Calcium gluconate (9% Ca):** 500 mg (45 mg Ca), 650 mg, 975 mg, 1g **Calcium lactate (13% Ca):** 325 mg (42 Ca), 650 mg **Calcium citrate:** (21% Ca) Tablet: 950 mg (200 mg Ca) **Calcium acetate:** (25% Ca) Capsule: 500 mg (125 mg Ca) **Tablet:** 250, 667, 1000 mg Calcium carbonate (40% Ca): Countless OTC proprietary preparations	CALCIUM KINETICS REGULATORS (G) Other Calcium Regulators (SG) **Cost:** Medium
CALCIUM SALTS, PARENTERAL Generic, Calcium Chloride, Calcium Gluconate, Calcium Gluceptate	**Cardiac Resuscitation:** IV(Chloride): 0.5–1 gm bolus. **Hypocalcemia:** IV(Chloride): 0.5–1 gm q24–72h (rate NOT > 1 ml/min). IV(Gluconate): 7–14 mEq (rate NOT > 2 ml/min of 10% CaGluc.). **Tetany (caused by hypocalcemia):** IV(Gluconate): 4.5–16 mEq(rate NOT > 2 ml/min). **Hypermagnesemia:** IV(Chloride): 0.5 gm (close clinical observation before additional doses). IV(Gluconate): 4.5–9 mEq. IV(Gluconate): 2–5 mEq. IV(Gluceptate): 1.1–4.4 gm (5–20 ml) (rate NOT > 2 ml/min). IV(Gluceptate): 0.44–1.1 gm (2–5 ml) into gluteus maximus.	**Calcium chloride: Injection:** 10% sln (10 ml) **Calcium gluconate: Injection:** 10% sln (10, 20 ml) **Calcium gluceptate: Injection:** 220 mg/ml (5, 50 ml)	CALCIUM KINETICS REGULATORS (G) Other Calcium Regulators (SG) **Cost:** Low
Calcium Chloride	See CALCIUM SALTS		
Calcium Gluceptate	See CALCIUM SALTS		
Calcium Gluconate	See CALCIUM SALTS		
Calderol	See CALCIFEDIOL		D Vitamin Precursor
Camphorated tincture of opium	See PAREGORIC		Narcotic (Antidiarrheal)
Camptosar	See IRINOTECAN		Cancer Chemotherapy
Cantil	See MEPENZOLATE		Anticholinergic
Capoten	See CAPTOPRIL		ACE Inhibitor

GENERIC NAME Trade Name	INDICATIONS AND DOSAGES	DOSE FORMS	GROUP (G)/SUBGROUP (SG) Relative Cost within Group
CAPOZIDE	**Hypertension:** Adjust dosage within limit imposed	**Tablet:** PO: Captopril/HCTZ: 50/25 mg, 25/25 mg, 50/15 mg, 25/15 mg	ACE INHIBITOR-DIURETIC COMBINATION
CAPREOMYCIN	**Tuberculosis (given in combination):** PO Adults (single dose/day): 15 mg/kg/d (max. dose 1,000 mg/d). Pediatric PO (single dose/day): 15 mg/kg/d (max. dose 1,000 mg/d).	**Injection:** (powder) 1 g per 10 ml	ANTITUBERCULOUS AND RELATED AGENTS (G) Antituberculous Second Line Agents (SG) **Cost:** Very High
CAPTOPRIL Capoten	**Hypertension:** PO: 25 mg bid or tid to start; 50–100 mg tid maintenance (max. dose 450 mg/d). **Congestive Heart Failure:** PO: 25 mg tid to start; 50–100 mg tid maintenance (max. dose 450 mg/d; 6.25–12.5 mg tid to start in hypotensive or hyponatremic patients).	**Tablet:** 12.5, 25, 50, 100 mg	VASODILATORS (G) ACE Inhibitors (SG) **Cost:** Low
Carafate	See SUCRALFATE		Antacid
CARBACHOL Miostat, Isoptocarbachol	**Produce Miosis:** Intraocular (Miostat): 0.5–2.0 ml. **Glaucoma:** Topical intrapalpebral (Isopto): 1–2 drops, 1–3 times/day.	**Miostat solution:** 0.01% **Isopto Solution:** 0.75, 1.5, 2.25, 3%	AGENTS USED IN THE TREATMENT OF GLAUCOMA (G) Parasympathomimetic (SG) **Cost:** Medium
CARBAMAZEPINE Generic, Tegretol	**Seizure Disorders:** PO: 200 mg bid to start, increase by up to 200 mg/d at weekly intervals (to max. dose 1,000–1,200 mg/d) in 3–4 doses. Pediatric PO (6–12 y.o.): 100 mg bid to start, increase by 100 mg/d to max. dose 1,000 mg/d in 3–4 doses when > 200 mg/d (dose can also be based on 20–30 mg/kg/d given in 3 or 4 divided doses). **Trigeminal Neuralgia:** PO: 100 mg bid for 1 day, increase by 100 mg q12h; usual maintenance 400–800 mg/d (max. dose 1,200 mg/d).	**Tablet:** 200 mg **Tablet:** (chewable) 100 mg **Suspension:** 100 mg/5 ml	ANTICONVULSANTS (G) Hydantoins and Equivalent (SG) **Cost:** Low
CARBENICILLIN Pyopen, Geopen, Geocillin	**Urinary Tract Infections:** PO: 382–764 mg q6h. **Prostatitis:** PO: 764 mg q6h.	**Tablet:** 382 mg	LACTAM ANTIBIOTICS (G) Extended Gram Negative and Other No/Marginal Effectiveness In Meningitis And No/Marginal Activity Vs. P. aeruginosa (SSG) **Cost:** Low
CARBIDOPA Lodosyn	Do not use as single agent. See Levodopa—Carbidopa combination.	**Tablet:** 25 mg	ANTIPARKINSONIAN AGENTS (G) Dopamine Precursors, Agonists And Related Agents (SG) **COST:** Medium
Carbocaine	See MEPIVACAINE		Local Anesthetic
CARBOPLATIN Paraplatin	CANCER CHEMOTHERAPY (G) Alkylating Agents (SG) Chelates of Platinum (SSG)		

GENERIC NAME Trade Name	INDICATIONS AND DOSAGES	DOSE FORMS	GROUP (G)/SUBGROUP (SG) Relative Cost within Group
CARBOPROST Hemabate, Prostin/15M, 15 methyl PGF2a	**Postpartum Bleeding:** IM: 250 mcg initially, then repeat q15 to 90 minutes as needed (max dose 2 mg [8 doses]). **Abortion:** IM: 250 mcg (1 ml) initially, then 250 mcg q 1.5–3.5 hours based on uterine response (max. individual dose—500 mcg); do not exceed 12 mg total dose over 2 days of treatment or 2 days of total treatment duration.	**Injection:** 250 mcg	CARDIOVASCULAR AGENTS(G) Vasoconstrictors and Oxytocics (SG) **Cost:** High
Cardabid	See NITROGLYCERIN		Vasodilator
Cardene	See NICARDIPINE		Calcium Channel Blocker
Cardioquin	See QUINIDINE		Antiarrhythmic
Cardizem	See DILTIAZEM		Calcium Channel Blocker
Cardura	See DOXAZOSIN		Alpha Adrenergic Blocker
CARISOPRODOL Generic, Soma, Soprodol, Rela	PO: 350 mg tid or QID.	**Tablet:** 350 mg	MUSCLE RELAXANTS (G) Sedative Hypnotics (SG) **Cost:** Low
CARMUSTINE BCNU	CANCER CHEMOTHERAPY (G) Alkylating Agents (SG) Nitrosoureas		
CARTEOLOL Ocupress, Cartrol	**Elevated IOP:** Instill 1 drop bid. **Hypertension:** PO: Initial 2.5mg qd, increase to 5–10mg qd if necessary. Maintenance: 2.5–5mg qd.	Solution: 1.0% **Tablet**: 2.5, 5 mg	AGENTS USED IN THE TREATMENT OF GLAUCOMA (G) Sympathoplegics (G) **Cost:** High Beta adrenergic receptor blockers, cardioselective (Beta 1) (SSG) **Cost:** Medium
Cartrol	See CARTEOLOL		Beta Adrenergic Blocker
CASCARA Generic, OTC, Cascara sagrada Available OTC as such and in many combinations.	**Laxative:** PO: 325 mg (tablet) qhs; or 5 ml (liquid).	**Tablet:** 325 mg **Liquid (fluid extract);** 5 ml/ dose	LAXATIVES AND BOWEL CLEANSERS (G) Irritant Laxatives (SG) **Cost:** Low
Casodex	See BICALUTAMIDE		Antiandrogen
CASTOR OIL Generic, OTC, Neoloid, Purge, Alphamul, Emulsoil, etc.	PO: 15–60 ml of liquid. Pediatric PO (6–12 yrs): 5–15 ml of liquid.	**Liquid:** in 60 and 120 ml **Emulsion:** 36.4%, 60%, 67%, 95% **Liquid:** 95%	LAXATIVES AND BOWEL CLEANSERS (G) Irritant Laxatives (SG) **Cost:** Low
Cataflam	See DICLOFENAC		NSAID, Ocular
Catapres	See CLONIDINE		Hypotensive (Central Sympathoplegic)
Catarase	See CHYMOTRYPSIN		Proteolytic Enzyme, Intraocular
Caverject	See ALPROSTADIL		Vasodilator

GENERIC NAME Trade Name	INDICATIONS AND DOSAGES	DOSE FORMS	GROUP (G)/SUBGROUP (SG) Relative Cost within Group
CCNU	See Lomustine		Cancer Chemotherapy
Ceclor	See CEFACLOR		Lactam Antibiotic
Cedax	See CEFTIBUTEN		Broad Spectrum Cephalosporin
CeeNu	Nitrosoureas		Cancer Chemotherapy
CEFACLOR Ceclor	**General Infections:** PO: 250–500 mg q8h. **Pediatric Infections:** Minor: 20 mg/kg/d given in 3 doses. Severe: 40 mg/kg/d given in 3 doses; max. dose 1 g/d.	**Capsule:** 250, 500 mg **Oral Suspension:** (powder) 125 mg/5 ml, 187 mg/5 ml, 250 mg/5 ml, 375 mg/ml	LACTAM ANTIBIOTICS (G) Benzyl Penicillins and First Generation Cephalosporins (SG) **Cost:** Medium
CEFADROXIL Generic, Duricef, Ultracef	**Urinary Tract Infections:** PO: 1–2 g/d in 1–2 doses. Pharyngitis, Tonsillitis (beta-hemolytic streptococci), **Skin Infections:** PO: 1 g/d in 1–2 divided doses (continue for minimum 10 days with beta-hemolytic strep). **Pediatric Infections:** Pediatric PO: 15 mg/kg bid.	**Capsule:** 500 mg **Tablet:** 1 g **Oral Suspension:** 25, 50, 100 mg/ml	LACTAM ANTIBIOTICS (G) Benzyl Penicillins and First Generation Cephalosporins (SG) **Cost:** Medium
Cefadyl	See CEPHAPIRIN		Lactam Antibiotic
CEFAMANDOLE Mandol	Administer IV or by deep IM injection. **General Infections:** IM, IV: 500 mg to 1g q4–8h (max. dose 2 g q4h). Pediatric IM, IV: 50–100 mg/kg/d, divided and given q4–8h. **Perioperative Prophylaxis:** IM, IV: 1–2 g IM or IV 30–60 minutes prior to surgery, followed with 1–2 g q6h for 1–2 days. **Uncomplicated UTI:** IM, IV: 500 mg q8h. Uncomplicated Pneumonia, Simple Cellulitis: IM, IV: 500 mg q6h.	**Powder for Injection:** 1, 2, 10 g	LACTAM ANTIBIOTICS (G) Wider Gram Negative Coverage With Activity vs. Gram Positives Retained; (SG) **Cost:** High
CEFAZOLIN Generic, Zolicef, Ancef, Kefzol	**Minor Infections:** IM, IV: 250–500 mg q8h. **Severe Infections:** IM, IV: 1–1.5g q6h (max. dose 12 g/d). **Pediatric Infections:** IM, IV: 25–100 mg/kg/d in 3–4 doses. **Surgical Prophylaxis:** IM, IV: 1 g 30–90 min before surgery; 500–1000 mg repeated q6–8h for 24 hours after surgery.	**Injection:** (powder) 250, 500 mg; 1, 5, 10, 20 g **Injection:** 500 mg in 5% Dextrose in water, 1 g in 5% Dextrose in water	LACTAM ANTIBIOTICS—PENICILLINS & CEPHALOSPORINS (G) Benzyl Penicillins and First Generation Cephalosporins (SG) Cephalosporins Equivalent To Benzyl Penicillins (SSG) **Cost:** High
CEFEPIME Maxipime	**Uncomplicated Skin, Pneumonic or UTI; Febrile Neutropenia (Labeled Uses):** IM: 0.5–1.0 gm q 12h. IV: 1–2 gm q 8–12h.		LACTAM ANTIBIOTICS—PENICILLINS & CEPHALOSPORINS (G) Wider Gram Negative Coverage With Activity vs. Gram Positives Retained; (SG) No/Marginal Effectiveness In Meningitis; Active vs. P. aeruginosa (SSG)

GENERIC NAME Trade Name	INDICATIONS AND DOSAGES	DOSE FORMS	GROUP (G)/SUBGROUP (SG) Relative Cost within Group
CEFIXIME Suprax	**Gonorrhea (uncomplicated), acute bronchitis, pharyngitis:** PO: 400 mg/d given as 1 dose or in 2 divided doses. **Otitis media:** PO(adults, children > 12 yrs): 400 mg/d given as 1 dose or in 2 divided doses, treat for 10 days. **Pediatric PO:** PO: 8 mg/kg/d in 1 dose or in 2 divided doses, treat for 10 days.	**Tablet:** 200, 400 mg **Powder (oral suspension):** 100 mg per 5 ml.	LACTAM ANTIBIOTICS (G) Wider Gram Negative Coverage with Activity vs. Gram Positives Retained; (SG) **Cost:** High
Cefizox	See CEFTIZOXIME		Lactam Antibiotic
CEFMETAZOLE Zefazone	**General Infections:** IV: 2 g q6–12 h for 5 to 14 days. **Perioperative Prophylaxis:** IV: 1 g 30–90 minutes prior to surgery, repeat at 8 and 16 hours. (Note: colorectal surgery requires a 2 gram dose).	**Powder for Injection:** 1, 2 g	LACTAM ANTIBIOTICS (G) Wider Gram Negative Coverage (SG)
Cefobid	See CEFOPERAZONE		Lactam Antibiotic
CEFONICID Monocid	**General Infections:** IM, IV: 1–2 g qd (give IM doses over 1 g at two sites). **Surgical Prophylaxis:** IM, IV: 1 g 60 min before surgery, then 1 g/d for 2 days.	**Injection:** (powder) 0.5, 1, 10 g	LACTAM ANTIBIOTICS—PENICILLINS & CEPHALOSPORINS (G) Wider Gram Negative Coverage with Activity vs. Gram Positives Retained; (SG) **Cost:** Very High
CEFOPERAZONE Cefobid	**General Infections:** IM, IV: 1–2 g q12h (max. dose 16 g/d in 2–4 divided doses)	**Injection:** 1, 2 g **Injection:** (powder) 1, 2 g	LACTAM ANTIBIOTICS (G) Extended Gram Negative and Other Coverage (SG) Effective In Meningitis and Some Activity vs. P. aeruginosa: **Cost:** High
Cefotan	See CEFOTETAN		Lactam Antibiotic
CEFOTAXIME Claforan	**General Infections:** IV, IM: 1–8 g/d in 2–6 divided doses (max. dose 2 g q4h IV). Pediatric (< 50 kgs,and > 1 year): IM, IV 50–180 mg/kg/d in 4–6 divided doses. **Sepsis:** IV: 2 g q6–8h. **Perioperative prophylaxis:** 1 g IV or IM 30–90 minutes prior to surgery.	**Injection:** 1, 2 g **Injection:** (powder) 1, 2 g	LACTAM ANTIBIOTICS—PENICILLINS & CEPHALOSPORINS (G) Extended Gram Negative and Other Coverage (SG) Effective In Meningitis and Some Activity vs. P. aeruginosa: **Cost:** High
CEFOTETAN Cefotan	**Urinary tract infections:** IM, IV: 500 mg q12h; or 1–2 g q12h—24 h for more serious infections. **Other infections:** IV, IM: 2–4 g q12–24 hours (max. dose: 6 g/d).	**Powder (for injection):** 1 g, 2g, 10g (contains 3.5 mEq sodium/g).	LACTAM ANTIBIOTICS—PENICILLINS & CEPHALOSPORINS (G) Wider Gram Negative Coverage with Activity vs. Gram Positives Retained; (SG) **Cost:** High

GENERIC NAME Trade Name	INDICATIONS AND DOSAGES	DOSE FORMS	GROUP (G)/SUBGROUP (SG) Relative Cost within Group
CEFOXITIN Mefoxin	**Infections:** IM, IV: 1 g q6–8h (mild); 6–8 g/d in 3–6 divided doses (severe); 12 g/d given in 4–6 divided doses (very severe) (give larger doses as IV). Pediatric IM, IV: 80–160 mg/kg/d in 4–6 doses (max. dose 12 g/d). **Gonorrhea:** IM: 2 g with 1 g PO probenecid (given 30 min before injection). IV: (disseminated infection) 1 g q6h for 7 days. **Acute Pelvic Inflammatory Disease:** IM: 2 g with 1 g PO probenecid given 30 min before injection, plus doxycycline 100 mg bid for 10–14 days. IV: (inpatient) 2 g q6h (plus 100 mg doxycycline IV q12h) for a minimum of 4 days and at least 2 days after clinical improvement; follow with doxycycline 100 mg bid for 10–14 days. **Surgical Prophylaxis:** IM, IV: 2 g 30–60 min before surgery; then 2 g q6h for 4 doses	**Injection:** (powder) 1, 2, 10 g **Injection:** 1 g in 5% Dextrose in Water, 2 g in 5% Dextrose in Water	LACTAM ANTIBIOTICS (G) Wider Gram Negative Coverage with Activity vs. Gram Positives Retained; (SG) **Cost:** High
CEFPODOXIME Vantin	**Pneumonia (community acquired):** PO: 200 mg q12h for 14 days. **Chronic Bronchitis:** PO: 200 mg q12h for 10 days. **Gonorrhea** (uncomplicated): PO: 200 mg single dose. **Pharyngitis, Tonsillitis:** PO: 100 mg q12h for 10 days. **Skin Infection:** PO: 400 mg q12h for 1–2 weeks. **UTI (uncomplicated):** PO: 100 mg q12 for 1 week.	**Tablet:** 100, 200 mg **Granules (Sup):** 50, 100 mg per ml	LACTAM ANTIBIOTICS (G) Benzyl Penicillins and First Generation Cephalosporins (SG) Cephalosporins Equivalent to Benzyl Penicillins (SSG)
CEFPROZIL Cefzil	**Pharyngitis, Tonsillitis:** PO: 500 mg qd for 10 days. **Acute Bronchitis:** PO: 500 mg q12h for 10 days. Skin infections (uncomplicated): PO: 250–500 mg q12h for 10 days.	**Tablet:** 250, 500 mg **Powder for suspension:** 125 mg & 250 mg per 5 ml when prepared	LACTAM ANTIBIOTICS (G) Benzyl Penicillins and First Generation Cephalosporins (SG) Cephalosporins Equivalent to Benzyl Penicillins (SSG)
CEFTAZIDIME Generic, Fortaz, Ceptaz, Tazicef, Tazidime	**General Infections:** IM, IV: 1000 mg q8–12h; max. dose 6 g/d. Pediatric IV: 30–50 mg/kg/d in 3 doses (max. dose 6 g/d). **Meningitis:** IV: 2 g q8h. **Urinary Tract Infections:** IM, IV (uncomplicated): 250 mg q12h. IV, IV (complicated): 500 mg q12h. **Uncomplicated Pneumonia:** IM, IV: 500–1000 mg q8h. **Bone, Joint Infections:** IV: 2 g q12h. **Injection:** 1.2 g	**Injection:** (powder) 0.5, 1, 2, 6, 10 g	LACTAM ANTIBIOTICS (G) Extended Gram Negative and Other Coverage: Wider Gram Negative Coverage; Activity (SG) No/Marginal Effectiveness In Meningitis; Some Activity vs. P. aeruginosa (SSG) **Cost:** High

GENERIC NAME Trade Name	INDICATIONS AND DOSAGES	DOSE FORMS	GROUP (G)/SUBGROUP (SG) Relative Cost within Group
CEFTIBUTEN Cedax	**Gonorrhea (uncomplicated), acute bronchitis, pharyngitis:** PO: 400 mg/d given as 1 dose or in 2 divided doses. **Otitis media:** PO (adults, children > 12 yrs): 400 mg/d given as 1 dose or in 2 divided doses, treat for 10 days. **Pediatric PO:** PO: 8 mg/kg/d in 1 dose or in 2 divided doses, treat for 10 days.	**Capsules:** 400 mg **Suspension:** 90, 180 m/5 ml	LACTAM ANTIBIOTICS (G) Wider Gram Negative Coverage with Activity vs. Gram Positives Retained; (SG) **Cost:** High
Ceftin	See CEFUROXIME		Lactam Antibiotic
CEFTIZOXIME Cefizox	**General Infections:** IM, IV: 1–2 g q8–12h (max. dose 12 g/d). Pediatric IM, IV: 50 mg/kg q6–8h (max. dose 200 mg/kg/d, do not exceed adult doses). **Urinary Tract Infections:** IM, IV : 500 mg q12h. **Pelvic Inflammatory Disease:** IV : 2 g q8h. **Uncomplicated Gonorrhea:** IM: 1 g single dose. **Sepsis:** IV : 6–12 g/d given in 3 divided doses.	**Injection:** 1, 2 g **Injection:** (powder) 0.5, 1, 2, 10 g	LACTAM ANTIBIOTICS (G) Extended Gram Negative and Other Coverage: Wider Gram Negative Coverage; Activity (SG) No/Marginal Effectiveness In Meningitis; Some Activity vs. P. aeruginosa: (SSG) **Cost:** High
CEFTRIAXONE Rocephin	**Infections:** IM, IV: 250–2,000 mg/d given in 1–2 doses; usual duration of treatment 4–14 days (max. dose 4 g/d). Pediatric IM, IV: 50–75 mg/kg/d given in 2 doses (max. dose 2 g/d). **Meningitis:** IV: 1–2 g q12h. Pediatric IV: 100 mg/kg/d (max. dose 4 g/d). **Gonococcal Infections:** IM, IV (Uncomplicated): 250 mg (single dose). IV, IV (Disseminated): 1g q24h. **Surgical Prophylaxis:** IM: 1 g 30–120 min prior to surgery.	**Injection:** 1, 2 g **Injection:** (powder) 0.25, 0.5, 1, 2, 10 g	LACTAM ANTIBIOTICS (G) Extended Gram Negative and Other Coverage: Wider Gram Negative Coverage; Activity (SG) Effective In Meningitis and Some Activity vs. P. aeruginosa (SSG) **Cost:** Very High

GENERIC NAME Trade Name	INDICATIONS AND DOSAGES	DOSE FORMS	GROUP (G)/SUBGROUP (SG) Relative Cost within Group
CEFUROXIME Zinacef, Ceftin, Kefurox	**General Infections:** PO: 250–500 mg bid. IV, IV: 750–1500 mg q8h for 5–10 days. Pediatric IM, IV: 50–100 mg/kg/d given in 3–4 doses (do not exceed adult doses). **Bacterial Meningitis:** IV: 9 g/d given q8h. Pediatric IV: 200–240 mg/kg/d to start in 3–4 doses. **Simple Gonococcal Infections:** PO: 1 g (single dose), give with 1 g PO probenecid. IV: 1.5 g (single dose), give split dose at two different sites with 1 g PO probenecid. **Surgical Prophylaxis:** IM, IV: 1500 mg (IV) 30–60 min before surgery, then 750 mg q8h postoperatively (IM or IV). **Urinary Tract Infection (uncomplicated):** PO: 125–250 bid. **Otitis Media:** PO: 250 mg bid. Pediatric PO: (2–12 yrs) 250 mg bid. Pediatric PO: (< 2 yrs) 125 mg bid.	**Injection:** (powder) 0.75 g, 1.5 g, 7.5 g/vial **Injection:** 750 mg, 1.5 g **Tablets:** 125, 250, 500 mg	LACTAM ANTIBIOTICS (G) Wider Gram Negative Coverage with Activity vs. Gram Positives Retained; (SG) Cephalosporins: Wider Gram Negative Coverage-Activity vs. Gram Positives Retained (SSG) **Cost:** Medium
Cefzil	See CEFPROZIL		Lactam Antibiotic
Cel-U-Jec	See BETAMETHASONE		Corticosteroid
Celestone	See BETAMETHASONE		Corticosteroid
Celontin	See METHSUXIMIDE		Anticonvulsant
Cena-K	See POTASSIUM CHLORIDE		
Cenocort	See TRIAMCINOLONE		Corticosteroid
Centrax	See PRAZEPAM		Sedative-Hypnotic
CEPHALEXIN Generic, Kefros, Keflex, Keflet	**General Infections:** PO: 250 mg q6–8h; max. (dose 4 g/d in divided doses). Pediatric PO: 25–100 mg/kg/d in 4 doses. **Streptococcal Skin Infections, Pharyngitis:** PO: 500 mg q12h, for beta-hemolytic strep treat 10 days minimum. **Otitis Media:** Pediatric PO: 75–100 mg/kg/d given in 4 divided doses.	**Tablet:** 250 mg, 500 mg, 1 g **Capsule:** 250, 500 mg **Oral Suspension:** 25, 50 mg/ml **Drops:** (pediatric) 100 mg/ml	LACTAM ANTIBIOTICS—PENICILLINS & CEPHALOSPORINS (G) Benzyl Penicillins and First Generation Cephalosporins (SG) Cephalosporins Equivalent to Benzyl Penicillins (SSG) **Cost:** Low

GENERIC NAME Trade Name	INDICATIONS AND DOSAGES	DOSE FORMS	GROUP (G)/SUBGROUP (SG) Relative Cost within Group
CEPHALOTHIN Generic, Keflin	**Infections:** IM, IV: 4–6 g/d in 4–6 divided doses (max. dose 2g q4h). **Pediatric Infections:** IM, IV: 80–160 mg/kg/d given in 4–6 divided doses. **Surgical Prophylaxis:** IV: 1–2 g 30–60 min before surgery; 1–2 g q6h for 24 hours after surgery. **Renal Impairment (maximum doses):** IV: 1–2 g to start; then 2 g q6h if creatinine clearance = 50–80 cc/min; 1.5 g q6h if 25–50 cc/min; 1 g q6h if 10–25 cc/min; 500 mg q6h if 2–10 cc/min; 500 mg q8h if < 2 cc/min.	**Injection:** (powder) 1, 2, 20 g **Injection:** 1g in 5% Dextrose, 2 g in 5% Dextrose	LACTAM ANTIBIOTICS—PENICILLINS & CEPHALOSPORINS (G) Benzyl Penicillins and First Generation Cephalosporins (SG) Cephalosporins Equivalent to Benzyl Penicillins (SSG) **Cost:** High
CEPHAPIRIN Generic, Cefadyl	**Infections:** IM, IV: 500 mg–1 g q4–6h; max. dose 12 g/d. Pediatric Infections: IM, IV: 40–80 mg/kg/d given in 4 divided doses. **Surgical Prophylaxis:** IM, IV: 1–2 g 30–60 min before surgery, 1–2 g during surgery; then q6h for 24 hours after surgery.	**Injection:** (powder) 500 mg, 1, 2, 4, 20 g	LACTAM ANTIBIOTICS (G) Benzyl Penicillins And First Generation Cephalosporins (SG) Cephalosporins Equivalent to Benzyl Penicillins (SSG) **Cost:** High
CEPHRADINE Generic, Velosef, Anspor	**Infections:** PO: 250 mg q6h or 500 mg q12h (Minor); 500 mg—1 g q12h (Severe). IV, IV: 2–4 g qd given in 4 divided doses (max. dose 8 g/d). Pediatric PO: 25–50 mg/kg/d in 2–4 doses (max. dose 4 g/d). Pediatric IV, IM: 50–100 mg/kg/d as 4 doses (do not exceed adult doses). **Otitis Media:** Pediatric PO: 75–100 md/kg/d given in 2–4 divided doses (max. dose 4g/d). **Surgical Prophylaxis:** IM, IV: 1 g 30–90 min before surgery; repeat q4–6h for 2 doses.	**Capsule:** 250, 500 mg **Oral Suspension:** 25, 50 mg/ml **Injection:** (powder) 250 mg, 500 mg, 1g, 2g	LACTAM ANTIBIOTICS (G) Benzyl Penicillins and First Generation Cephalosporins (SG) Cephalosporins Equivalent to Benzyl Penicillins (SSG) **Cost:** Medium
Ceptaz	See CEFTAZIDIME		Lactam Antibiotic
Ceredase	See ALGLUCERASE		Enzyme Used in Gaucher's
Cerespan	See PAPAVERINE		Vasodilator
Cerubidine	See DAUNORUBICIN		Cancer Chemotherapy
CETIRIZINE Zyrtec	**Allergic Rhinitis, Urticaria:** PO: 5–20 mg daily	**Tablet:** 5, 10 mg	ANTI-INFLAMMATORY ETC (G) Antihistamine (H1) Antagonist (SG) **Cost:** High
Chenix	See CHENODIOL		Dissolve Gallstones
Chenodeoxy-cholic Acid	See CHENODIOL		Dissolve Gallstones

GENERIC NAME Trade Name	INDICATIONS AND DOSAGES	DOSE FORMS	GROUP (G)/SUBGROUP (SG) Relative Cost within Group
CHENODIOL Chenodeoxy-cholic Acid, Chenix	**Dissolution of Radiolucent Gallstones:** PO: 250 mg bid initially (for 2 weeks), then each week increase dose by 250 mg/day; maintenance dose 13–16 mg/kg/day (if diarrhea occurs, decrease dose until symptoms abate then leave at previously acceptable dose). Discontinue if no gallstone resolution after 18 months of use.	**Tablet:** 250 mg	GASTROINTESTINAL AGENTS (G) Miscellaneous GI Agents (SG) Gallstone Dissolving Agents (SSG)
Chibroxin	See NORFLOXACIN		Quinolone Antibacterial
CHLORAMBUCIL Leukeran	CANCER CHEMOTHERAPY (G) Alkylating Agents (SG) Nitrogen Mustards (SSG)		
Chlor-Trimeton	See CHLORPHENIRAMINE		Antihistamine
CHLORAL HYDRATE Generic, Noctec	**Hypnotic:** PO: 500–1000 mg (max. dose: 2 gm/d). **Sedative:** PO: 250 mg tid. Pediatric PO: 25 mg/kg/day (max. dose: 50 mg/kg/d; not to exceed 1 gm per single dose).	**Capsule:** 250, 500 mg **Syrup:** 250 mg/5 ml, 500 mg/5 ml **Suppositories:** 324, 500, 648 mg	CNS AGENTS (G) Sedative-Hypnotics (SG) Ultrashort-Acting Hypnotics (SSG) **Cost:** Medium
CHLORAMPHEN-ICOL Generic, Chlo-romycetin	**Typhoid, Rickettsia:** PO, IV: (give IV over 1 minute) 50 mg/kg/d in divided doses q6h; max. dose 100 mg/kg/d, (therapeutic levels: peak 10–20 mcg/ml; trough 5–10 mcg/ml). Pediatric PO, IV: (give IV over 1 minute) 50–75 mg/kg/d in divided doses q6h. **Meningitis:** Pediatric PO, IV: (give IV over 1 minute) 50–100 mg/kg/d in divided doses q6h. **Topical:** Apply 1 to 4 times daily to infected area. Cover with sterile bandage as appropriate.	**Capsule:** 250 mg **Oral Suspension:** 150 mg/5 ml **Injection:** (powder) 100 mg/ml when reconstituted **Solution:** 0.5% **Powder for solution:** 25 mg **Ointment:** 1%	ANTI-INFECTIOUS AGENTS (G) Miscellaneous Antibacterials (SG) **Cost:** Low OPHTHALMIC AGENTS (G) Ophthalmic Anti-Infective Agents (G) Antibacterial (SG) **Cost:** Medium
CHLORDIAZE-POXIDE Generic, Lib-rium, Libritabs, A-poxide, Others	**Sedation:** PO: 5–10 mg tid or QID (max. dose 40 mg/d; up to 100 mg/day may be given for severe anxiety states). IV: 50–100 mg to start, then 25–50 mg q6–8h PRN; (max. dose 300 mg/d). **Alcohol Withdrawal:** IV, IM: 50–100 mg to start, repeat q2–4h PRN (max. recommended dose 300 mg/d). PO: 50–100 mg with repeated doses PRN (max. dose 300 mg/d). **Preoperative Sedation:** IM: 50–100 mg 1 hour before surgery.	**Capsule:** 5, 10, 25 mg **Injection:** 100 mg **Tablet:** 5, 10, 25 mg	CNS AGENTS (G) Sedative-Hypnotics (SG) Long-Acting Sedatives (SG) **Cost:** Low
Chloromycetin	See CHLORAMPHENICOL		Antibiotic

GENERIC NAME Trade Name	INDICATIONS AND DOSAGES	DOSE FORMS	GROUP (G)/SUBGROUP (SG) Relative Cost within Group
CHLOROMY-CETIN HYDRO-CORTISONE	2 qtt in the affected eye(s) q 3 h. Continue dosing day and night for the first 48 h, after which the interval between applications may be increased. Treatment should continue for 48 h after the eye appears normal.		**Powder for Ophthalmic Suspension:** chloramphenicol (12.5 mg), hydrocortisone acetate (25 mg) in vials with diluent
CHLOROPRO-CAINE Nesacaine	**Infiltration:** 1–2%. Peripheral Nerve Block: 1–2%	**Injection:** 1, 2, 3%	LOCAL ANESTHETICS (G) Injectable Only (SG) **Cost:** Medium
CHLOROQUINE Generic, Aralen, Nivaquine, Roquine	**Acute Malaria, Extraintestinal Amebiasis:** PO: 1g (600 mg base) daily, use for 2 days, followed by 500 mg/d (300 mg base) use for 2–3 weeks. IV (HCL): 4–5 ml/d (200–250 mg; 160–200 mg base), use for 10–12 days (convert to PO when possible). **Malaria Chemoprophylaxis:** PO: 500 mg phosphate (300 mg base) once/wk (begin therapy 2 weeks prior to exposure, if possible; however, if dose is begun only 1 week before exposure, as the first dose give 600 mg base in 2 divided doses 6 hours apart) (after leaving exposed area manufacturer recommends continuing suppressive therapy for 8 weeks; other authorities hold that only 4 weeks is required post exposure). Pediatric PO: 5 mg base/kg per week; (max. dose 300 mg base/wk) (begin therapy 2 weeks prior to exposure, after leaving exposed area manufacturer recommends continuing suppressive therapy for 8 weeks; other authorities hold that only 4 weeks is required post exposure).	**Tablet:** 250 mg (= 150 mg base), 500 mg (= 300 mg base) as phospate **Injection:** 50 mg/ml (= 40 mg base) HCl	ANTI-INFECTIOUS AGENTS (G) Antiparasitic Agents (SG) **Cost:** Low
CHLOROTHIA-ZIDE Generic, Diuril	**Hypertension:** PO: Initially 0.5 to 1g/day; Maintenance 0.5 to 2g/day. **Edema:** PO, IV: 0.5 to 1g qd or bid.	**Tablet:** 250, 500 mg **Oral Suspension:** 250 mg/ 5ml **Injection:** (powder) 500 mg	RENAL AGENTS (G) Sodium Diuretics (SG) Thiazide Diuretics (SSG) **Cost:** Low

GENERIC NAME Trade Name	INDICATIONS AND DOSAGES	DOSE FORMS	GROUP (G)/SUBGROUP (SG) Relative Cost within Group
CHLOROTRIANISENE Tace	**Menopausal Symptoms:** PO: 12–25 mg/d (Treat for first 21 days of each month or treat continuously with added progestin. **Atrophic Vaginitis and Related Conditions:** PO: 12–25 mg/d (cyclic treatment: treat for 20 days, then stop for 10 days, then repeat), treat for 30–60 days. **Hypogonadism:** PO: 12–25 mg/d (cyclic treatment: treat for 20 days, then stop for 10 days, then repeat); (IM progesterone, 100 mg) or an oral progestin may be given during last 5 days of therapy. Begin next cycle on day 5 of uterine bleeding. **Prostatic Cancer:** PO: 12–25 mg/d. **Prevention of Postpartum Breast Enlargement:** PO: 12 mg QID for 7 days (alternative schedule: 50 mg q6h for 6 doses) give first dose within 8 hours of delivery.	**Capsule:** 12, 25 mg	ENDOCRINE AGENTS (G) Estrogens (SG) **Cost:** High
CHLORPHENESIN CARBAMATE Maolate	PO: initial 800 mg tid. Maintenance can be reduced to 400 mg QID or less.	**Tablet:** 400 mg	MUSCLE RELAXANTS (G) Sedative Hypnotics (SG) **Cost:** Medium
CHLORPHENIRAMINE OTC, Generic, Chlor-Trimeton	**Allergic Reactions (Type 1):** PO: 4 mg q4–6h (max. dose 24 mg/d). Pediatric (6–12 yrs) PO: 2 mg q 4–6h, (max. dose 12 mg/d). Pediatric (2–6 yrs) PO: 1 mg q 4–6h, (max. dose 4 mg/d). PO: (Ext'd release) 8–12 mg q8–12h (max. dose 24mg/d).	**Tablet:** 4, 8, 12 mg **Tablet:** (chewable) 2 mg **Tablet:** (Ext'd release) 8, 12 mg **Capsule:** 12 mg **Capsule:** (Ext'd release) 8, 12 mg **Syrup:** 2 mg/ 5 ml **Injection:** 10, 100 mg/ml	ANTI-INFLAMMATORY ETC (G) Antihistamines (H1 Antagonists) (SG) Antihistamines with Mild Sedation (SSG) **Cost:** Low

GENERIC NAME Trade Name	INDICATIONS AND DOSAGES	DOSE FORMS	GROUP (G)/SUBGROUP (SG) Relative Cost within Group
CHLORPROMA-ZINE Generic, Thora-zine, CPZ	**Psychotic Disorders (Adults):** PO (outpatients): 10–25 mg tid to start; 25–100 mg tid maintenance (max. dose 400 mg/d). PO (inpatients): 25 mg tid to start; 25–100 mg tid maintenance (max. dose 800 mg/d). IV: 25 mg, can repeat with 25–50 mg in 1 hour; over several days increase to a max. 400 mg q4–6h, then PO maintenance. **Severe Agitation:** IM: 25 mg to start, can repeat once with 25 mg one hour after initial injection; may gradually increase over days up to max. dose = 400 mg q4–6h; begin PO maintenance as soon as feasible (usually no advantage to doses exceeding 1000 mg/d). **Nausea and Vomiting:** PO: 10–25 mg q4–6h PRN. IV: 25 mg to start; then 25–50 mg q3–4h PRN (only if no hypotension). Rectal: 50–100 mg q6–8h. Pediatric PO: 0.25 mg/pound q4–6h PRN. Pediatric Rectal: 0.5 mg/pound q6–8h PRN. Pediatric IM: 0.25 mg/pound q6–8h (max. dose [< 5 yrs] = 40 mg/d; max. dose [5–12 yrs] = 75 mg/d). **Intractable Hiccups:** PO: 25–50 mg q6–8h.	**Tablet:** 10, 25, 50, 100, 200 mg **Capsule:** (Ext'd release) 30, 75, 150, 200, 300 mg **Syrup:** 10 mg/5 ml **Concentrate:** 30 mg/ml, 100 mg/ml **Injection:** 25 mg/ml **Suppositories:** 25, 100 mg	CNS AGENTS (G) Antipsychotics (G) Moderate Extrapyramidal Effects (SG) **Cost:** Low
CHLORPROP-AMIDE [illegible], Dia-binese	**Diabetes (NIDDM):** PO: [illegible] mg/d (max. dose 750 mg/d); in older patients start out at 100–125 mg/d.	**Tablet:** 100, 250 mg	[illegible] Antidiabetic Agents (SG) Sulfonylurea (SSG) **Cost:** Low
CHLORPRO-THIXENE Taractan	**Psychotic Disorders:** PO: Adult 25–50 mg tid or QID to start; increase as needed (max. dose 600 mg/day) Geriatric: 10–25 mg tid or QID to start Pediatric (> 6 yrs): 10–25 mg tid or QID to start IM: (> 12 yrs) 25–50 mg; up to tid or QID.	**Tablet:** 10, 25, 50, 100 mg **Concentrate:** 20 mg/ml **Injection:** 12.5 mg/ml	CNS AGENTS (G) Antipsychotics (SG) Agents Causing Moderate Extrapyramidal Side Effects (SSG) **Cost:** High
CHLORTETRACY-CLINE Generic, Aureo-mycin	Apply 1 to 4 times daily to infected area. Cover with sterile bandage as appropriate.	**Ointment (Topical):** 3% **Ointment: (Ophthalmic)** 1%	OPHTHALMIC ANTI-INFECTIVE AGENTS (G) Antibacterial (SG) **Cost:** Medium
CHLORTHALI-DONE Generic, Hygro-ton, Thalitone	**Hypertension:** PO: Initially 25 mg qd: Maintenance 25–100 mg qd. **Edema:** PO: Initially 50–100 mg/d; Maintenance 50–200 mg/d.	**Tablet:** 15, 25, 50, 100 mg	RENAL AGENTS (G) Sodium Diuretics (SG) Thiazide Diuretics (SG) **Cost:** Low

GENERIC NAME Trade Name	INDICATIONS AND DOSAGES	DOSE FORMS	GROUP (G)/SUBGROUP (SG) Relative Cost within Group
CHLORZOXA-ZONE Generic, Parafon Forte	PO: initial dose 500 mg tid or QID. maintenance 250 mg tid or QID (max. dose 750 mg QID).	**Tablet:** 250, 500 mg **Caplet:** 250, 500 mg	CNS AGENTS (G) Muscle Relaxants (SG) Sedative Hypnotics (SG) **Cost:** Medium
Cholac	See LACTULOSE		Laxative Used in Hepatic Failure
Choledyl	See OXTRIPHYLLINE		Xanthine Bronchodilator
CHOLESTYRA-MINE Questran, Questran Light	PO: 4 g 1 to 6 times daily.	**Powder:** 4 g cholestyramine per 9 g powder **Bar:** 4 g cholestyramine per bar **Oral Suspension:** (powder) 4 g cholestyramine resin per 5 g powder	LIPID LOWERING DRUGS (G) Bile Acid Binding Resins (SG) **Cost:** High
Chooz	See CALCIUM CARBONATE		Antacid
Chronulac	See LACTULOSE		Laxative, Hepatic Failure
CHYMOTRYPSIN Catarase, Zolyse	**Enzymatic Zonulysis (cataract extraction):** Posterior Chamber: Irrigate with 0.5 to 2 ml of solution (after pupillary dilation), may repeat 2 or 3 times with 2–4 minutes between instillations.	**Ophthalmic solution:** 150, 300 units with 2 ml sodium chloride diluent; 750 units per vial with 9 ml blanched salt solution diluent.	OPHTHALMIC AGENTS (G) Adjuncts To Surgery (SG) **Cost:** High
Cibacalcin	See CALCITONIN—HUMAN		Inhibit Osteoclastic Activity
CICLOPIROX Loprox	Topical: Apply bid; rethink diagnosis if no improvement after 4 weeks.	**Cream:** 1% **Lotion:** 1%	DERMATOLOGIC AGENTS (G) Topical Anti-Infectious Agents (SG) Topical Fungicides (SSG) **Cost:** Moderate
CIDOFOVIR Vistide	**CMV Retinitis:** IV: 5 mg/kg/week for two weeks, then 3–5 mg/kg q2weeks		ANTI-INFECTIOUS AGENTS (G) Antivirals, systemic (SG)
Ciloxan	See CIPROFLOXACIN		Lactam Antibiotic

GENERIC NAME Trade Name	INDICATIONS AND DOSAGES	DOSE FORMS	GROUP (G)/SUBGROUP (SG) Relative Cost within Group
CIMETIDINE Generic, OTC, Tagamet	**Duodenal/Gastric Ulcer (Acute):** PO: 300 mg QID (with meals and hs); or 400 mg bid; (max. dose 2400 mg/d); or 800 mg qhs. Continue 4–6 weeks for ulcer. **Ulcer (Prophylaxis/Maintenance):** PO: 400 mg qhs. IV, IV: 300 mg q6–8h; infuse IV over 15–20 min. (max. dose 2400 mg/d). **Above with Impaired Renal Function:** PO, IM, IV: 300 mg q8–12h; may accumulate. **GE Reflex with Erosions, Hypersecretory States:** PO: 300 mg QID, given ac and hs (max. dose: 2400 mg/day). IV, IV: 300 mg q6–8h; infuse IV over 15–20 min. (max. dose 2,400 mg/d).	**Tablet:** 200, 300, 400, 800 mg **Injection:** 300 mg (as HCL) per 2 ml, 300 mg (as HCL) in 50 ml **Liquid:** 300 mg (as HCL) per 5 ml	GASTROINTESTINAL AGENTS (G) Inhibitors of Gastric Acid Secretion (SG) H2 Antagonists (SSG) **Cost:** Low
Cin-Quin	See QUINIDINE		Antiarrhythmic
Cinobac	See CINOXACIN		Quinolone Antibacterial
CINOXACIN Cinobac	**Urinary Tract Infections:** PO: 1 g/d in 2–4 doses for 7–14 days.	**Capsule:** 250, 500 mg	SULFONAMIDES AND CLINICALLY SIMILAR AGENTS (G) Non-Sulfonamide Urinary Tract Agents (SG) **Cost:** High
Cipro	See CIPROFLOXACIN		Quinolone Antibacterial
CIPROFLOXACIN Cipro, Ciloxan	**Infections:** PO: 500–750 mg q12h. UTI 250 mg q12h **Conjunctivitis:** [illegible] 1–2 drops q2h (while awake) for 2 days, then q4h for 5 days. **Corneal Ulcer:** Apply to conjunctival sac 2 drops q15 min. for 6 hours, then q30 min., until the end of day #1; then apply 2 drops q1h on 2nd day. Days 3–14 use 2 drops q4h.	**Tablet:** 250, 500, 750 mg (Cipro) **Injection:** [illegible] 200, 400 mg in vials and bags. (Cipro) **Solution:** 3.5 mg/ml (Ciloxan)	ANTI-INFECTIOUS AGENTS (G) Quinolones (SG) OPHTHALMIC AGENTS (G) Antibacterial (SG) **Cost:** High
CISAPRIDE Propulsid	**Gastroesophageal Reflux with Nocturnal Heartburn:** PO: 10–20 mg QID at least 15 min ac and at hs.	**Tablet:** 10, 20 mg	GASTROINTESTINAL AGENTS(G) Antiemetics (SG) Antiemetics (Minor) (SG) **Cost:** Medium
CISPLATIN Platinol, DDP	CANCER CHEMOTHERAPY (G) Alkylating Agents (SG) Chelates of Platinum (SSG)		
Citanest	See PRILOCAINE		Local Anesthetic
Citracal	See ORAL CALCIUM SALTS		
Citrovorum Factor	See LEUCOVORIN		Active Form of Folate
Citrucel	See METHYLCELLULOSE		Bulk Laxative
CLADRIBINE Leustatin	CANCER CHEMOTHERAPY (G) Antimetabolites (SG) Pyrimidine Analogues (SSG)		
Claforan	See CEFOTAXIME		Lactam Antibiotic

GENERIC NAME Trade Name	INDICATIONS AND DOSAGES	DOSE FORMS	GROUP (G)/SUBGROUP (SG) Relative Cost within Group
CLARITHRO-MYCIN Biaxin	**Infections (Pharyngitis, Bronchitis, Sinusitis, etc.):** PO: 250–500 mg q12h. **Mycobacterial Infections (including MAC):** PO: 500 mg bid. Pediatric PO: 7.5 mg/kg bid (max. dose 500 mg bid).	**Tablet:** 250, 500 mg **Granules:** (for oral suspension) 125 mg/5 ml, 250 mg/5 ml	ANTI-INFECTIOUS AGENTS (G) Macrolide Antibiotics (SG) **Cost:** High
Claritin	See LORATADINE		Antihistamine
CLEMASTINE OTC, Generic, Tavist	**Allergic (Type I) Reaction:** PO: 1.34–2.68 mg q8–12h (max. dose 8.04 mg/d).	**Tablet:** 1.34, 2.68 mg **Syrup:** 0.67 mg/ 5 ml	ANTI-INFLAMMATORY, ETC (G) Antihistamines (H1 Antagonists) (SG) Antihistamines with Mild Sedation (SG) **Cost:** High
Cleocin	See CLINDAMYCIN		Macrolide Antibiotic
CLIDINIUM Quarzan	**Peptic Ulcer:** PO: 2.5–5 mg q6–8h. **Geriatric:** PO: 2.5 mg tid before meals.	**Capsule:** 2.5, 5 mg	AUTONOMIC NS AGENTS (G) Parasympatholytics (SG) Parasympatholytics, Quaternary Amines (SSG) **Cost:** High
CLINDAMYCIN Cleocin	**Bacterial Infections:** PO: 150–300 mg q6h; max. dose 450 mg q6h. Pediatric PO: (HCl form) 8–16 mg/kg/d given in 3–4 divided doses (max. dose 20 mg/kg/d). Pediatric PO: (palmitate form) 8–12 mg/kg/d given in 3–4 divided doses (max. dose 25 mg/kg/d). IM, IV: 0.6–2.7 g/d given in 2–4 divided doses (max. dose: 4.8 g/d; single IM injections > 600 mg not recommended). **Pelvic Inflammatory Disease (Acute):** IV: 900 mg q8h (plus IM or IV gentamicin loading dose of 2 mg/kg, followed by gentamicin 1.5 mg/kg q8h; see gentamicin remarks above) continue for 48 hours after clinical improvement; following hospital discharge treat with PO doxycycline 100 mg bid for 10–14 days. **Topical:** Apply thin coating bid **Vaginal Antibacterial:** 1 applicatorful qhs for 7d	**Capsule:** 75, 150, 300 mg **Injection:** 150 mg/ml **Granules:** (for oral solution) 75 mg/ 5ml (as palmitate)	ANTI-INFECTIOUS AGENTS (G) Macrolide Antibiotics (SG) **Cost:** Low
Clinoril	See SULINDAC		Non-Narcotic Analgetic
CLOBETASOL Temovate	Apply to affected area sparingly 2 times a day. Maximum 50 grams per week.	Highest Potency: **Ointment:** 0.05%. **Cream:** 0.05%. **Gel:** 0.05%. **Scalp application:** 0.05%.	DERMATOLOGIC AGENTS (G) Anti-Inflammatory Steroids, Topical (SG) **Cost:** Medium

GENERIC NAME Trade Name	INDICATIONS AND DOSAGES	DOSE FORMS	GROUP (G)/SUBGROUP (SG) Relative Cost within Group
CLOFIBRATE Generic, Atromid-S	**Hyperlipidemia:** PO: 2 gm/d in divided doses (lower doses may be effective).	**Capsule:** 500 ml	METABOLIC AGENTS (G) Lipid Lowering Drugs (SG) Other Lipid Lowering Agents (SSG) **Cost:** High
Clomid	See CLOMIPHENE		Stimulate Ovulation
CLOMIPHENE Clomid, Serophene, Milophene	**Initial therapy:** PO: 50 mg/day for 5 days; if ineffective may give second course of treatment of 100 mg/day for 5 days (may start in as little as 30 days after first dose); a third and final is permissible.	**Tablet:** 50 mg	ENDOCRINE AGENTS (G) Anterior Pituitary Hormones or Equivalent (SG)
CLOMIPRAMINE Anafranil	**Obsessive Compulsive Disorder:** PO: 25 mg qd to start, increase over 2 weeks to 100 mg/d (max. dose 250 mg/d).	**Capsule:** 25, 50, 75 mg.	CNS AGENTS (G) Tricyclic Antidepressants (SG) **Cost:** Medium
CLONAZEPAM Generic, Klonopin	**Hypnotic:** PO: Not labeled for this use. Approved for use only against a petit mal variant.		CNS AGENTS (G) Sedative-Hypnotic (SG) Ultrashort-Acting Hypnotics (SSG)
CLONIDINE Generic, Catapres	**Hypertension:** PO: 0.1 mg bid or tid initially; 0.2–0.8 mg/d maintenance in 2–4 doses (max. dose 2.4 mg/d). Transdermal: initial dose 0.1 mg patch qweek; may increase to 0.2 or 0.2 mg patch q week as needed (assess effect of each dosage after 1–2 weeks).	**Tablet:** 0.1, 0.2, 0.3 mg **Transdermal Patches:** Catapres-TTS-1 (0.1 mg/d, 3.5 cm. sq.); Catapres-TTS-2 (0.2 mg/d, 7.0 cm. sq.), Catapres-TTS-3 (0.3 mg/d, 10.5 cm. sq.)	CV AGENTS (G) SYMPATHOPLEGICS (SG) Centrally-Acting Adrenergic Inhibitors (SSG) **Cost:** PO: Low, Patch**:** Medium
CLORAZEPATE Generic, Tranxene	**Alcohol Withdrawal:** PO: 30 mg to start, then 15 mg bid-QID (max dose 90mg/day; begin tapering after second day to reach a dose of 7.5 to 15 mg/day—discontinue when stable). **Anxiety:** PO: 30 mg/d given in two or more doses (max dose: 60 mg/day). **Partial Seizures (adjunct to other anti-epileptics):** PO: 7.5 mg tid to start, increase by 7.5 mg/week (max dose: 90 mg/d). Pediatric PO (9–12 y/o): 7.5 mg bid to start, increase by 7.5 mg/week (max dose: 60 mg/d).	**Capsule:** 3.75, 7.5, 15 mg **Tablet:** 3.75, 7.5, 11.25, 15, 22.5 mg	CNS AGENTS (G) Sedative-Hypnotics (SG) Intermediate-Acting Sedative Hypnotics (SSG) **Cost:** Low
CLOTRIMAZOLE Generic, OTC, Lotrimin, Mycelex	Topical: Massage into affected area bid, for four weeks .	**Cream:** 1%. **Lotion:** 1%. **Powder: Spray: Solution:** 1%.	DERMATOLOGIC AGENTS (G) Topical Fungicides (SG) **Cost:** Medium
CLOXACILLIN Generic, Tegopen	**Infections:** PO: 250–500 mg q6h. Pediatric PO: 50–100 mg/kg/d given in 4 divided doses (max dose 4g/d).	**Capsule:** 250, 500 mg **Oral Solution:** (powder) 25 mg/ml	LACTAM ANTIBIOTICS (G) Penicillins: resistant to staphylococcal lactamase (SG) **Cost:** Low

GENERIC NAME Trade Name	INDICATIONS AND DOSAGES	DOSE FORMS	GROUP (G)/SUBGROUP (SG) Relative Cost within Group
CLOZAPINE Clozaril	PO: Initial 25 mg qd or bid daily dosage increments of 25–50 mg to achieve target dose of 300–450 mg/ day by end of 2 weeks (increments not to exceed 100 mg).	**Tablet:** 25, 100	CNS AGENTS (G) Atypical Antipsychotics (SG) **Cost:** Very High
Clozaril	See CLOZAPINE		Atypical Antipsychotic
COAGULANT FACTOR IX (HUMAN)	All are concentrated human plasma fractions MEONINE is purified with a monoclonal antibody and does not contain the adventitious factors found in the other preps. ALPHA NINE SD is virusfiltered. KONYNE 80, BEBULIN AND PROPLEX T are heat treated. Primary indication is Hemophilia B	Consult the label for each lot.	ANTICOAGULANTS AND COAGULANTS (G) Clotting Factors (SG)
COCAINE Generic	Topical: 1–10% (max. single dose should not exceed 1mg/kg: concentrations greater than 4% may cause systemic toxic reaction).	**Solution:** (topical) 40, 100 mg/ml **Solution:** (topical) 4%, 10% **Tablet:** (soluble) 135 mg **Powder:** 5,25 g	LOCAL ANESTHETICS (G) Topical (Mucosal) Only (SG) **Cost:** High
CODEINE Generic, Methylmorphine	**Analgesia:** PO, IM, IV, SC: 15–60 mg q4–6h (max. dose 360 mg/d). **Antitussive:** PO: 10–20 mg q4–6h (max. dose 120 mg/d). Pediatric PO: (6–12 yrs). 5–10 mg q4–6h (max. dose 60 mg/d). Pediatric PO: (2–6 yrs): 2.5–5 mg q4–6h (max. dose 30 mg/d).	**Injection:** 30, 60 mg **Tablet:** 15, 30, 60 mg **Soluble Tablet:** 15, 30, 60 mg	CNS AGENTS (G) Narcotic Analgesics And Related Agents (SG) Of Lowest Potency (SSG) **Cost:** Low
Cogentin	See BENZTROPINE		Anticholinergic
Colace	See DOCUSATE		Stool Softener
Colbenemid	See colchicine and probenecid		Gout
COLCHICINE Generic	**Acute Attacks:** PO: 1–1.2 mg initial dose, then 0.5–1.2 mg q1–2h (max. dose 4–8 mg/attack). Wait 3 days prior to initiating a second course of therapy. IV: 2 mg to start, then 0.5 mg q6h PRN (max. dose 4 mg/d); NOT in D5W. **Gouty Attack, Prophylaxis:** PO: 0.5–1 mg qd or bid (often given w/uricosuric OR other agent).	**Tablet:** 0.5, 0.6 mg **Injection:** 1 mg/ ml	METABOLIC AGENTS (G) Agents Used in The Treatment of Gout (SG) **Cost:** Medium
Colestid	See COLESTIPOL		Bile Acid Binding Resin

GENERIC NAME Trade Name	INDICATIONS AND DOSAGES	DOSE FORMS	GROUP (G)/SUBGROUP (SG) Relative Cost within Group
COLESTIPOL Colestid	**Hyperlipemia:** PO: 5 g once or twice daily initially, then maintenance of 5–30 g/day given as one or more doses (to increase dose, add 5 g daily at 1 or 2 month intervals).	**Granules:** In 300 and 500 g bottles and 5 g packets	METABOLIC AGENTS (G) Lipid Lowering Drugs (SG) Bile Acid Binding Resins (SSG) **Cost:** High
COLFOSCERIL Exosurf Neonatal, DPPC with Dispersant	**Prophylactic Treatment (low BW and lung immaturity):** Intratracheal: 5 ml/kg initial dose, repeat at 12 and 24 h. **Rescue Treatment (RDS):** Intratracheal: 5 ml/kg initial dose as soon as possible after birth, repeat in 12 h.	**Lyophilized Powder:** (for injection) 108 mg colfosceril palmitate to make up 10 ml.	RESPIRATORY AGENTS (G) Lung Surfactant (SG)
COLISTI-METHATE Coly-Mycin M	**Bacterial Infections:** IM, IV (Inject IV over 3–5 minutes): 2.5–5 mg/kg/d in 2–4 doses; (max. dose 5 mg/kg/d).	**Injection:** 150 mg colistin (as colistimethate sodium) for reconstruction	ANTI-INFECTIOUS AGENTS (G) Miscellaneous Antibacterials (SG) Polymyxins (SSG) **Cost:** Very High
COLISTIN Coly-Mycin S	**Bacterial Infections:** PO: 5–15 mg/kg/d given in 3 divided doses.	**Oral Suspension:** (powder) 25 mg colistin (as sulfate) per 5 ml when reconstituted	ANTI-INFECTIOUS AGENTS (G) Miscellaneous Antibacterials (SG) Polymyxins (SSG) **Cost:** Low
Coly-Mycin M	See COLISTIMETHATE		Polymyxin Antibiotic
CALAMYCIN S, OTIC	5 instilled qtt into the affected ear(s) tid—QID.		**Otic Suspension (per cc):** neomycin sulfate (4 71 mg, equivalent to 3.3 mg neomycin base), colistin sulfate (3 mg) hydrocortisone acetate (10 mg = 1%)
Colyte	See POLYETHYLENE GLYCOL-ELECTROLYTE SOLUTIONS		Bowel Cleanser
COMBIPRES	**Hypertension:** A clonidine-diuretic combination: PO: Adjust dose within the limits imposed.	**Tablets:** Clonidine/ Chlorthalidone: 0.1/15 mg, 0.2/ 15 mg, 0.3/15 mg.	CENTRAL SYMPATHOLYTIC (G) AND SODIUM DIURETIC (G)
Compal	See DIHYDROCODEINE		Narcotic Analgetic
Compazine	See PROCHLORPERAZINE		Antipsychotic
Concentraid	See DESMOPRESSIN		Antidiuretic Hormone
Condylox	See PODOFILOX		Lyse Warts/Papillomas

GENERIC NAME Trade Name	INDICATIONS AND DOSAGES	DOSE FORMS	GROUP (G)/SUBGROUP (SG) Relative Cost within Group
CONJUGATED ESTROGENS Premarin	**Estrogen Replacement (Maintenance):** 0.625 mg/d. 1.25 mg/d for acute menopausal symptoms 0.3 initially if pt nauseated. Treat for first 21 d of each month or give continuously with added progestin. **Atrophic Vaginitis and Related Conditions:** PO: 0.3–1.25 mg/d to start, adjust dose by clinical response. **Hypogonadism:** PO: 2.5–7.5 mg/d in 3–4 doses (**Cyclic Treatment:** Treat for 20 days, then stop for 10 days, then repeat cycle if needed to induce bleeding), if bleeding occurs prior to end of the 10 days, start a 20 day cycle of treatment with combined estrogen-progestin (estrogen dose 2.5–7.5 mg/d, give progestin during last 5 days of the 20 days). **Breast Engorgement (postpartum):** PO: 3.75 mg q4h for 5 doses **Abnormal Uterine Bleeding:** IV, IM: 25 mg given once, repeat in 6–12 hours if needed. **Prostatic Cancer Palliation:** PO: 1.25–2.5 mg tid.	**Tablet:** 0.3, 0.625, 1.25, 2.5 mg. **Injection:** 25 mg/5 ml vial.	ENDOCRINE AGENTS (G) Estrogens (SG) **Cost:** High
Constilac	See LACTULOSE		Laxative. Hepatic Failure
Copaxone	See GLATIRAMER		Relapsing Multiple Sclerosis
Cordarone	See AMIODARONE		Antiarrhythmic
Cordran	See FLURANDRENOLIDE		Corticosteroid
Corgard	See NADOLOL		Beta Adrenergic Blocker
Cortef	See HYDROCORTISONE		Corticosteroid
CORTICOTROPIN Generic, Acthar, ACTH	**ACTH-Responsive Conditions:** IM, SC: 20–40 units QID. IM, SC (repository form): 40–80 units q24 to q72h. Multiple Sclerosis: IM: 80–120 units/d, treat for 2 to 3 weeks.	**Injection:** (powder) 25, 40 units per vial **Injection:** (repository) 40 & 80 units/ml See also COSYNTROPIN	ENDOCRINE AGENTS (G) Anterior Pituitary Hormones (SG) **Cost:** Low
Cortisol	See HYDROCORTISONE		Corticosteroid, topical
CORTISONE Generic	**Addison's:** PO: 10–37.5 mg with fludrocortisone	**Tablet:** 5, 10, 25 mg **Injection: (Suspension):** IM 50 mg/ml	ENDOCRINE AGENTS (G) Anti-Inflammatory (Glucocorticoid) Steroid (SG)

GENERIC NAME Trade Name	INDICATIONS AND DOSAGES	DOSE FORMS	GROUP (G)/SUBGROUP (SG) Relative Cost within Group
CORTISPORIN	**Ophthalmic Suspension:** 1–2 drops into the affected eye(s) q3–4 h. **Ophthalmic Ointment:** 0.25 to 0.5 inch ribbon applied q3–4 h. **Otic Solution, Suspension:** 4 drops in the affected ear(s) tid to QID. Keep in ear 5 min. before allowing to drain out (may use cotton wick and re-wet with medication q4h—replace wick q24h). **Topical Cream, Ointment:** apply bid—QID. (Use a thin coat and rub in as appropriate).		**Ophthalmic Suspension (per cc):** polymyxin B sulfate (10,000 Units), neomycin sulfate (equal to 3.5 mg of neomycin base), hydrocortisone 10 mg (=1%) **Ophthalmic Ointment (per g):** polymyxin B sulfate (10,000 Units), neomycin sulfate (equal to 3.5 mg of neomycin base), bacitracin zinc (400 Units), hydrocortisone 10 mg (=1%) **Otic Solution and Suspension (per cc):** neomycin sulfate (equal to 3.5 mg of neomycin base), polymyxin B sulfate (10,000 Units), hydrocortisone 10 mg (=1%) **Topical Cream (per g):** polymyxin B sulfate (10,000 Units), neomycin sulfate (equal to 3.5 mg of neomycin base), hydrocortisone acetate 5 mg (=0.5%) **Topical Ointment** (per g): polymyxin B sulfate (5,000 Units), neomycin sulfate (equal to 3.5 mg of neomycin base), bacitracin zinc (400 Units), hydrocortisone 10 mg (=1%)
Cortrosyn	See COSYNTROPIN		Corticotropin
Corvert	See IBUTILIDE		Antiarrhythmic
CORZIDE 40/5, 80/5	**Hypertension:** PO: Beta blocker diuretic Combination. Adjust dose as fixed proportion permits.	**Tablet:** Combination of nadolol/bendroflumethiazide, 40/5 mg or 80/5	CARDIOVASCULAR AGENTS (G) Beta-Adrenergic Receptor Blocker (SG) and Sodium Diuretic (SG)
Cosmegen	See DACTINOMYCIN		Cancer Chemotherapy
COSYNTROPIN Corticotropin, Cortrosyn, ACTH Recombinant	**Test of Adrenal Function:** IM, IV: 0.25 given as a single dose (normal response is > 20 mcg/dl of plasma cortisol, if response blunted suggests secondary adrenal insufficiency).	**Injection:** (powder) 0.25 mg/vial	ENDOCRINE AGENTS (G) Anterior Pituitary Hormones (SG) **Cost:** Low
Cotrim	See TRIMETHOPRIM SULFAMETHOXAZOLE		Antibacterial
Coumadin	See WARFARIN SODIUM		Anticoagulant
Cozaar	See LOSARTAN		Vasodilator
CPZ	See CHLORPROMAZINE		Anticoagulant
Cristi 1000	See CYANOCOBALAMIN		B_{12}
Crixivan	See INDINAVIR		Protease Inhibitor
Cromoglycate	See CROMOLYN		Mast Cell Stabilizer

GENERIC NAME Trade Name	INDICATIONS AND DOSAGES	DOSE FORMS	GROUP (G)/SUBGROUP (SG) Relative Cost within Group
CROMOLYN OTC, Cromoglycate, Intal, Gastrocrom, Nasalcrom	**Asthma:** Inhalation (capsules, nebulizer): 20 mg inhaled QID to start (use at regular intervals). **Exercise induced asthma:** Inhalation (capsules, nebulizer): 20 mg inhaled no more than 60 min. prior to exercise. **Allergic rhinitis (prevention and tx.):** Intranasal (soln.): 1 spray each nostril 3–6 times/day. **Mastocytosis:** PO: 200 mg QID(give 30 min. ac and hs). Pediatric PO: 100 mg QID(give 30 min. ac and hs).	**Capsule (for oral use only):** 100 mg **Capsule:** (for inhalation only) 20 mg **Nasal Solution:** 40 mg/ml (each spray delivers 5.2 mg) **Aerosol Spray:** each puff delivers 800 mcg **Inhalation:** 20 mg/2ml **Solution:** (for nebulizer only) 20 mg per amp	RESPIRATORY AGENTS (G) Antiallergic Agents, Nonsteroidal (SG) **Cost:** Medium
CROTAMITON Eurax	**Scabies:** Topical: Apply to all skin surfaces and repeat at 24 hours; remove at 48 hours by thorough washing. Repeat in 7–10 days if necessary. Change bed clothing and linen in the morning after the first application. **Pruritus:** Topical: Gently rub into affected areas until absorbed, repeat PRN.	**Cream:** 10% **Lotion:** 10%	DERMATOLOGIC AGENTS (G) Topical Anti-Infectious Agents (SG) (Ecto) Parasiticidal Agents (SSG) **Cost:** Low
Cruex	See UNDECYLENIC ACID		Fungicide, topical
Crystamine	See CYANOCOBALAMIN		B_{12}
Crysticillin	See PENICILLIN G PROCAINE		Lactam Antibiotic
Crystodigin	See DIGITOXIN		Cardiac Glycoside
Cuprimine	See PENICILLAMINE		Chelating Agent, Antirheumatic
Curretab	See MEDROXYPROGESTERONE		Progestin
CYANOCOBAL-AMIN Generic, Vitamin B_{12}, **Cyomin, Crystamine, Cristi 1000, Rubesol 1000**	**Pernicious Anemia:** IM, Deep SC: 100 mcg qd for 6 or 7 days, then 100 mcg qod for 7 doses, then 100 mcg q3–4days for 2–3wks (monitor reticulocyte and other hematologic indices to assess effectiveness of therapy); chronic maintenance 100 mcg/month for life (as appropriate, give w/ folic acid). **Vitamin B_{12} Deficiency:** Oral: Up to 1000 mcg/day (oral not usually recommended). IV or SC: 30 mcg qd for 5 to 10 days, then100 to 200 mcg qmonth, give w/ folic acid for serious deficiency. **Schilling Test (flushing dose):** IM: 1000 mcg.	**Injection:** 100, 1000 mcg per ml. **Tablets:** 25, 50, 100, 250, 500, 1,000 mcg (OTC).	METABOLIC AGENTS (G) Vitamins (SG) **Cost:** Low
Cyantin	See NITROFURANTOIN		Antibacterial

GENERIC NAME Trade Name	INDICATIONS AND DOSAGES	DOSE FORMS	GROUP (G)/SUBGROUP (SG) Relative Cost within Group
CYCLANDELATE Generic, Cyclan, Cyclospasmol	PO: 1.2–1.6 g per day given in divided doses before meals and at bedtime; then maintenance, dose of 400–800 mg/day given in 2–4 divided doses. Tablet: 200, 400 mg	**Capsule:** 200, 400 mg	CARDIOVASCULAR AGENTS (G) Vasodilators (SG) Post-Arteriolar (Antianginal and related agents) (SG) **Cost:** Low
CYCLIZINE OTC, Generic, Marezine	**Motion Sickness:** PO: 50 mg hour before departure; repeat q4–6h; max. dose 200 mg/d. IV: 50 mg q4–6h PRN. Pediatric PO (6–12 yrs): 25 mg; tid.	**Tablet:** 50 mg **Injection:** 50 mg/ml	ANTI-INFLAMMATORY ETC (G) Antihistamines (H1 Antagonists) (SG) Motion Sickness Prevention (SSG) **Cost:** High
CYCLOBENZA-PRINE Generic, Flexeril	PO: 20–40 mg/day in 3 divided doses (max. dose 60 mg/day; do not use longer than 2 or 3 weeks)	**Tablet:** 10 mg	CNS AGENTS (G) Muscle Relaxants (SG) Other, Negligible Compounds (SSG) **Cost:** Medium
Cyclocort	See AMCINONIDE		Corticosteroid
Cyclogyl	See CYCLOPENTOLATE		Mydriatic
Cyclan	See CYCLANDELATE		Vasodilator
CYCLOPENTO-LATE Generic, Cyclogyl	**Pupillary Dilation:** Intraocular: Adults: Instill 1 or 2 drops of 0.5%, 1% or 2% solution into eye(s), repeat in 5 to 10 minutes prn.	**Solution:** 0.5, 1, 2%.	OPHTHALMIC AGENTS (G) Mydriatics (SG) Cycloplegic Mydriatics (SSG) **Cost:** Low
CYCLOPHOSPHA-MIDE Generic, Cy-toxan, Endoxan	CANCER CHEMOTHERAPY (G) Alkylating Agents (SG) Nitrogen Mustards (SSG)		
CYCLOSERINE Seromycin	**Tuberculosis (given in combination):** PO Adult: 10–15 mg/kg/d given in 2–4 doses (max. dose 1,000 mg/d). Pediatric PO:10–20 mg/kg/d (max. dose 1,000 mg/d).	**Capsule:** 250 mg	ANTI-INFECTIOUS AGENTS (G) Antituberculous Second Line Agents (SG) **Cost:** Medium
Cyclosporine	See CYCLOSPORINE-A		Immunosuppressant
CYCLOSPORINE-A Cyclosporine, Sandimmune, Neoral	**Suppress Rejection Reaction:** PO: 15 mg/kg/day (range 14–18 mg/kg/d), start 4–12 hours prior to transplantation; then continue post-op for 1–2 weeks; then taper by 5% per week to maintenance dose of 5–10 mg/kg/d. IV: 5–6 mg/kg/day (give as slow infusion over 2–6 hours) start infusion 4–12 hours prior to transplantation; then continue the same dose daily until patient can be switched to oral doses.	**Capsules:** 25, 100 mg. **Oral solution:** 100 mg/ml. **IV solution:** 50 mg/ml.	ANTI-INFLAMMATORY, ETC. (G) Immunomodulators (SG)
Cycrin	See MEDROXYPROGESTERONE		Progestin
Cyklokapron	See TRANEXAMIC ACID		Hemostatic
Cylert	See PEMOLINE		Sympathomimetic Stimulant
Cyomin	See CYANOCOBALAMIN		B_{12}

GENERIC NAME Trade Name	INDICATIONS AND DOSAGES	DOSE FORMS	GROUP (G)/SUBGROUP (SG) Relative Cost within Group
CYPROHEPTA-DINE Generic, Peri-actin	**Stimulate Weight Gain:** PO: adults: initially 4 mg tid, maintenance 4–20 mg daily (max. dose 32 mg/d; do not exceed 0.5 mg/kg/day (0.23 mg/lb/day). Pediatric (2–7 yrs) PO: 2 mg bid or tid (max. dose 12 mg/d). Pediatric (7–14 yrs) PO: 4 mg bid or tid (max. dose 16 mg/d).	**Tablet:** 4 mg **Syrup:** 2 mg/ 5 ml	ANTI-INFLAMMATORY, ETC. (G) Antihistamines (H1 Antagonists) (SG) Antihistamines, Miscellaneous (SSG) **Cost:** Low
Cytadren	See AMINOGLUTETHIMIDE		Inhibit Glucocorticoid Synthesis
CYTARABINE Generic, Cytosine Arabinoside, Cytosar	CANCER CHEMOTHERAPY (G) Antimetabolites (SG) Pyrimidine Analogues (SSG)		
Cytomel	See LIOTHYRONINE (T3)		Thyroid Replacement
Cytosar	See CYTARABINE		Cancer Chemotherapy
Cytosine Arabinoside	See CYTARABINE		Cancer Chemotherapy
Cytotec	See MISOPROSTOL		Protect Against Ulcers From NSAIDs
Cytovene	See GANCICLOVIR		Antiviral
Cytoxan	See CYCLOPHOSPHAMIDE		Cancer Chemotherapy
D.H.E.45	See DIHYDROERGOTAMINE		Vasoconstrictor
DACARBAZINE Generic DTIC	CANCER CHEMOTHERAPY (G) Alkylating Agents (SG) Other Alkylating Agents (SSG)		
DACTINOMYCIN Actinomycin D Cosmegen	CANCER CHEMOTHERAPY (G) React With DNA (SG) Antibiotics (SSG)		
Dalalone Dalalone-LA	See DEXAMETHASONE		Corticosteroid
Dalgan	See DEZOCINE		Narcotic Analgetic
Dalmane	See FLURAZEPAM		Hypnotic,short acting
DANAZOL Danocrine	**Endometriosis:** PO: 100–400 mg bid, initially; then 100–200 mg bid, continue therapy for 3–6 months (max. duration 9 months). **Fibrocystic Breast Disease:** PO: 50–200 mg bid. **Hereditary Angioedema:** PO: 200 mg bid or tid initially, then taper dose by 50% every 1–3 months to lowest effective dose (monitor tapering closely).	**Capsule:** 50, 100, 200 mg	ENDOCRINE AGENTS (G) Androgenic/Anabolic Steroids (SG)
Danassol	See METHENAMINE		Antibacterial, Urinary
Danocrine	See DANAZOL		Androgen/Anabolic
Dantrium	See DANTROLENE		Muscle Relaxant

GENERIC NAME Trade Name	INDICATIONS AND DOSAGES	DOSE FORMS	GROUP (G)/SUBGROUP (SG) Relative Cost within Group
DANTROLENE Dantrium	**Spasticity:** PO: Adults initial dose 25 mg qd: increase to 25 mg 2–4 times daily. **Malignant Hyperthermia:** IV (push): 1 mg/kg until symptoms subside or a max. dose of 10 mg/kg has been reached. PO: (post-crisis follow-up) 4–8 mg/kg/day orally in 4 divided doses for 1 to 3 days. **Preoperative Prophylaxis:** PO: 4–8 mg/kg/day in 3 or 4 divided doses for one or two days prior to surgery; IV: 2.5 mg/kg approx. 75 minutes before procedure (give over 60 minutes).	**Capsule:** 25, 50 100 mg **Injection:** (powder) 20 mg/ vial	CNS AGENTS (G) Muscle Relaxants (SG) Miscellaneous Muscle Relaxant (SSG) **Cost:** High
DAPIPRAZOLE Rev-Eyes	**Reversal of Iatrogenic Mydriasis:** Into conjunctival sac: 2 drops initially, then 2 more drops in 5 minutes.	**Powder:** (lyophilized) 25 mg	OPHTHALMIC AGENTS (G) Agents Used in The Treatment of Glaucoma (SG) Alpha Adrenergic Blocking Agent (SSG)
DAPSONE Dapsone	**Dermatitis Herpetiformis:** PO: 50 mg/d initially, maintenance 50–300 mg/d. **Leprosy (intermediate type):** PO: 50–100 mg/d (given with rifampin for 6 months 600 mg/d), treat for 3 years minimum. **Leprosy (Lepromatous type):** PO: 100 mg/d, treat for a minimum of 10 years.	**Tablet:** 25 mg, 100 mg	ANTI-INFECTIOUS AGENTS (G) Antituberculous And Related Agents (SG) Agents For Atypical Mycobacteria (SSG) **Cost:** High
Daranide	See DICHLORPHENAMIDE		Carbonic Anhydrase Inhibitor
Daraprim	See PYRIMETHAMINE		Antimalarial
Darbid	See ISOPROPAMIDE		Anticholinergic
Daricon	See OXYPHENCYCLIMINE		Anticholinergic
Darvocet-N	See PROPOXYPHENE		APAP with propoxyphene
Darvon	See PROPOXYPHENE		Legally a narcotic analgetic
Darvon Compound-65	See Propoxyphene.		ASA-Caffeine-Propoxyphene
Daunomycin	See DAUNORUBICIN		Cancer Chemotherapy
DAUNORUBICIN Daunomycin Cerubidine	CANCER CHEMOTHERAPY (G) React With DNA (SG) Antibiotics (SSG)		
Daypro	See OXAPROZIN		Non-Narcotic Analgetic
DDAVP	See DESMOPRESSIN		Antidiuretic
ddI	See DIDANOSINE		Antiviral
Deamino-arginine vasopressin	See DESMOPRESSIN		Antidiuretic
Deca-Durabolin	See NANDROLONE		Androgen/Anabolic
Decadron	See DEXAMETHASONE		Corticosteroid

GENERIC NAME Trade Name	INDICATIONS AND DOSAGES	DOSE FORMS	GROUP (G)/SUBGROUP (SG) Relative Cost within Group
Decadron W/ Xylocaine	**Bursitis:** Intrabursal: Initially give 0.5 to 0.75 cc by injection. Repeat q4–7 d, PRN. **Tenosynovitis:** Intrasynovial: Initially give 0.1 to 0.25 cc by injection. Repeat q4–7 d, PRN.		**Injection (per cc):** dexamethasone sodium phosphate (4 mg), lidocaine HCl (10 mg)
Declomycin	See DEMECLOCYCLINE		Tetracycline Antibiotic
DEFEROXAMINE Desferal	**Acute iron intox:** IM: 1 g initially then 0.5 g q4h for two times then q4–12 h PRN. **Chronic iron overload:** IM 0.5–1.0 g daily. (max dose = 6 g/d).	**Powder (for injection):** 500 mg	ANTIDOTES & AGENTS USED IN POISONINGS (G)
Delacurarine	See TUBOCURARINE		Curariform
Deltalin	See ERGOCALCIFEROL(D2)		D Vitamin Precursor
Delatestryl	See TESTOSTERONE ENANTHATE		Androgen/Anabolic
DELAVIRDINE Rescriptor	**AIDS:** PO: With other agents, 400 mg tid.	**Tablet:** 100 mg	ANTI-INFECTIOUS AGENTS (G) Antivirals, Systemic (G)
Delestrogen	See ESTRADIOL VALERATE		Estrogen
Deltasone	See PREDNISONE		Corticosteroid
Demadex	See TORSEMIDE		Sodium Diuretic
DEMECLOCY-CLINE Declomycin	**Infection:** PO: 150 mg q6h; or 300 mg q12h. PO (Pediatric > 8 yrs only): 6–12 mg/kg given in 2–4 divided doses. **Gonorrhea (Penicillin Sensitive Patients):** PO: 600 mg to start; then 300 mg q12h (for 4 days or to 3 g total).	**Capsule:** 150 mg **Tablet:** 150, 300 mg	ANTI-INFECTIOUS AGENTS (G) Tetracyclines (SG) **Cost:** Very High
Demerol	See MEPERIDINE		Narcotic Analgetic
Denavir	See PENCICLOVIR		Antiviral, Topical
Dendrid	See IDOXURIDINE		Antiviral
Depakene	See VALPROIC ACID		Anticonvulsant
Depakote	See VALPROIC ACID		Anticonvulsant
Depen	See D-PENICILLAMINE		Chelating Agent, Antirheumatic
dep Gynogen	See ESTRADIOL CYPIONATE		Estrogen
Depo-Medrol	See METHYLPREDNISOLONE		Corticosteroid
Depo-Testosterone	See TESTOSTERONE CYPIONATE		Androgen/Anabolic
Depogen	See ESTRADIOL CYPIONATE		Estrogen
Depoject	See METHYLPREDNISOLONE		Corticosteroid
Desenex	See TOLNAFTATE		Fungicide
Desenex	See UNDECYLENIC ACID		Fungicide
Desferal	See DEFEROXAMINE		Iron Chelator
DESIPRAMINE Generic, Norpramin, Pertofrane	**Endogenous Depression:** PO: 100–200 mg/d to start in 1–3 doses; maintenance < 300 mg/d. Geriatric/adolescent PO: 25–100 mg/d (max. dose 150 mg/d).	**Tablet:** 10, 25, 50, 75, 100, 150 mg **Capsule:** 25, 50 mg	CNS AGENTS (G) Tricyclic Antidepressants (SG) **Cost:** Low

GENERIC NAME Trade Name	INDICATIONS AND DOSAGES	DOSE FORMS	GROUP (G)/SUBGROUP (SG) Relative Cost within Group
DESMOPRESSIN Deamino-arginine vasopressin, DDAVP, Concentraid	**Diabetes Insipidus:** IV, SC: 2–4 microg/d (0.5–1 ml/d) in 2 divided doses. Nasal: 0.1–0.4 ml/d in 1–2 doses. Pediatric Nasal (3 mo–12 y.o): 0.05–0.3 ml/d in 1–2 doses.	**Nasal Spray:** 0.1 mg equivalent to 400 IU arginine vasopressin: 0.1 mg/ml **Injection:** 4 mg/ml.	ENDOCRINE AGENTS (G) Posterior Pituitary Hormones (Antidiuretic) (SG)
DESONIDE Tridesilon, DesOwen	Apply to affected area 2 to 4 times a day. Medium Potency:	**Ointment:** 0.05%. **Cream:** 0.05%. **Lotion:** 0.05%.	ANTI-INFLAMMATORY STEROIDS, TOPICAL (G) **Cost:** Medium
DesOwen	See DESONIDE		Corticosteroid, Topical
DESOXIMETA-SONE Generic, Top-icort	Apply to affected area 2 to 4 times a day.	**Ointment:** 0.25%. **Cream:** 0.05%, 0.25%. **Gel:** 0.05%.	DERMATOLOGIC AGENTS (G) Anti-Inflammatory Steroids, Topical (SG) **Cost:** Medium
Desoxyephedrine	See METHAMPHETAMINE See L-DESOXYEPHEDRINE		Sympathomimetic Stimulant Nasal Vasoconstrictor
Desoxyn	See METHAMPHETAMINE		Sympathomimetic Stimulant
Desoxyphenobar-bital	See PRIMIDONE		Anticonvulsant, Sedative
Desquam-X	See BENZOYL PEROXIDE		Keratolytic (Acne)
Desyrel	See TRAZODONE		TCA Antidepressants
DEXACIDIN	**Ophthalmic:** Apply a small amount (about 0.5 in.) into the conjunctival sac tid–QID.		**Ophthalmic Ointment (per g):** neomycin sulfate (equal to 3.5 mg of neomycin base), polymyxin B sulfate (10,000 Units), dexamethasone (1 mg)
Dexameth	See DEXAMETHASONE		Corticosteroid
DEXAMETHA-SONE Generic, Deca-dron, Dexameth, Dala-lone-LA, Dalalone, De-xone, Hexadrol	PO: 0.75–9 mg/d. IV: (acetate): 8–16 mg q1–3 weeks. Intraarticular (acetate): 0.8–16 mg/injection. Intraarticular (phosphate): 0.4–4.0 mg/injection. IV (phosphate): **Cerebral edema:** 10 mg initially then 4 mg IM q6 hrs. **Adrenal suppression test.**	**Tablet:** 0.25, 0.5, 0.75, 1, 1.5, 2, 4, 6 mg **Elixir:** 0.5 mg/5 ml **Oral Solution:** 0.5 mg/5 ml **Acetate (suspension):** 8, 16/ml **Phosphate (solution):** 4, 10, 20, 24/ml	ENDOCRINE AGENTS (G) Anti-Inflammatory Steroids (SG) **Cost:** Low
DEXCHLORPHE-NIRAMINE Generic, Po-laramine	**Allergic (Type I) Reactions:** PO: 2 mg q4–6h PO: (ext'd release) 4–6 mg qhs or bid.	**Tablet:** 2 mg **Tablet:** (ext'd release) 4 mg, 6 mg **Syrup:** 2 mg/5 ml	ANTI-INFLAMMATORY AGENTS (G) Antihistamines (H1 Antagonists) (SG) With Mild Sedation (SSG) **Cost:** Low
Dexedrine	See DEXTROAMPHETAMINE		Stimulant
DEXFENFLURA-MINE Redux	**Obesity:** 15 mg 1–2 times daily	**Tablet:** 15 mg	CNS AGENTS (G) Stimulants (SG) Diet Pill, Atypical (SSG)
Dexone	See DEXAMETHASONE		Corticosteroid

GENERIC NAME Trade Name	INDICATIONS AND DOSAGES	DOSE FORMS	GROUP (G)/SUBGROUP (SG) Relative Cost within Group
DEXRAZOXANE Zinecard	CANCER CHEMOTHERAPY (G) Cardioprotective (SG)		
DEXTROAMPHETAMINE Generic, Dexedrine	**Narcolepsy:** PO: 10 mg/d to start (initial dose on awakening with 1 or 2 additional doses at 4–6 hour intervals); increase 10 mg/d q1week; maintenance 5–60 mg/d. **Attention Deficit:** PO: Pediatric (3–5 yrs): 2.5 mg/d to start; increase by 2.5 mg/d q1week PRN; use lowest effective dose. Pediatric PO (>5 yrs): 5 mg q12–24h to start; increase by 5 mg/d q1week; maintenance 10–40 mg/d.	**Tablet:** 5, 10 mg **Capsule:** (Ext'd release) 5, 10, 15 mg **Elixir:** 5 mg/5 ml	CNS AGENTS (G) Sympathomimetic Stimulants (SG) Schedule II Agents (SSG) **Cost:** Medium
DEXTROMETHORPHAN Generic, OTC,	In many proprietary mixtures. **Liquid, Syrup and Lozenges:** PO: (Adults and children > 12 yrs): 10–30 mg q4–8h (max. 120 mg/24 hours). Pediatric PO: (6 to 12 yrs): 5–10 mg q4h or 15 mg q6–8h (max. 60 mg/24 hours). Pediatric PO: (2 to 6 yrs)-Syrup: 2.5 to 7.5 mg every 4 to 8 hours (max. 30 mg/hours). PO: (Sustained action liquid): 60 mg q12h. Pediatric PO: (6 to 12 yrs): 30 mg q12h. Pediatric PO: (2 to 5 yrs): 15 mg q12h.	**Capsule:** 30 mg **Liquid:** 10 mg/ 15 ml, 3.5 mg/ 5 ml, 7.5 mg/ 5 ml, 15 mg/ 5 ml methorphan HBr/5ml. **Syrup:** 10 mg/ 5ml, 15 mg/ 15 ml **Lozenges:** 2.5 mg, 5 mg, 7.5 mg	RESPIRATORY AGENTS (G) Antitussives (SG) **Cost:** Low
DEZOCINE Dalgan	IM: 5–10 mg q3–6h (max. individual dose 20 mg; max. daily dose 120 mg/d). IV: 2.5–10 mg q2–4h.	**Injection:** 5, 10, 15 mg/ml	NARCOTIC ANALGESICS AND RELATED AGENTS (G) Mixed Agonist-Antagonist Effects (SG)
DHT	See DIHYDROTACHYSTEROL		Vit D Substitute
DiaBeta	See GLYBURIDE		Oral Antidiabetic
Diabinese	See CHLORPROPAMIDE		Oral Antidiabetic
Diaceles	See NITROGLYCERIN		Vasodilator
Dialose	See DOCUSATE		Stool Softener
Diamox	See ACETAZOLAMIDE		Carbonic Anhydrase Inhibitor
Diaqua	See HYDROCHLOROTHIAZIDE		Sodium Diuretic

GENERIC NAME Trade Name	INDICATIONS AND DOSAGES	DOSE FORMS	GROUP (G)/SUBGROUP (SG) Relative Cost within Group
DIAZEPAM Generic, Valium	**Sedation, Anxiety:** PO: 2–10 mg q6–12h. PO (Ext'd release): 15–30 mg/d. Pediatric PO: 1–2.5 mg q6–8h. IV, IM: 2–5 mg q3–4h PRN **Alcohol Withdrawal:** PO: 10 mg, (3–4 doses given over 24 hours), then 5 mg q6–8h PRN. IV, IM: 10 mg, repeat once at 3–4 hours. **Muscle Spasms:** IV, IM: 5–10 mg, repeat q3–4h (once). PO: 2–10 mg q6–8h (max. dose 30 mg/d). Pre-Procedure Sedation: IV: 5–15 mg immediately prior to procedure (reduce concurrent narcotic dosage by 1/3 or more). IV: 5–10 mg 30 min prior to procedure (reduce concurrent narcotic dosage by 1/3 or more). **Seizures:** IV, IM: 5–10 mg to start, repeat q10–15min PRN (max. dose: 30 mg; may repeat this dosage in 2–4 hours if needed).	**Tablet:** 2, 5, 10 mg **Capsule:** (Ext'd release) 15 mg **Injection:** 5 mg/ ml **Liquid:** 5 mg/ 5 ml, 5 mg/ ml	CNS AGENTS (G) Sedative-Hypnotics (SG) Intermediate-Acting Sedative Hypnotics (SSG) **Cost:** Low
DIAZOXIDE Hyperstat, Proglycem	**Hypertensive Emergency:** IV: 1–3 mg/kg (max single dose: 150 mg; give RAPIDLY in < 30 sec. to supine patient), may repeat q 5–15 min until BP acceptable; repeat q4–24 hours as needed (do not administer for > 10 days). **Hypoglycemia (due to hyper inoulism):** PO: 3–8 mg/kg/d given in 2 or 3 divided doses.	**Capsule:** 50 mg **Oral Suspension:** 50 mg/ml **Injection:** 15 mg/ml, 300 mg/ 20 ml	CV AGENTS (G) Vasodilators (SG) Arteriolar Dilators and Miscellaneous Agents (SSG) **Cost:** Very High
Dibent	See DICYCLOMINE		Anticholinergic
Dibenzyline	See PHENOXYBENZAMINE		Alpha Adrenergic Blocker
DIBUCAINE Generic, Nupercaine	Apply to the affected area as needed.	**Ointment:** 1% **Cream:** 0.5%	LOCAL ANESTHETICS (G) Topical (Mucosal) Only (SG) **Cost:** Low
DICHLORPHE-NAMIDE Daranide	**Glaucoma:** PO: 100–200 mg to start, then 100 mg q12h; maintenance 25–50 mg q8–12h.	**Tablet:** 50 mg	AGENTS USED IN THE TREAT-MENT OF GLAUCOMA (G) Carbonic Anhydrase Inhibitors (SG) **Cost:** Medium
DICLOFENAC Voltaren (Na Salt), Cataflam (K salt)	**Osteoarthritis:** PO: 100–150 mg/d given as 2 or 3 divided doses. **Rheumatoid arthritis:** 150–200 mg/d given in 3 or 4 divided doses. **Dysmenorrhea:** PO: 50 mg tid (max dose first day 200 mg/d; thereafter 150 mg/d).	**Tablet:** 50 mg **Tablet:** (Enteric) 25, 50 75 mg	CNS AGENTS (G) Non-Narcotic Analgesics (SG) Aspirin and Related NSAIDs (SSG) **Cost:** High

GENERIC NAME Trade Name	INDICATIONS AND DOSAGES	DOSE FORMS	GROUP (G)/SUBGROUP (SG) Relative Cost within Group
DICLOXACILLIN Generic, Dycill, Dynapen, Pathocil, Veracillin	**Mild to Moderate Infections:** PO Adults and pediatric (> 40 kg): 125 mg q6h. Pediatric (<40 kg) PO: 12.5 mg/kg/d, given in 4 divided doses. **Severe Infections:** PO Adults and pediatric (> 40 kg): 250 mg q6h. Pediatric (<40 kg) PO: 25 mg/kg/d given in 4 divided doses.	**Capsule:** 125, 250, 500 mg **Oral Suspension:** (powder) 62.5 mg/5 ml reconstituted	ANTI-INFECTIOUS AGENTS (G) Lactam Antibiotics (SG) Penicillins: Resistant To Staphylococcal Lactamase (SG) **Cost:** Medium
DICUMAROL Generic	**Anticoagulation:** PO: 200–300 mg for 1 day, then 25–200 mg/d (dose to maintain prothrombin activity at 20 to 30% of normal level).	**Tablet:** 25 mg	METABOLIC AGENTS (G) Anticoagulants And Coagulants (SG) Inhibitors of Prothrombin Synthesis (SSG) **Cost:** Low
DICYCLOMINE Generic, Bentyl, Dibent, Byclomine, A-Spaz, Or-Tyl	**Irritable Bowel, Hypermotility:** PO: 20 mg QID; maintenance 40 mg q6h. IV: 20 mg q6h; then PO maintenance.	**Tablet:** 10, 20 mg **Injection:** 10 mg/ml **Syrup:** 2 mg/ml	AUTONOMIC NS AGENTS (G) Parasympatholytics (SG) Parasympatholytics, Tertiary Amines (SSG) **Cost:** Low
DIDANOSINE Videx, ddl, Dideoxyinosine	**Advanced HIV Infection:** PO (> 59 kgs): 200 mg bid (tablets); 250 mg bid (buffered powder). PO (< 60 kgs): 125 mg bid (tablets); 167 mg bid (buffered powder).	**Tablet:** 25 50, 100, 150 mg. **Powder for Oral Solution:** (pediatric) 2, 4 g. **Powder for Oral Solution:** (buffered) 100, 167, 250, 375 mg.	ANTI-INFECTIOUS AGENTS (G) Antiviral Agents, Systemic (SG) **Cost:** Medium
Didrex	See BENZPHETAMINE		Diet Pill
Didronel	See ETIDRONATE		Inhibit Osteoclasts
DIENESTROL Generic, DV cream	**Atrophic vaginitis:**	**Vaginal cream:** 0.01%, 30, 78 g.	ENDOCRINE AGENTS (G) Estrogens (SG)
DIETHYLPROPION Generic, Tenuate	**Exogenous Obesity:** PO: 25 mg tid (1 hour before meals). PO (Ext'd Release): 75 mg take midmorning.	**Tablet:** 25 mg **Tablet:** (Ext'd release) 75 mg	CNS AGENTS (G) Sympathomimetic Stimulants (SG) Other Schedule 3 or 4 "Diet Pills" (SSG) **Cost:** Medium
DIETHYLSTILBESTROL (DES) Generic	**Prostatic Cancer:** PO: 1–3 mg/d to start; taper to 1 mg/d as clinically appropriate. **Post-Coital Contraception** (unlabeled use), PO: 25 mg bid for 5 days, must start < 72 hours after coitus.	**Tablets:** 1, 5 mg	ENDOCRINE AGENTS (G) Estrogens (SG) **Cost:** Low
Differin	See ADAPALENE		Keratolytic (Acne)
DIFLORASONE Generic, Maxiflor	Apply to affected area 1–3 times a day.	**Ointment:** 0.05%. **Cream:** 0.05%.	ANTI-INFLAMMATORY ETC (G) Anti-Inflammatory Steroids (SG) **Cost:** High
Diflucan	See FLUCONAZOLE		Antifungal, systemic

GENERIC NAME Trade Name	INDICATIONS AND DOSAGES	DOSE FORMS	GROUP (G)/SUBGROUP (SG) Relative Cost within Group
DIFLUNISAL Generic, Dolobid	**Pain:** PO: 1,000 mg to start, then 500 mg q8–12h (max. dose 1500 mg/d).	**Tablet:** 250, 500 mg	ANTI-INFLAMMATORY AGENTS (G) Non-Narcotic Analgesics (SG) Aspirin and related NSAIDs (SSG) Other Salicylates (SSG) **Cost:** Medium
Digibind	See DIGOXIN IMMUNE Fab		Digoxin Antibody
DIGITOXIN Generic, Crystodigin	PO: 0.6 mg first dose; then 0.4 mg second dose in 4 to 6 hours after first dose, then 0.2 mg q6–8h for 2–3 doses; maintenance 0.05–0.3 mg/d.	**Tablet:** 0.1, 0.2 mg	CV AGENTS (G) Cardiotonic Glycosides And Related (SG) **Cost:** Low
DIGOXIN Generic, Lanoxin, Lanoxicaps	PO (tablet): 0.5–0.75 mg to start; 0.125–0.5 mg/day maintenance, use serum levels to adjust dose. IV: single dose—400–600 mcg to start; (dose range: 8–15 mcg/kg); 0.1–0.375 mg maintenance. Many other dosing schemes exist.	**Tablet:** 0.125, 0.25, 0.5 mg **Capsule:** 0.05, 0.1, 0.2 mg **Elixir:** 0.05 mg/ml **Elixir (pediatric):** 0.05 mg/ml **Injection:** 0.25 mg/ml **Injection (pediatric):** 0.1 mg/ml	CV AGENTS (G) Cardiotonic Glycosides And Related (SG) **Cost:** Low
DIGOXIN IMMUNE FAB Digibind	**Digoxin Intoxication (known amount):** Each 40 mg(content of one vial) binds the equivalent of 0.6 mg of digoxin or digitoxin. Administer Digibind over 30 minutes through a 0.22 micrometer membrane filter. **Digoxin Intoxication (unknown amount):** IV: give 20 vials (760 mg) of Digibind for life-threatening ingestions. Give 6 vials (228 mg) for reversal of chronic toxicity in adults.	**Injection:** 40 mg per vial	CV AGENTS (G) Cardiotonic Glycosides And Related (SG) **Cost:** An orphan drug. Supply must be arranged.
DIHYDROCOD-EINE Generic, Com-pal; Synalgos-DC	**Pain:** Synalgos-DC: 2 capsules q4h PRN.	Mixture only dose forms. Synalgos-DC Capsules: 16 mg dihydro-codeine, 356.4 mg aspirin, 30 mg caffeine.	CNS AGENTS (G) Narcotic Analgesics And Related Agents (SG) Narcotic Analgesics of Lowest Potency (SSG) **Cost:** Low
DIHYDROERGO-TAMINE D.H.E. 45	**Migraine Headaches:** IM: 1 mg at headache onset, repeat qhour PRN up to a max dose of 3 mg. IV: Administer up to 2 mg at headache onset (max dose: 6 mg/week).	**Injection:** 1 mg/ml	CV AGENTS (G) Vasoconstrictors and Oxytocics (SG) **Cost:** High
Dihydro-morphine	See HYDROMORPHONE		Narcotic Analgetic

GENERIC NAME Trade Name	INDICATIONS AND DOSAGES	DOSE FORMS	GROUP (G)/SUBGROUP (SG) Relative Cost within Group
DIHYDRO-TACHYSTEROL Generic, DHT, Hytakerol	**Tetany, Hypoparathyroidism:** PO: 0.8–2.4 mg/daily initially, then maintenance of 0.2–1mg/d PRN (usual dose is 0.6 mg/d).	**Tablet:** 0.125, 0.2, 0.4 mg **Intensol:** (solution) 0.2 mg/ml **Capsule:** 0.125 mg **Oral Solution:** 0.25 mg/ml	METABOLIC AGENTS (G) Calcium Kinetics Regulators (SG) D Vitamins and Related Agents (SSG) **Cost:** High
Dihydroxychole-calciferol (1,25)	See CALCITRIOL		D Vitamin Prodrug
Diiodo-hydroxyquin	See IODOQUINOL		Antiparasitic Agents
Dilacor	See DILTIAZEM		Calcium Channel Blocker
Dilantin	See PHENYTOIN		Anticonvulsant
Dilatrate	See ISOSORBIDE DINITRATE		Vasodilator
Dilaudid	See HYDROMORPHONE		Narcotic Analgetic
Dilin	See DYPHYLLINE		Bronchodilator
Dilor	See DYPHYLLINE		Bronchodilator
DILTIAZEM Generic, Dilacor, Cardizem, Tiazac	**Chronic Stable and Vasospastic Angina:** **Hypertension:** **Supraventricular Tachycardia:** See discussion Section 1	**Tablet:** **Capsule:** (Ext'd release) 60, 90, 120, 180, 240, 300, 360 mg **Injection:**	CV AGENTS (G) Vasodilators (SG) Calcium Channel Blockers (SSG) **Cost:** Low
DIMENHYDRINATE OTC, Generic, Dramamine, Dramocen,	**Motion Sickness:** PO: 50–100 mg q4–6h; max. dose 400 mg/d. IV: 50 mg q6h PRN. IV: 50 mg in 10 ml saline over 2 min. Pediatric PO (6–12 yrs): 25–50 mg q6–8h; max. dose 150 mg/d. Pediatric PO (2–6 yrs): 12.5–25 mg q6–8h; max. dose 75 mg/d. Pediatric (6–12 yrs) IM: 1.25 mg/kg q6h (max. dose 300 mg/d).	**Tablet:** 50 mg **Tablet:** (chewable) 50 mg **Capsule:** 50 mg **Injection:** 50 mg/ml **Liquid:** 12.5 mg/4 ml, 12.5 mg/5 ml, 15.62 mg/5 ml	ANTIINFLAMMATORY ETC (G) Antihistamines (H1 Antagonists) (SG) Motion Sickness Prevention (SSG) **Cost:** Low
DIMERCAPROL British anti-Lewisite	**Mercury poisoning acute:** Deep IM: 5 mg/kg to start followed by 2.5 mg/kg 1–2 times daily for 10 days.	**Injection (in oil):** 100 mg/ml	ANTIDOTES AND AGENTS USED IN POISONINGS (G)
Dimetane	See BROMPHENIRAMINE		Antihistamine
DIMETHYL SULFOXIDE DMSO Rimso-50	**Interstitial Cystitis:** Instill 50 ml into bladder	**Solution:** 50% aqueous	
DINOPROSTONE Prepidil, Prostaglandin E2, Prostin E2	**Abortion:** 1 suppository intravaginally q3–5h until uterus empties or 2 days.	**Vaginal Suppository:** 20 mg **Gel:** 0.5 mg (in 2.5 cc Syringes)	CV AGENTS (G) Vasoconstrictors And Oxytocics (SG) **Cost:** High
Dioval	See ESTRADIOL VALERATE		Estrogen
Diovan	See VALSARTAN		Angiotensin II Receptor Blocker
Dipentum	See OLSALAZINE		Prodrug for 5-ASA
Diphen	See DIPHENHYDRAMINE		Antihistamine

GENERIC NAME Trade Name	INDICATIONS AND DOSAGES	DOSE FORMS	GROUP (G)/SUBGROUP (SG) Relative Cost within Group
DIPHENHYDRA-MINE Generic, OTC, Benadryl, Fenyl-hist, Nyto-l,others	**Type 1 Allergic Reactions:** PO: 25–50 mg 1 or 2 times/d	**Capsule:** 25, 50 mg **Injection:** 10, 50 mg/ml **Elixir:** 12.5 mg/5 ml **Syrup:** 12.5 mg/5 ml	**Parkinsonism, Drug-Induced Extrapyramidal Disorders:** PO: 25–50 mg IV: 10–25 mg **OTC "Sleep Aid"** ANTI-INFLAMMATORY, ETC (G) Antihistamines (H1 Antagonists) (SG) Antihistamines with Sedation Prominent (SG) CNS AGENTS (G) Antiparkinsonian Agents (SG) Anticholinergics and Related Agents (SSG) **Cost:** Low
DIFENOXIN WITH ATROPINE Generic, Motofen	**Diarrhea:** PO: Initially 2 tabs, then 1 tab after each BM.	**Tablet:** Difenoxin (1 mg), atropine (0.025 mg)	GASTROINTESTINAL AGENTS (G) Anti-Diarrheal Agents (SG) Weak Narcotic **Cost:** Low
DIPHENOXYLATE WITH ATROPINE Generic, Lomotil, Logen, Lonox	**Diarrhea:** PO: 10 cc or 2 tabs QID until control of diarrhea is achieved. Pediatric PO (2–12 yrs): 0.3–0.4 mg/kg (of diphenoxylate)/day given in 4 divided doses.	**Liquid (per 5 cc):** diphenoxylate (2.5 mg), atropine (0.025 mg), alcohol (15%) **Tablet:** diphenoxylate (2.5 mg), atropine (0.025 mg)	GASTROINTESTINAL AGENTS (G) Anti-Diarrheal Agents (SG) Weak Narcotic **Cost:** Low
Diphenylhydantoin	See PHENYTOIN		Anticonvulsant
DIPIVEFRIN Generic, Propine	**Elevated IOP:** Instill 1 drop bid.	**Solution:** 0.25% (2.8 [2.5 mg base] mg/ml); 0.5% (5.6 [5 mg base] mg/ml).	OPHTHALMIC AGENTS (G) Agents Used In The Treatment Of Glaucoma (SG) Sympathomimetic (SG) **Cost:** Medium
Diprolene	See BETAMETHASONE DIPROPIONATE		Corticosteroid
DIPYRIDAMOLE Generic, Persantine	**Post Valve Replacement:** PO: 75 to 100 mg QID.	**Tablet:** 25, 50, 75 mg	METABOLIC AGENTS (G) Anticoagulants And Coagulants (SG) Antiplatelet Agents (SG) **Cost:** Medium
DIRITHROMYCIN Dynabac	**Uncomplicated URI or Skin Infections:** **Mycobacterial Infections (including MAC):** PO: 500 mg daily.	**Tablet:** 250 mg	ANTI-INFECTIOUS AGENTS (G) Macrolide Antibiotics (SG) **Cost:** High
Disalcid	See SALSALATE		Non-Narcotic Analgetic

GENERIC NAME Trade Name	INDICATIONS AND DOSAGES	DOSE FORMS	GROUP (G)/SUBGROUP (SG) Relative Cost within Group
DISOPYRAMIDE Generic, Norpace	**Ventricular Arrhythmias:** PO: 100–150 mg q6h, maintenance range 400–800 mg/d given in 4 divided doses (initial loading dose 300 mg, then maintenance).	**Capsule:** 100, 150 mg **Capsule:** (Ext'd release) 100, 150 mg	ANTIARRHYTHMIC AGENTS (G) Group I Antiarrhythmic Agents (SG) **Cost:** Medium
Dithranol	See ANTHRALIN		Keratoplastic (Tar)
Ditropan	See OXYBUTYNIN		Anticholinergic
Diucardin	See HYDROFLUMETHIAZIDE		Sodium Diuretic
DIUPRES 250, 500	**Hypertension:** A combination PO: 1–2 tablets qd.		**Tablet:** Reserpine/Chlorothiazide: 0.125/250mg, 0.125/500mg CENTRAL SYMPATHOLYTIC (G) and SODIUM DIURETIC (G)
Diurese	See TRICHLORMETHIAZIDE		Sodium Diuretic
Diuril	See CHLOROTHIAZIDE		Sodium Diuretic
Divalproex	See VALPROIC ACID		Anticonvulsant
DMSO	See DIMETHYL SULFOXIDE		Interstitial Cystitis
DOBUTAMINE Dobutrex	**Shock:** IV: The usual range of doses is 2.0–20 mcg/kg/min (max. dose 40 mcg/kg/min).	**Injection:** 250 mg in 20 ml vials	ANS AGENTS (G) Sympathomimetics (G) Sympathomimetics, with Unselective Beta 1 and 2 Agonists (SG) **Cost:** Very High
Dobutrex	See DOBUTAMINE		Beta Adrenergic Agonist
DOCUSATE Generic, OTC, Dioctyl sodium sulfosuccinate, Colace, DSS, Dialose, Many others	**Constipation:** PO: 50–500 mg. Pediatric (6–12 yrs): 40–120 mg. Pediatric (3–6 yrs): 20–60 mg.	**Tablet:** 100 mg **Capsule:** 50, 100, 240, 250 mg **Syrup:** 50 mg/ 15 ml, 60 mg/ 15 ml **Liquid:** 150 mg/ 15 ml **Solution:** 50 mg/ml	GASTROINTESTINAL AGENTS (G) Laxatives And Bowel Cleansers (SG) Fecal Softener (Emulsifier) (SSG) **Cost:** Low
Dolobid	See DIFLUNISAL		Non-Narcotic Analgetic
Dolophine	See METHADONE		Narcotic Analgetic
DONEPEZIL Aricept	**Alzheimer's Disease:** PO: Initially 5 mg hs increasing to 10 mg after 4–6 weeks	**Tablet:** 5, 10 mg	CNS AGENTS (G) Cholinergic Agents (SG) Cholinesterase Inhibitor, Central (SSG) **Cost:** Moderate
DONNATAL	PO: 1–2 capsules (or tablets) tid or QID. PO: 5–10 cc tid or QID.		**Capsule,Tablet or Elixir:** atropine sulfate, scopolamine HBr, hyoscyamine sulfate, phenobarbital (16.2 mg) **Tablets ER:** As above with phenobarbital (48.6 mg)

GENERIC NAME Trade Name	INDICATIONS AND DOSAGES	DOSE FORMS	GROUP (G)/SUBGROUP (SG) Relative Cost within Group
DOPAMINE Generic, Intropin, Dopastat	**Shock Persisting After Volume Replacement:** IV: 1–5 mcg/kg/min initially, then increase gradually in 2 mcg/kg/min increments until satisfactory perfusion is obtained (max. dose: 20 mcg/kg/min).	**Injection:** 0.8, 1.6, 3.2, 40, 80, 160 mg/ml	ANS AGENTS (G) Sympathomimetics (SG) Sympathomimetics, Mixed Alpha And Beta Agonist Effects (SSG) **Cost:** High
Dopar	See LEVODOPA		Dopamine Precursor
Dopastat	See DOPAMINE		Sympathomimetic
Doral	See QUAZEPAM		Sedative Hypnotic
Doriden	See GLUTETHIMIDE		Sedative Hypnotic
DORNASE ALFA Pulmozyme	**Cystic fibrosis:** Nebulizer Inhalation: 2.5 mg single-use amp inhaled once daily (some have used 2.5 mg twice/day).	**Solution:** (for inhalation) 1 mg/ml in 2.5 ml amps.	RESPIRATORY AGENTS (G) Expectorants and Mucolytic Agents (SG)
Doryx	See DOXYCYCLINE		Tetracycline Antibiotic
DORZOLAMIDE Trusopt	**Glaucoma:** Intraocular: 1 drop 2% tid	**Ophthalmic Drops:** 2%	OPHTHALMIC AGENTS (G) USED IN THE TREATMENT OF GLAUCOMA (SG) Carbonic Anhydrase Inhibitor (SSG) **COST:** Expensive
Dostinex	See CABERGOLINE		Decrease prolactin secretion
Dovonex	See CALCIPOTRIENE		D Vitamin
DOXAZOCIN Cardura	**Hypertension:** Initial dose 1mg once daily, maintenance dose range 1–16 mg/d (doses > 4 mg may cause significant postural effects).	**Tablet:** 1, 2, 4, 8 mg	SYMPATHOPLEGICS (G) Alpha Adrenergic Receptor Blockers (SG) **Cost:** Medium
DOXEPIN Generic, Adapin, Sinequan	**Endogenous Depression:** PO: 25–150 mg/d to start in 1–3 doses; maintenance 75–150 mg/d (max. dose 300 mg/d).	**Capsule:** 10, 25, 50, 75, 100, 150 mg **Liquid:** 10 mg/ml	CNS AGENTS (G) Tricyclic Antidepressants (SG) **Cost:** Low
DOXIDAN	PO: 1–2 capsule qd, for up to 1 week.	**Capsule:** phenolphthalein (65 mg), docusate (60 mg)	
DOXORUBICIN Generic, Adriamycin	CANCER CHEMOTHERAPY (G) React With DNA (SG) Antibiotics (SSG)		

GENERIC NAME Trade Name	INDICATIONS AND DOSAGES	DOSE FORMS	GROUP (G)/SUBGROUP (SG) Relative Cost within Group
DOXYCYCLINE Generic, Vibramycin, Monodox, Doryx	**Bacterial Infections:** PO: 100 mg q12h for 1 day; then 100–200 mg/d in 1–2 doses (higher dose for chronic urinary tract infections). Pediatric (> 8 yrs, < 45 kgs) PO: 2.2 mg/kg q12h for 1 day; then 2.2 mg/kg/d in 1–2 doses (max. dose 4.4 mg/kg/d). **Acute Gonococcal Infection:** PO: 100 mg bid for 7 days (this follows initial parenteral treatment with lactam antibiotics and probenecid). **Adjunct in Pelvic Inflammatory Disease:** PO: 100 mg bid for 10–14 days (this follows initial parenteral treatment with ceftriaxone (or other lactam antibiotics and probenecid). IV: 100 mg bid (this is given with parenteral treatment with ceftriaxone (or other lactam antibiotics and probenecid); give IV infusion over 1–4 hours. **Chlamydia (Urethral, Endocervical, Rectal), Female Urethral Syndrome, Post-Rape Prophylaxis:** PO: 100 mg bid for 7 days. **"Traveler's Diarrhea" Prophylaxis (off label use):** PO: 100 mg/d. **Sexually Transmitted Epididymitis:** PO: 100 mg bid for 10 days (this follows initial parenteral treatment with lactam antibiotics and probenecid). **Lymphogranuloma Venereum:** PO: 100 mg bid for a minimum of 14 days. **Primary/Secondary Syphilis:** PO: 300 mg/d in divided doses for a minimum of 10 days.	**Tablet:** 100 mg **Injection:** (powder) 100, 200 mg **Oral Suspension:** (powder) 25 mg per 5 ml when reconstituted **Syrup:** 50 mg/ 5 ml	ANTI-INFECTIOUS AGENTS (G) Tetracyclines (SG) **Cost:** Low
DPH	See PHENYTOIN		Anticonvulsant
Dramamine	See DIMENHYDRINATE		Antihistamine
Dramocen	See DIMENHYDRINATE		Antihistamine
Drisdol	See ERGOCALCIFEROL (D2)		D Vitamin Prodrug
Drithocreme	See ANTHRALIN		Keratoplastic (Tar)
DRONABINOL tetrahydro-cannabinol, (delta-9), Marinol, THC	**Anorexia:** PO: Initially 2.5 mg bid or as tolerated (max. dose: 20 mg/d) **Nausea/vomiting:** PO: 5 mg/sq. meter on the day prior to chemotherapy, then 2.5 mg/sq. meter 1–3 prior to chemotherapy and then 2.5–10 mg/sq. meter bid.	**Capsules:** 2.5,5, 10 mg	CNS AGENTS (G) Sedative-Hypnotics (SG) Long-Acting Sedatives (SSG) **Cost:** Medium
Droxone	See DYPHYLLINE		Xanthine Equivalent
DSS	See DOCUSATE		Stool Softener
Dulcolax	See BISACODYL		Irritant Laxative

GENERIC NAME Trade Name	INDICATIONS AND DOSAGES	DOSE FORMS	GROUP (G)/SUBGROUP (SG) Relative Cost within Group
DUO-MEDIHALER	**Acute Bronchospasm:** Inhalation: 1 puff, may repeat once in 2–5 minutes; then maintenance dose of 1–2 puffs 4–6 times /d.		**Aerosol:** isoproterenol HCl (160 mcg), phenylephrine bitartrate (240 pg)/spray
Duphalac	See LACTULOSE		Laxative Removes Ammonia
Dura-Estrin	See ESTRADIOL CYPIONATE		Estrogen
Dura-Tabs	See QUINIDINE		Antiarrhythmic
Durabolin	See NANDROLONE		Androgen /Anabolic
Duragen	See ESTRADIOL VALERATE		Estrogen
Duragesic (transdermal patch)	See FENTANYL		Narcotic Analgetic
Duralutin	See HYDROXYPROGESTERONE		Progestin
Duranest	See ETIDOCAINE		Local Anesthetic
Duraquin	See QUINIDINE		Antiarrhythmic
Duratest-100	See TESTOSTERONE CYPIONATE		Androgen/Anabolic
Durathate	See TESTOSTERONE ENANTHATE		Androgen/Anabolic
Duricef	See CEFADROXIL		LACTAM ANTIBIOTIC
Duricef	See CEFADROXIL		Lactam Antibiotic
Duvoid	See BETHANECHOL		Cholinergic
DVcream	See DIENESTROL		Estrogen
DYAZIDE	PO: 1–2 capsule qd.		**Capsule:** triamterene (37.5 mg), hydrochlorothiazide (25 mg)
Dycill	See DICLOXACILLIN		Lactam Antiblotic
Dyclone	See DYCLONINE		Local Anesthetic
DYCLONINE OTC, Dyclone, Sucrets		**Topical:** 0.5–1% **Solution:** 0.5, 1%	LOCAL ANESTHETICS (G) Topical (Mucosal) Only (SG) **Cost:** Medium
Dydrozide-50	See HYDROCHLOROTHIAZIDE		Sodium Diuretic
Dyflex	See DYPHYLLINE		Bronchodilator
Dymelor	See ACETOHEXAMIDE		Oral Antidiabetic
Dynacin	See MINOCYCLINE		Tetracycline Antibiotic
DynaCirc	See ISRADIPINE		Calcium Channel Blockers
Dynapen	See DICLOXACILLIN		Lactam Antibiotic
DYPHYLLINE Generic, Lufyllin, many others	**Bronchodilation:** PO: Up to 15 mg/kg q6h. **Acute Bronchospasm:** IM: 250–500 mg injected SLOWLY (max. dose 15 mg/kg q6h).	**Tablet:** 200, 400 mg **Elixir:** 100 mg/ 15 ml, 160 mg/ 15 ml **Injection:** 250 mg/ml	CV AGENTS (G) Xanthines (SG) **Cost:** Low
Dyrenium	See TRIAMTERENE		Potassium Sparing Diuretic
E-Mycin	See ERYTHROMYCIN		Macrolide Antibiotic
E-PILO-1,2,3,4,6	**Ophthalmic:** 1–2 qtt into affected eye(s) up to QID.		**Ophthalmic Solution:** Epinephrine bitartrate (1%) with pilocarpine 1, 2, 3, 4 or 6%

GENERIC NAME Trade Name	INDICATIONS AND DOSAGES	DOSE FORMS	GROUP (G)/SUBGROUP (SG) Relative Cost within Group
E.E.S.	See ERYTHROMYCIN ETHYL SUCCINATE		Macrolide Antibiotic
Easprin	See ASPIRIN		Non-Narcotic Analgetic
ECONAZOLE Spectazole	**Tinea (pedis, cruris, corporis and versicolor):** Topical: apply once daily (treat pedis for four weeks, others for two weeks). **Cutaneous Candidiasis:** Topical: apply to affected and surrounding skin areas bid (treat for two weeks).	**Cream:** 1%.	DERMATOLOGIC AGENTS (G) Topical Anti-Infectious Agents (SG) Topical Fungicides (SG) **Cost:** Medium
Ecotrin	See ASPIRIN		Non-Narcotic Analgetic
Edecrin	See ETHACRYNIC ACID		Non-Sulfonamide Loop Diuretic
EDETATE CALCIUM DISODIUM Calcium disodium versenate	**Acute or Chronic Lead Intoxication:** IM (Maximum): dose 35 mg/kg bid, less in mild cases.	**Injection:** 200 mg/ml	ANTIDOTES AND AGENTS USED IN POISONINGS (G)
EDROPHONIUM Tensilon, Enlon, Reversol	**Reversal of Non-Depolarizing Neuro-Muscular Blockade:** IV: 10 mg given over 1 min, repeat q5–10 min prn (max. dose 40 mg); plus atropine, observe closely. **Myasthenia Gravis—Diagnosis:** IV: 2 mg initially; then 8 mg at 45 sec. if no response to initial dose (if a cholinergic reaction occurs with initial dose, discontinue test and administer atropine IV: 0.4–0.5 mg). Test may be repeated after 30 min if necessary. IV: 10 mg (if a cholinergic reaction occurs, may give 2 mg at 30 min to verify). Other cholinesterase medications should be withdrawn 8h prior to the diagnostic test. Equipment for support of respiration should be available.	**Injection:** 10 mg/ml	AUTONOMIC NS AGENTS (SG) Cholinergic Agents (SSG) Cholinesterase Inhibitors, Reversible (SSG) **Cost:** Medium
Effexor	See VENLAFAXINE		Aminergic Stimulant
EFLORNITHINE Ornidyl	Sleeping Sickness (T. brucei Gambiense): IV: 100 mg/kg/dose given q6h, treat for 14 days. (Give IV over at least 45 minutes).	**Injection: Concentrate:** 200 mg per ml	ANTI-INFECTIOUS AGENTS (G) Antiparasitic Agents (SG)
Elavil	See AMITRIPTYLINE		TCA Antidepressant
Elimite	See PERMETHRIN		Ectoparasiticide
Elixophyllin	See THEOPHYLLINE		Bronchodilator, Xanthine
ELIXOPHYLLIN-GG	**Bronchospasm:** PO: Initial dose 6 mg/kg; then reduce to 3 mg/kg q6h for 2 doses; maintenance does 3 mg/kg q8h (dose based on theophylline content).		**Liquid** (per 15 cc): theophylline anhydrous (100 mg), guaifenesin (100 mg)
ELIXOPHYLLIN-KI	**Bronchospasm:** PO: Initial dose 6 mg/kg (dose based on theophylline content); then reduce to 3 mg/kg q6h for 2 doses; maintenance does 3 mg/kg q8h.		**Elixir** (per 15 cc): theophylline anhydrous (80 mg), potassium iodide (130 mg), alcohol (10%)

GENERIC NAME Trade Name	INDICATIONS AND DOSAGES	DOSE FORMS	GROUP (G)/SUBGROUP (SG) Relative Cost within Group
Elmiron	See PENTOSTATIN POLYSULFATE		Interstitial Cystitis
Elspar	See ASPARAGINASE		Cancer Chemotherapy
EMCYT	See ESTRAMUSTINE		Cancer Chemotherapy
Emete-con	See BENZQUINAMIDE		Antinauseant
Eminase	See ANISTREPLASE		Thrombolytic
Emitrip	See AMITRIPTYLINE		TCA Antidepressant
EMPIRIN W/ CODEINE	See Part III		
Emulsoil	See CASTOR OIL		Irritant Laxative
ENALAPRIL Vasotec	**Hypertension:** PO: 5 mg qd to start; 10–40 mg/d maintenance in 1–2 doses. PO (patient on diuretics): 2.5 mg test dose, observe until BP stable. IV: 1.25 mg q6h (give SLOWLY over 5 minutes); doses up to 5 mg q6h have been tolerated. **Congestive Heart Failure:** PO: 2.5 mg qd or bid to start; 5–20 mg/d maintenance in 2 doses (max dose: 40 mg/d).	**Tablet:** 2.5, 5, 10, 20 mg **Injection:** 1.25 mg/ml	CV AGENTS (G) Vasodilators (SG) ACE Inhibitors (SSG) **Cost:** Medium
Endep	See AMITRIPTYLINE		TCA Antidepressant
Endoxan	See CYCLOPHOSPHAMIDE		Cancer Chemotherapy
Enduron	See METHYCLOTHIAZIDE		Sodium Diuretic
Enlon	See EDROPHONIUM		Cholinesterase Inhibitor
ENOVID 5 mg **ENOVID** 10 mg	**Hypermenorrhea:** PO: 1 tablet qd (give from 5th through 24th days of menstrual cycle). **Endometriosis:** PO: 1 tablet qd for 2 weeks, beginning on 5th day of menstrual cycle. Increase by 1 tablet at q2 weeks, up to 20 mg/d.		**Tablet:** mestranol (150 mcg), norethynodrel (9.85 mg) OR mestranol (75 mcg), norethynodrel (5 mg)
ENOXACIN Penetrex	**Urinary Tract Infections:** PO: (uncomplicated) 200 mg q12h for 7 days; (complicated) 400 mg q12h for 14 days. **Gonorrhea (uncomplicated):** PO: 400 mg given as a single dose.	**Tablet:** 200, 400 mg	ANTI-INFECTIOUS AGENTS (G) Quinolone Antibacterial (SG) **Cost:** High
ENOXAPARIN Lovenox, Low Molecular Weight Heparin	**DVT Prophylaxis (post-hip or knee replacement):** SC: 30 mg q12h.	**Injection:** 30mg/0.3ml	METABOLIC AGENTS (G) Anticoagulants And Coagulants (SG) Heparin and Related Agents (SSG)
Enulose	See LACTULOSE		Hepatic Failure, Laxative

GENERIC NAME Trade Name	INDICATIONS AND DOSAGES	DOSE FORMS	GROUP (G)/SUBGROUP (SG) Relative Cost within Group
EPHEDRINE Generic	**Pressor Agent in Hypotension:** PO: 25–50 mg 2–3 times per day. IV, SC: 25–50 mg q3–4h. IV: 5–25 mg slow PUSH; may be repeated after 10–15 min (do not exceed 150 mg in 24 hours). Pediatric PO, IV, SC: 3 mg/kg/day or 25–100 mg/square meter/day divided into 4 to 6 doses. Give IV slowly. **Asthma:** PO: 25–50 mg 2–3 times per day. Pediatric IM, IV, SC: 3 mg/kg/day or 25–100 mg/square meter/day divided into 4 to 6 doses. Give IV slowly.	**Injection:** 25, 50, mg/ml	AUTONOMIC NS AGENTS(G) SYMPATHOMIMETICS (SG) Mixed Alpha and Beta Agonist Effects (SSG) **Cost:** Medium
EPINEPHRINE Generic, Adrenalin	**Cardiac Arrest** IV: 1 mg (10 ml of 1:10,000 solution) initially, then 0.5 mg q3–5 min. **Anaphylaxis:** SC: (mild reactions) 0.3–0.5 ml of aqueous epinephrine (1:1,000, 1 mg/ml). May repeat q 15–30 min for 2–3 doses. Pediatric SC: (mild reactions) 0.01 ml/kg of aqueous epinephrine (1:1,000, 1 mg/ml). May repeat q 15–30 min for 2–3 doses. IM or IV (adult): (severe anaphylactic reactions) 0.3–0.5 ml of aqueous epinephrine (1:1,000, 1 mg/ml). May repeat q 15–30 min for 2–3 doses.	**Solution:** 0.1%, 0.25%, 0.5%, 1%, 2% **Injection Solution:** 0.1% (1:1000), 0.25%, 0.5%, 1%, 2%	AUTONOMIC NS AGENTS (G) Sympathomimetics (SG) Mixed Alpha and Beta Agonist Effects (SSG) **Cost:** Medium
Epivir	See LAMIVUDINE		Reverse Transcriptase Inhibitor
EPO	See EPOETIN ALPHA		Hematopoietic Hormone
EPOETIN ALPHA Erythropoietin Recombinant, Epogen, Procrit, EPO	**Chronic Renal Failure (**starting dose): IV, SC: 50–100 U/kg 3 times/week (target hematocrit [HCT] range = 30–36%; decrease dose if Hct increases > 4% in any 2 week period; increase dose if Hct does not increase by 5 or 6% after 8 weeks and is below target range). **Maintenance Dose** (dialysis patients): IV, SC: 75 U/kg 3 times/week (range = 12.5–525 U/kg 3 times/week). **Maintenance Dose** (nondialysis patients): IV, SC: 75–150 U/kg per week. **Anemia from Malignancy:** SC: 150 U/kg 3 times/week. **Anemia from Zidovudine Treatment:** SC: 100 U/kg 3 times/week for 8 weeks.	**Injection:** 2,000, 3,000, 4,000, 10,000 units/ml.	ANTI-INFLAMMATORY ETC AGENTS (G) Hemopoietic Colony—Stimulating Factors (SG)
Epogen	See EPOETIN ALPHA		Hematopoietic Hormone
EPOPROSTENOL Flolan	**Primary Pulmonary Hypertension:** Available only after prescriber signs contract to underwrite cost		VASODILATOR (G)
Equagesic	PO: 1–2 tablet tid, PRN pain.		**Tablet:** aspirin (325 mg), meprobamate (200 mg)
Equanil	See MEPROBAMATE		Sedative Hypnotic
Ercaf (Ergotamine a component)	See ERGOTAMINE		Vasoconstrictor (Migraine)

GENERIC NAME Trade Name	INDICATIONS AND DOSAGES	DOSE FORMS	GROUP (G)/SUBGROUP (SG) Relative Cost within Group
Ergamisol	See LEVAMISOLE		Immunomodulator
ERGOCALCIFEROL OTC, Generic, D2, Calciferol, Drisdol, Deltalin	**RDA:** PO (<25 yrs): 400 IU/d. PO (>24 yrs): 200 IU/d. **Vit. D Resistant Rickets:** PO, IM: 12,000–500,000 IU/d. **Hypophosphatemia (familial):** PO, IM: 10,000–80,000 IU/d (give with phosphate equivalent to 1–2 g of phosphorous). **Hypoparathyroidism:** PO, IM: 50,000–200,000 IU/d (give with calcium salt equivalent to 3 g calcium). Ergocalciferol (D2)	**Tablet:** 50,000 IU **Capsule:** 50,000 IU **Liquid:** 8,000 IU per ml **Injection:** 500,000 IU per ml Cholecalciferol (D3) **Tablet:** 400, 1000 IU D3	METABOLIC AGENTS (G) Calcium Kinetics Regulators (SG) D Vitamins and Related Agents (SSG) **Cost:** Medium
ERGONOVINE Generic, Ergotrate	**Control of Postpartum Bleeding:** IM: 0.2 mg q2–4 hrs PRN. PO, SL: 0.2–0.4 mg q6–12h PRN	**Tablet:** 0.2 mg **Injection:** 0.2 mg per ml	CARDIOVASCULAR AGENTS (G) Vasoconstrictors And Oxytocics (SG)
Ergostat	See ERGOTAMINE		Vasoconstrictor
ERGOTAMINE Generic	**Migraine Headaches:** SL: 2 mg at attack onset; then 2 mg q30 min PRN (max. dose 6 mg/d or 10 mg/week). Inhalation: 1 puff at onset; then 1 puff q5 min PRN (max. dose 6 puffs/d or 15 puffs/week). **Combination Agents:** Cafergot, Ercaf, Wigraine: 2 tablets at attack onset, then 1 tablet q30 min PRN (max. dose: 6 tablets per attack; do not exceed 10 tablets/week). Catatine Supps, Cafergot Supps (max dose: 2 suppositories per attack; do not exceed 5 suppositories /week).	**Tablet:** (sublingual) 2 mg **Aerosol (Medihaler):** 9 mg/ml (delivers 0.36 mg/puff) **Injection:** 1 mg/ml **Combinations:** Cafergot, Ercaf, Wigraine: (combination Tablets: 1 mg ergotamine; 100 mg caffeine). Cafatine Supps, Cafergot Supps: (combination suppositories: 2 mg ergotamine; 100 mg caffeine).	CV AGENTS (G) VASOCONSTRICTORS AND OXYTOCICS (G) **Cost:** Low
Ergotrate	See ERGONOVINE		Oxytocic/Vasoconstrictor
Ery-Tab	See ERYTHROMYCIN		Macrolide Antibiotic
Eryc	See ERYTHROMYCIN		Macrolide Antibiotic
ERYTHROMYCIN STEARATE Generic, Erythrocin Stearate	**Infections:** PO: 250–500 mg QID Pediatric: PO: 30–50 mg/kg/d in four doses.	**Tablet:** 250, 500 mg	ANTI-INFECTIOUS AGENTS (G) Macrolide Antibiotics (SG)
ERYTHROMYCIN ETHYLSUCCINATE Generic, E.E.S.	As for erythromycin stearate except that potency is less and 400 mg must be given for same effect as 250 mg of other forms.	**Tablet:** 200 mg chewable, 400mg **Suspension:** 100,200,400 mg/5 ml Powder for Suspension: 200, 400 mg/5 ml when prepared	ANTI-INFECTIOUS AGENTS (G) Macrolide Antibiotics (SG)

GENERIC NAME Trade Name	INDICATIONS AND DOSAGES	DOSE FORMS	GROUP (G)/SUBGROUP (SG) Relative Cost within Group
ERYTHROMYCIN (Base) Generic, EryC, E-Mycin, Ery-Tab,	**Infections:** PO: As for stearate. The base is acid labile and salts better absorbed	**Capsule:** 250 mg **Tablet:** (Coated) 250, 333, 500 mg	
ERYTHROMYCIN ESTOLATE Generic, Ilosone,	**Infections:** As for stearate	**Tablet:** 500 mg **Capsule:** 250 mg **Suspension:** 125 mg/5ml, 250 mg/5ml	ANTI-INFECTIOUS AGENTS (G) Macrolide Antibiotics (SG)
ERYTHROMYCIN LACTOBIONATE (IV) Generic	**Severe Infections:** 15–20 mg/kg/d is continuous infusion or 20–60 m infusion q 6h.	**Lactobionate Injection:** (powder) 0.5, 1 g per vial	ANTI-INFECTIOUS AGENTS (G) Macrolide Antibiotics (SG)
Erythropoietin Recombinant	See EPOETIN ALPHA		Hematopoietic Hormone
Eserine	See PHYSOSTIGMINE		Cholinesterase Inhibitor
Esidrix	See HYDROCHLOROTHIAZIDE		Sodium Diuretic
ESIMIL	PO: 2 tabs qd. Dosage may be increased at weekly intervals.	**Tablet:** guanethidine (10 mg), hydrochlorothiazide (25 mg)	
Eskalith	See LITHIUM		Control mania
ESMOLOL Brevibloc	**Supraventricular Tachycardia:** IV: 50 to 200 mcg/kg/min, average dose = 100 mcg/kg/min. Loading dose = 500 mcg/kg/min for 1 min, then give a 4 minute maintenance infusion of 50 mcg/kg/min for 4 minutes; if needed, increase the maintenance infusion upwards by 25 to 50 mcg/kg/min at 5 to 10 minute intervals to a maximum of 300 UCG/kg/min.	**Injection:** 10 mg/ml, 250 mg/ml	SYMPATHOPLEGICS (G) Beta Adrenergic Receptor Blockers (SG) Cardioselective (Beta 1) (SSG) **Cost:** Very High
ESTAZOLAM ProSom	**Hypnotic:** PO: 1 mg hs (max. dose 2 mg hs).	**Tablet:** 1, 2 mg	CNS AGENTS (G) Sedative-Hypnotics (G) Short Acting Hypnotics (SG) **Cost:** Medium
ESTERIFIED ESTROGENS Estratab, Menest	**Menopausal Symptoms, Atrophic Vaginitis and Related Conditions:** PO: 0.3–1.25 mg/d to start; adjust to lowest effective dose and stop treatment when possible. **Hypogonadism (female):** PO: 2.5–7.5 mg/d in 3–4 doses (cyclic treatment: treat for 20 days, then stop for 10 days, then repeat cycle if needed to induce bleeding), if bleeding occurs before end of the 10 days, start a 20-day cycle of treatment with combined estrogen-progestin (estrogen dose 2.5–7.5 mg/d, give progestin during last 5 days of the 20 days). **Ovarian Replacement:** PO: 1.25 mg/d (cyclic treatment: treat for 20 days, then stop for 10 days, then repeat cycle) **Prostatic Cancer:** PO: 1.25–2.5 mg tid.	**Tablet:** 0.3, 0.625, 1.25, 2.5 mg.	ENDOCRINE AGENTS (G) Estrogens (SG) **Cost:** Medium

GENERIC NAME Trade Name	INDICATIONS AND DOSAGES	DOSE FORMS	GROUP (G)/SUBGROUP (SG) Relative Cost within Group
Estinyl	See ETHINYL ESTRADIOL		Estrogen
Estra-D	See ESTRADIOL CYPIONATE		Estrogen
Estrace	See ESTRADIOL		Estrogen
Estraderm	See ESTRADIOL		Estrogen
ESTRADIOL Generic, Estrace, Estraderm	**Menopausal Symptoms, Female Hypogonadism, Estrogen Replacement:** PO: 1–2 mg/d (cyclic treatment: treat for first 21 days of each month, then stop for 1 week, then repeat cycle). Transdermal: 0.5 mg system 2 times/ week (cyclic treatment: treat for 3 weeks, then stop for 1 week, then repeat cycle), (use lowest effective dose; attempt taper or discontinuation at 3–6 month intervals). **Osteoporosis Prophylaxis:** PO: 0.5 mg/d (cyclic treatment: treat for 3 weeks, then stop for 1 week, then repeat cycle). **Prostatic Cancer:** PO: 1–2 mg tid.	Estrace **Patches** (Estraderm: Mg/ d estradiol delivered to patient = 0.05 or 0.1 for patches sized (sq. cm): 10 and 20 respectively (total estradiol content/patch (mg): 4 and 8 respectively).	ENDOCRINE AGENTS (G) Estrogens (SG) **Cost:** High
ESTRADIOL CYPIONATE Generic, Depogen, depGynogen, Dura-Estrin, Estra-D, Estro-Cyp, Estroject-L.A	**Menopausal Symptoms:** IM: 1–5 mg q 3–4 wks. Post-Menopausal Estrogen Replacement: IM: 1.5–2 mg q4 wks.	**Injection:** 5 mg/ ml in oil	ENDOCRINE AGENTS (G) Estrogens (SG) **Cost:** Medium
ESTRADIOL VALERATE Generic, Duragen, Dioval, Delestrogen	**Menopausal Symptoms, Atrophic Vaginitis, Estrogen Replacement:** IM: 10–20 mg q4 wks. **Prostatic Cancer:** IM: 30 mg q1–2 wks.	**Injection IM:** 10, 20, 40 mg/ ml in oil	ENDOCRINE AGENTS (G) Estrogens (SG) **Cost:** Medium
ESTRAMUSTINE Estrogen-Mustard Conjugate EMCYT	CANCER CHEMOTHERAPY (G) Alkylating Agents (SG) Nitrogen Mustards (SSG)		
Estratab	See ESTERIFIED ESTROGENS		Estrogen
Estro-Cyp	See ESTRADIOL CYPIONATE		Estrogen
Estroject-L.A.	See ESTRADIOL CYPIONATE		Estrogen
ESTRONE Aquest, Estronol	**Abnormal Uterine Bleeding:** IM: 2–5 mg/d for several days. **Estrogen Replacement:** IM: 0.1–1 mg/wk given qd or in divided doses (max. dose 2 mg/wk). **Prostatic Cancer Palliation:** IM: 2–4 mg given 2–3 times/wk.	Injection: 2, 5 mg/ml	ENDOCRINE AGENTS (G) Estrogens (SG) **Cost:** Medium

GENERIC NAME Trade Name	INDICATIONS AND DOSAGES	DOSE FORMS	GROUP (G)/SUBGROUP (SG) Relative Cost within Group
Estronol	See ESTRONE		Estrogen
ESTROPIPATE Generic, Piperazine Estrone Sulfate, Ogen, Ortho-Est	**Menopausal Symptoms, Atrophic Vaginitis and Related Conditions:** PO: 0.625–5 mg/d initially (cyclic treatment: treat for 20 days, then stop for 10 days, then repeat cycle). **Hypogonadism (female):** PO: 1.25–7.5 mg/d (cyclic treatment: treat for 20 days, then stop for 10 days, then repeat cycle if needed to induce bleeding), if withdrawal bleeding fails to occur, add a progestin during last week of the 20 day estropipate treatment. **Osteoporosis Prophylaxis:** PO: 0.625 mg/d, (cyclic treatment: treat for 21 days, then stop for 10 days, then repeat cycle).	**Tablet:** 0.625, 1.25, 2.5, 5 mg	ENDOCRINE AGENTS (G) Estrogens (SG) **Cost:** High
Estrovis	See QUINESTROL		Estrogen
ETHACRYNIC ACID Edecrin	**Edema:** PO: 50mg/d qAM to start, 25–400 mg/d maintenance as 1–2 doses. IV: (give slowly over several minutes) 0.5–1 mg/kg or may give 50 mg/d as 1 dose.	**Tablet:** 25, 50 mg **Injection:** (powder) 50 mg per vial	RENAL AGENTS (G) Sodium Diuretics (G) Potent ("Loop") Diuretics (SG) **Cost:** Medium
ETHAMBUTOL Myambutol	**Tuberculosis (Initial Therapy, given in combination):** Adults (single dose/day): 15–25 mg/kg/d (max. dose 2,500 mg/d). Adults (two doses/week): 50 mg/kg twice per week (max. dose 2,500 mg/week). Pediatric (single dose/day): 15–25 mg/kg/d (max. dose 2,500 mg/d). Pediatric (two doses/week): 50 mg/kg/week (max. dose 2,500 mg/week). **Tuberculosis (with Previous Therapy):** PO: 25 mg/kg/d once every 24 hours.	**Tablet:** 100, 400 mg	ANTI-INFECTIOUS AGENTS(G) Antituberculous And Related Agents (G) Agents of First Choice (SG) **Cost:** Low
ETHCHLOR-VYNOL Placidyl	**Hypnotic:** PO: 500–750 mg	**Capsule:** 200, 500, 750 mg	CNS AGENT (D) Sedative-Hypnotics (G) Short Acting Hypnotics (SG) **Cost:** Medium

GENERIC NAME Trade Name	INDICATIONS AND DOSAGES	DOSE FORMS	GROUP (G)/SUBGROUP (SG) Relative Cost within Group
ETHINYL ESTRADIOL Generic, Ethinyl Estradiol, Estinyl	**Menopause Symptoms and Maintenance:** PO: 0.02–1.5 mg/d to start. Treat first 21 days each month. May add progestin and treat continuously. **Late Menopause Symptoms:** PO: 0.02 mg/d to start continue for a few cycles; then 0.05 mg/d. May add progestin and treat continuously. **Female Hypogonadism:** PO: 0.05 mg qd to tid for 2 weeks within one cycle, then add progesterone in last half of cycle; treat for 3–6 months and stop for 2 months while evaluating need for ongoing therapy. **Prostatic Cancer Palliation:** PO: 0.15–2 mg tid.	**Tablet:** 0.02, 0.05, 0.5 mg.	ENDOCRINE AGENTS (G) Estrogens (SG) **Cost:** Low
Ethyol	See AMIFOSTINE		Reduce Cisplatin Toxicity
ETHIONAMIDE Trecator	**Tuberculosis (given in combination):** PO Adults: 7–15 mg/kg/d given in 4 doses q6h (max. dose 1,000 mg/d). Pediatric PO (single dose/day): 15–20 mg/kg/d (max. dose 1,000 mg/d).	**Tablet:** 250 mg	ANTI-INFECTIOUS AGENTS (G) Antituberculous And Related Agents (SG) Antituberculous Second Line Agents (SSG) **Cost:** Medium
Ethmozine	See MORICIZINE		Antiarrhythmic
ETHOSUXIMIDE Zarontin	**Seizure Disorders:** PO: 500 mg/d to start in 1–2 doses, increase by 250 mg/d q4–7d (max. dose 1,500 mg/d). Pediatric PO (3–6 y.o.): 250 mg/d to start; 20 mg/kg/d maintenance.	**Capsule:** 250 mg **Syrup:** 50 mg/ml	CNS AGENTS (G) Anticonvulsants (SG) Succinimides (SSG) **Cost:** High
ETHOTOIN Peganone	**Seizure Disorders:** PO: Up to 1,000 mg/d to start in 4–6 doses; maintenance 2,000–3,000 mg/d. Pediatric PO: Up to 750 mg/d to start; maintenance 500–2,000 mg/d (max. dose 3,000 mg/d).	**Tablet:** 250, 500 mg	ANTICONVULSANTS (G) Hydantoins and Equivalent (SG) **Cost:** Medium
Ethyl aminobenzoate	See BENZOCAINE		Local Anesthetic, Topical
ETIDOCAINE Duranest	Infiltration: 1.5% Peripheral Nerve Block: 1% Dental Alveolar Nerve Block: 1.5%	**Injection:** 1% **Injection:** (with epinephrine) 1%, 1.5%	GENERAL AND LOCAL ANESTHESIA (G) Local Anesthetics (SG) Injectable or Topical (Mucosal) (SSG) **Cost:** Medium

GENERIC NAME Trade Name	INDICATIONS AND DOSAGES	DOSE FORMS	GROUP (G)/SUBGROUP (SG) Relative Cost within Group
ETIDRONATE Didronel, Didronel IV	**Paget's disease:** PO: 5–10 mg/kg/day initially (do not exceed 6 months of therapy at this dose or, 3 months of therapy at 11–20 mg/kg/day) (max. dose 20 mg/kg/d). **Hypercalcemia Associated w/ Malignancy:** IV: 7.5 mg/kg/d for 3 days in a row (give SLOWLY over a minimum of 2h); begin PO etidronate (20 mg/kg/d) on day following last day of infusion and continue PO for 30 days. (Initial IV doses have been continued up to 7d but occurrence of hypocalcemia more common.)	**Tablet:** 200, 400 mg **Injection:** 300 mg per amp	METABOLIC AGENTS (G) Calcium Kinetics Regulators (SG) Other Calcium Regulators (SSG) **Cost:** High
ETODOLAC Lodine	**Arthritic Condition:** Initially 800–1200 mg/day in divided doses (max. dose 1200 mg/day). maintenance 600–1200 mg/day. **Pain:** 200–400 mg q6–8h (do not exceed 1200 mg/day).	**Tablet:** 400 mg **Capsule:** 200, 300 mg	NON-NARCOTIC ANALGESICS (G) Aspirin and Related NSAIDs (SG) **Cost:** High
ETOMIDATE Amidate	**Induction of General Anesthesia:** IV: 0.2 to 0.6 mg/kg given over 30 to 60 seconds (usual dose 0.3 mg/kg).	**Injection:** 2 mg/ml	GENERAL ANESTHETICS (G) Agents For Induction (SG)
ETOPOSIDE VP-16 VePesid	CANCER CHEMOTHERAPY (G) Mitotic Spindle Inhibitors (SG) Other Mitotic Spindle Inhibitors (SSG)		
ETRAFON 2/25 2/10 4/25	Depression: Combination of an antipsychotic and a TCA.	**Tablet:** contain perphenazine 2, 2 or 4 mg and amitriptyline 25, 10 or 25 mg	
ETRETINATE Tegison	**Severe, Unresponsive Psoriasis:** PO: 0.75 to 1 mg/kg/day in divided doses (do not exceed 1.5 mg/kg/day), maintenance dose 0.5 to 0.75 mg/kg/day (begin maintenance after 8 to 16 weeks).	**Capsule:** 10, 25 mg	DERMATOLOGIC AGENTS (G) Keratolytic And Keratoplastic Agents (SG) Antipsoriatic Agents (SSG) **Cost:** Low
Eulexin	See FLUTAMIDE		Androgen Antagonist
Eurax	See CROTAMITON		Ectoparasiticide
Euthroid	See LIOTRIX		Thyroid Replacement
Everone-200	See TESTOSTERONE ENANTHATE		Androgen/Anabolic
Ex-Lax	See PHENOLPHTHALEIN		Irritant Laxative
Exelderm	See SULCONAZOLE		Antifungal, Topical
Exna	See BENZTHIAZIDE		Sodium Diuretic
Exosurf Neonatal	See COLFOSCERIL		Lung Surfactant
FAMCICLOVIR Famvir	**Herpes Zoster:** PO: 500 mg q8h for 7 days.	**Tablet:** 500 mg	ANTI-INFECTIOUS AGENTS (G) Antiviral Agents, Systemic (SG)

GENERIC NAME Trade Name	INDICATIONS AND DOSAGES	DOSE FORMS	GROUP (G)/SUBGROUP (SG) Relative Cost within Group
FAMOTIDINE Pepcid, OTC	**Active Duodenal/Benign Gastric Ulcer:** PO: 40 mg/d at hs (effect usually seen in 4 weeks); or 20 mg bid. IV: 20 mg SLOWLY (infuse over > 2 min) q12h. **Hypersecretion:** PO: 20 mg QID (doses up to 160 mg have been used). GE reflux with or without erosions and esophagitis: PO: 20–40 mg bid (Treat for 6–12 weeks).	**Tablet:** 20, 40 mg **Oral Suspension:** (powder) 40 mg/5 ml when reconstituted **Injection:** 10 mg/ml	GASTROINTESTINAL AGENTS (G) Inhibitors Of Gastric Acid Secretion (SG) H2 Antagonists (SG)
Famvir	See FAMCICLOVIR		Antiviral
Fansidar	See SULFADOXINE PYRIMETHAMINE		Antimalarial
Fastin	See PHENTERMINE		Diet Pill
Feldene	See PIROXICAM		Non-Narcotic Analgetic
FELODIPINE Plendil	**Hypertension:** See discussion, Part 1	**Tablet:** (Ext'd release) 5, 10 mg	CARDIOVASCULAR AGENTS (G) Vasodilators (SG) Calcium Channel Blockers (SG) **Cost:** Low
Femotrone	See PROGESTERONE		Progestin
Femstat	See BUTOCONAZOLE		Antifungal
FENFLURAMINE Pondimin	**Exogenous Obesity:** PO: The labeled "usual" dose is 20 mg tid; increase 20 mg/d q week depending on effects; maintenance 60–120 mg/d.	**Tablet:** 20 mg	CNS AGENTS (G) Stimulants (SG) Other Schedule 3 or 4 "Diet Pills" (SSG) Atypical Diet Pill (SSG) **Cost:** Medium
FENOPROFEN Generic, Nalfon	**Arthritic Conditions:** PO: 300–600 mg q6–8h; max. dose 3200 mg/d. **Pain:** PO: 200 mg q4–6h.	**Capsule:** 200, 300 mg **Tablet:** 600 mg	ANTI-INFLAMMATORY, ETC (G) Aspirin and Related NSAIDs (SG) **Cost:** Medium
FENTANYL Generic, Sublimaze, Duragesic (Transdermal patch), Oralet (Lozenge)	**Preprocedure Sedation Adjunct:** IM,IV: 0.05–0.1 mg 30–60 min prior to procedure. Transmucosal (Oral, adults > 50 kg): give lozenge to suck on 20–40 minutes prior to desired effect. **Chronic Pain:** Transdermal: 1 patch q72h PRN (nominal delivery rate of 25 mcg/h); in non-opioid-tolerant patients begin with smallest patch and assess analgesic potency after the first 24 hours; may increase initial dose after 3 days but subsequent increases should be made only q6days (max. dose frequency = 1 patch q48h—multiple patches may be used for delivery rates > 100 mcg/h when appropriate).	**Injection:** 0.05 mg/ml. **Duragesic Transdermal** (size & Fentanyl content): 10 sq.cm & 2.5 mg; 20 sq.cm & 5 mg; 30 sq.cm & 7.5 mg; 40 sq.cm & 10 mg. **Transmucosal Lozenge** (Oralet): 200 mcg, 300 mcg, 400 mcg.	NARCOTIC ANALGESICS (G) Intermediate Potency (SG) **Cost:** Very High

GENERIC NAME Trade Name	INDICATIONS AND DOSAGES	DOSE FORMS	GROUP (G)/SUBGROUP (SG) Relative Cost within Group
Fentanyl-Droperidol Combination Generic, Innovar.		**Injection:** (0.05 mg/ml fentanyl, 2.5 mg droperidol) in 2,5 ml amps.	GENERAL ANESTHETICS (G) Preprocedural Agents (Conscious Sedation) (SG) Antipsychotic-Opiate Combination (SSG) **Cost:** High
Fenylhist	See DIPHENHYDRAMINE		Antihistamine
Feosol	See FERROUS SULFATE		Ferrous Ion
Feostat	See FERROUS FUMARATE		Ferrous Ion
Fergon	See FERROUS GLUCONATE		Ferrous Ion
FERROUS FUMARATE Generic, Fumerin, Fumiron, Feostat 33% iron	**Iron Replacement:** PO: 100 mg/d.	**Tablet:** 63 mg, 195 mg, 200 mg, 324 mg, 325 mg, 350 mg **Tablet:** (chewable) 100 mg **Capsule:** (Ext'd release) 325 mg **Suspension:** 100 mg, per 5 ml. **Drops:** 45 mg per 0.6 ml	METABOLIC AGENTS (G) Specific ions (SG) **Cost:** Medium
FERROUS GLUCONATE Generic, Fergon, Simron	**Iron Replacement in Deficiency States:** Gluconate = 11.6% elemental iron. PO: 300 mg/d.	**Tablet:** 300 mg, 320 mg, 325 mg. **Tablet:** (Ext'd release) 320 mg. **Capsule:** (soft gel) 86 mg **Elixir:** 300 mg per 5 ml.	METABOLIC AGENTS (G) Specific Ions (G) **Cost:** Low
FERROUS SULFATE Generic, Feosol	**Iron Replacement in Deficiency States:** Sulfate = 20% elemental iron. PO: 100 to 200 mg (2 to 3 mg/kg) elemental iron daily in 3 to 4 divided doses. Pediatric PO: (2 to 12 yrs): 3mg/kg/day in 3 to 4 divided doses. Pediatric PO: (6 mo. to 2 yrs): up to 6 mg/kg/day in 3 to 4 divided doses. PO (pregnancy): 30 mg/d. PO (Ext'd release): 525 mg qd or bid.	**Tablet:** 195 mg, 300 mg, 324 mg. **Tablet:** (Ext'd release) 525 mg . **Capsule:** 250 mg. **Syrup:** 90 mg, per 5 ml. **Elixir:** 220 mg per 5 ml. **Drops:** 75 mg per 0.6 ml.	SPECIFIC IONS (G) **Cost:** Low
Feverall	See ACETAMINOPHEN		Non-Narcotic Analgesic
FEXOFENADINE Allegra	**Type I Allergic Reactions:** (allergic rhinitis: 60 mg 1–3x/d)	**Capsules:** 60 mg	ANTI-INFLAMMATORY ETC AGENTS (G) Antihistamines H1 Antagonists (SG) Non-sedating (SSG) **Cost:** High

GENERIC NAME Trade Name	INDICATIONS AND DOSAGES	DOSE FORMS	GROUP (G)/SUBGROUP (SG) Relative Cost within Group
FILGRASTIM Neupogen, granulocyte colony-stimulating factor, G-CSF	**Myeloid Recovery After Chemotherapy:** IV, SC: 5 mcg/kg/d as a single dose. Increase 5 mcg/kg for each cycle of therapy depending on nadir of absolute neutrophil count. **Congenital Neutropenia:** SC: 6 mcg/kg bid. **Idiopathic or Cyclic Neutropenia:** SC: 5 mcg/kg/d.	**Injection:** 300 mcg/ml.	ANTI-INFLAMMATORY AGENTS (G) Hemopoietic Colony—Stimulating Factors (SG)
FINASTERIDE Proscar	**Symptomatic BPH:** Probably ineffective PO: 5 mg qd	**Tablets:** 5 mg	ENDOCRINE AGENTS (G) Testosterone Antagonist (SG) **Cost:** High
FIORINAL	Proprietary analgesic mixture containing, often unrecognized, a barbiturate sedative.		
Flagyl	See METRONIDAZOLE		Antimicrobial
Fleet Phospho-Soda	See SODIUM PHOSPHATE		Saline laxative
Flexeril	See CYCLOBENZAPRINE		Muscle Relaxant
Flexon	See ORPHENADRINE		Muscle Relaxant
Florinef	See FLUDROCORTISONE		Corticosteroid
Floxin	See OFLOXACIN		Quinolone Antibacterial
FLOXURIDINE **FUDR** **QUAD**	Cancer Chemotherapy (G) Antimetabolites (SG) Pyrimidine Analogues (SSG)		
FLUCONAZOLE Diflucan	**Candidiasis (Oropharyngeal, Esophageal):** PO, IV: 200 mg (day 1), then 100 mg qd (max. dose 400 mg/d, treat for three weeks minimum and for two weeks post-symptomatic improvement). **Candidiasis (UTI, other):** PO, IV: 50–200 mg/d (max. dose 400 mg/d). **Cryptococcal Meningitis:** PO, IV: 400 mg (day 1), then 200 mg qd (max. dose 400 mg/d, treat for 10–12 weeks after CSF cultures negative). Cryptococcal meningitis (HIV patients, relapse prevention): PO, IV: 200 mg qd.	**Tablet:** 50, 100, 200 mg **Oral Suspension:** (powder) 10 mg/ml, 40 mg/ml when reconstituted **Injection:** 200 mg/100 ml, 400 mg/200 ml	ANTI-INFECTIOUS AGENTS (G) Systemic Antifungal Agents (SG) **Cost:** High
FLUCYTOSINE Alkaban, 5-FC	**Fungal Infections:** PO: 50–150 mg/kg/d in 4 doses (ingest capsules over 15 minutes to minimize nausea).	**Capsule:** 250, 500 mg	ANTI-INFECTIOUS AGENTS (G) Systemic Antifungal Agents (SG) **Cost:** Low
Fludara	See FLUDARABINE		
FLUDARABINE Fludara	CANCER CHEMOTHERAPY (G) Antimetabolites (SG) Pyrimidine Analogues (SSG)		

GENERIC NAME Trade Name	INDICATIONS AND DOSAGES	DOSE FORMS	GROUP (G)/SUBGROUP (SG) Relative Cost within Group
FLUDROCORTI-SONE Florinef	**Addison's disease:** PO: 0.1 mg/day (doses range from 0.1 mg 3 times/ week to 0.2 mg/day). PO (Alternate dose): 0.05–0.1 mg/day.	**Tablet:** 0.1 mg	ENDOCRINE AGENTS (G) Mineralocorticoids (SG) **Cost:** Low
Flumadine	See RIMANTADINE		Antiviral
FLUMAZENIL Romazicon	**Reverse The Sedation of Benzodiazepines:** In therapeutic situation: 0.4–1.0 mg IV in 0.2 mg increments. Overdose in street use: 1–3 mg (in divided doses).	**Injection:** 0.1 mg/ml	ANTIDOTES AND AGENTS USED POISONINGS (G)
FLUNISOLIDE Intranasal (Nasalide), Deep (AeroBid)	**Bronchial Asthma:** Inhalation: 2 puffs (500 mcg) bid (max. dose 8 puffs/day [=2,000 mcg]). Children (6 to 15 yrs): 2 puffs bid (max. dose 4 puffs/day [=1,000 mcg]). **Rhinitis, Nasal Polyps:** Intranasal: 2 sprays (50 mcg) in each nostril bid initially, may increase to tid PRN (max. dose 16 sprays/day [= 400 mcg/day]). Pediatric Intranasal: 1 spray in each nostril tid [= 200 mcg/day].	**Intranasal Spray (Nasalide):** approx. 25 mcg flunisolide is delivered each spray. **Aerosol (Aero-Bid):** approx. 250 mcg is delivered by each puff.	RESPIRATORY AGENTS (G) Anti-inflammatory Steroids (SG) **Cost:** Medium
FLUOCINOLONE ACETONIDE Generic, Fluonid	Apply to affected area 2 to 4 times a day.	**Ointment:** 0.025%. **Cream:** 0.01.025%. **Cream (Synalar—HP):** 0.2%. **Solution:** 0.01%. **Shampoo:** 0.01%. **Oil:** 0.01%.	DERMATOLOGIC AGENTS (G) Anti-Inflammatory Steroids, Topical (SG) **Cost:** Medium
FLUOCINONIDE Generic	Apply to affected area 2 to 4 times a day. Maximum 50 grams per week.	**Cream:** 0.05%. **Ointment:** 0.05%. **Solution:** 0.05%. **Gel:** 0.05%.	DERMATOLOGIC AGENTS (G) Anti-Inflammatory Steroids, Topical (SG) **Cost:** Medium
Fluonid	See FLUOCINOLONE ACETONIDE		Corticosteroid
FLUOROMETHO-LONE Generic, FML, FML Forte	**Solution, Suspension:** 1 or 2 drops into the conjunctival sac qh during the day and q2h during the night. **Ointment:** apply thin coating QID-tid to start, after response noted apply bid then qd.	**Suspension:** 0.1%, 0.25% **Ointment:** 0.1%	OPHTHALMIC AGENTS (G) Anti-Inflammatory Steroids (SG) **Cost:** High
FLUOROURACIL Generic, Adrucil	5-FUCANCER CHEMOTHERAPY (G) Antimetabolites (SG) Pyrimidine Analogues (SSG)		
FLUOXETINE Prozac	**Depression, Obsessive-Compulsive Disorder:** Initial 20 mg qAM (do not exceed a max. dose of 80 mg/day).	**Capsules:** 10, 20 mg **Liquid:** 4 mg/ml	CNS AGENTS (G) OTHER AMINERGIC STIMULANTS (G) Specific Serotonin Uptake Inhibitors (SSRI) (SG) **Cost:** Medium

GENERIC NAME Trade Name	INDICATIONS AND DOSAGES	DOSE FORMS	GROUP (G)/SUBGROUP (SG) Relative Cost within Group
FLUOXYMEST-ERONE Halotestin	**Androgen Replacement Therapy:** PO: 5–20 mg/day	**Tablet:** 2, 5, 10 mg	ENDOCRINE AGENTS (G) Androgenic/Anabolic Steroids (SG) **Cost:** Medium
FLUPHENAZINE Generic, Prolixin, Permitil	**Psychotic Disorders:** PO: 0.5–10 mg/d in 3–4 doses (max. dose 20 mg/d); usual maintenance = 1–5 mg/d. Geriatric PO: 1–2.5 mg/d initial dose. IV: 1.25 mg to start; 2.5–10 mg/d maintenance in 3–4 doses. PO (Tab's): 1, 2.5, 5, 10 mg	**Liquid:** 5 mg/ml **Elixir:** 2.5 mg/ 5 ml **Injection:** 2.5, 5 mg/ml	CNS AGENTS (G) Antipsychotics (SG) Prominent Extrapyramidal Effects (SSG) **Cost:** Low
FLURANDRENO-LIDE Cordran	Apply to affected area 2 to 3 times a day.	**Ointment:** 0.025%, 0.05%. **Cream:** 0.025%, 0.05%. **Lotion:** 0.05%. **Tape:** 4 mcg per square cm.	DERMATOLOGIC AGENTS (G) Anti-Inflammatory Steroids, Topical (SG) **Cost:** High
FLURAZEPAM Generic, Dalmane	**Hypnotic:** PO: 15–30 mg at hs. (Start at lower doses in geriatric and debilitated pts.)	**Tablet:** 15, 30 mg	CNS AGENTS (G) Sedative-Hypnotics (SG) Short Acting Hypnotics (SG) **Cost:** Low
FLURBIPROFEN Generic, Ansaid	**Arthritic Conditions:** PO: 200–300 mg/d; given as 2–4 doses (max single dose 100 mg).	**Tablet:** 50, 100 mg	ANTI-INFLAMMATORY AGENTS (G) Non-Narcotic Analgesics (SG) Aspirin and Related NSAIDs (SG) **Cost:** Medium
FLUTAMIDE Eulexin	**Metastatic Ca of Prostate (in Combination with LHRH Antagonist):** PO: 2 capsules q8h, i.e., 750 mg/d.	**Capsule:** 125 mg	ENDOCRINE AGENTS (G) Testosterone Antagonist (SG)
FLUVASTATIN Lescol	PO: 20 mg q hs initially, then maintenance 20 to 40 mg/day as a single or divided dose (the latter may improve HDL-C slightly).	**Capsule:** 20, 40 mg	METABOLIC AGENTS (G) Lipid Lowering Drugs (SG) HMG-CoA Reductase Inhibitors (SG) **Cost:** Medium
FLUVOXAMINE Luvox	**Obsessive Compulsive State:** PO: 100 mg bid	**Tablet:** 50, 100 mg	CNS AGENTS (G) Aminergic Stimulant (SG) SSRI (SSG)
FOLIC ACID Generic, Pteroylglutamic Acid, Folvite, Folacin	**Usual Therapeutic Dosage:** PO: up to 1 mg daily. **Maintenance Doses:** PO (Pregnancy and lactation): 0.8 mg/day. PO (Adults and children > 4 yrs): 0.4 mg/day. PO (Children < 4 yrs): up to 0.3 mg/day. PO (Infants): 0.1 mg/day. **RDA:** PO (men): 0.15–0.2 mg/d. PO (women): 0.15–0.18 mg/d.	**Tablet:** 0.4, 0.8 mg (OTC), 1 mg **Injection:** 5 mg/ml	METABOLIC AGENTS (G) Vitamins (SG) **Cost:** Low
Folacin	See FOLIC ACID		
Folinic Acid	See LEUCOVORIN		Folate Active Form
Folvite	See FOLIC ACID		Vitamin
Fortaz	See CEFTAZIDIME		Lactam Antibiotic

GENERIC NAME Trade Name	INDICATIONS AND DOSAGES	DOSE FORMS	GROUP (G)/SUBGROUP (SG) Relative Cost within Group
Fosamax	See ALENDRONATE		Inhibit Osteoclasts
FOSCARNET Foscavir	**CMV Retinitis**: IV: 60 mg/kg (infused at a constant rate, at a minimum of one hour) q8h for 2–3 weeks to start; maintenance 90–120 mg/kg/day infused over 2 hours (higher maintenance doses used if retinitis progresses and if tolerated; initial dosage may be repeated as well).	**Injection:** 24 mg/ml	OPHTHALMIC AGENTS (G) Antiviral Agents (SG)
Foscavir	See FOSCARNET		Antiviral
FOSFOMYCIN Monurol	**Uncomplicated UTI in women:** PO: Single 3 gm dose	**Sachet:** 3 gm	ANTI-INFECTIOUS AGENTS (G) Non-Sulfonamide Urinary Tract Agent (SG)
FOSINOPRIL Monopril	**Hypertension:** PO: 10 mg qd to start; 20–40 mg/d maintenance in 1–2 doses (max dose 80 mg/d). PO (patient on diuretics): 10 mg qd to start, observe until BP stable.	**Tablet:** 10, 20 mg	CV AGENTS (G) Vasodilators (G) ACE Inhibitors (SG) **Cost:** Medium
FOSPHENYTOIN Cerebyx	**When Parenteral Phenytoin Is Indicated:** IV: Initially 10–20 mg/kg of phenytoin equivalent (drug is so labeled), then 4–6 mg/kg/d	**Injection:** 500 mg phenytoin in 10 ml, 100 mg in 2 ml for dilution	CNS AGENTS (G) Anticonvulsant (SG)
FUDR	See FLOXURIDINE		
Fulvicin-U/F	See GRISEOFULVIN		Antifungal, systemic
Fumerin	See FERROUS FUMARATE		Ferrous Ion
Fumiron	See FERROUS FUMARATE		Ferrous Ion
Fungizone	See AMPHOTERICIN B		Antifungal
Fungoid	See TRIACETIN		Antifungal, Topical
Furadantin	See NITROFURANTOIN		Antibacterial
FUROSEMIDE Generic, Lasix	**Peripheral Edema:** PO: 20–80 mg/d qAM to start (increase by 20–40 mg q6–8h if no response); 20–600 mg/d maintenance as 1–2 doses. IV, IM: 20–40 mg initial dose, repeat once in 2 hours; may increase by 20 mg 2 hours later until desired effect is seen. May repeat the last dose given once or twice per day until adequate diuresis is obtained (infuse IV doses over 1–2 min). **Acute Pulmonary Edema:** IV: 40 mg (infuse over 1–2 min); may give 80 mg in 1 hour if no response to initial dose. **Renal Failure:** PO: 80–2500 mg/d as 1–4 doses IV: 40–1000 mg/d as 1–8 doses (give 1000 mg dose over 30 minutes or more). **Hypertension:** PO: 40 mg bid.	**Tablet:** 20, 40, 80 mg **Injection:** 10 mg/ml **Oral Solution:** 10 mg/ml, 40 mg/5 ml	RENAL AGENTS (G) Sodium Diuretics (G) Potent ("Loop") Diuretics (SG) **Cost:** Low
G-CSF	See FILGRASTIM		Granulocyte Stimulation
G-well	See LINDANE		Ectoparasiticide

GENERIC NAME Trade Name	INDICATIONS AND DOSAGES	DOSE FORMS	GROUP (G)/SUBGROUP (SG) Relative Cost within Group
GABAPENTIN Neurontin	**Partial and Generalized Seizures:** PO: 900–1800 mg per day given in 3 divided doses. (To decrease side effects, give first dose at hs and gradually raise dose over first 3 days [doses up to 2400–3600 mg/day have been tolerated].)	**Capsule:** 100, 300, 400 mg	CNS AGENTS ANTICONVULSANTS (SG) Miscellaneous Anticonvulsants (SSG)
GALACTOSIDASE ALPHA-D OTC, Alpha-D-Galactosidase, Beano	PO: 3 to 8 qtt per average sized meal.	**Liquid:** >= 175 galactose units per 5-drop dosage.	GASTROINTESTINAL (G) Enzymes (SG)
Gamulin Rh	See RHo(D)IMMUNE GLOBULIN		RH Antibody
GANCICLOVIR Cytovene	**CMV Retinitis (systemic tx):** IV: 5 mg/kg (infused over 1 hour) q12h (for 14–21 days) to start; followed by 5 mg/kg/day IV infusion (given over 1 hour) 7 days a week.	**Powder for injection:** (lyophilized) 500 mg/vial.	OPHTHALMIC AGENTS (G) Antiviral Agents (SG)
Gantanol	See SULFAMETHOXAZOLE		Sulfonamide Antibacterial
Gantrisin	See SULFISOXAZOLE		Sulfonamide Antibacterial
Garamycin	See GENTAMICIN		Aminoglycoside
Gastrocrom	See CROMOLYN		Mast Cell Inhibitor
Gelumina	See ALUMINUM HYDROXIDE GEL		Reduce Phosphate Level
Gelusil	See ALUMINUM HYDROXIDE with MAGNESIUM TRISILICATE		Antacid
GEMFIBROZIL Generic, Lopid	**Hyperlipidemia:** PO: 450–600 mg bid,1/2 hour prior to AM and PM meals (max. dose: 1500 mg/d).	**Capsule:** 300 mg **Tablet:** 600 mg	METABOLIC AGENTS (G) LIPID LOWERING DRUGS (G) Other Lipid Lowering Agents (SG) **Cost:** High
Genabid	See PAPAVERINE		Vasodilator
GENTAMICIN Generic, Garamycin, Jenamicin	**Severe infections:** IM, IV: 3–5 mg/kg/d in 3–4 doses after an initial loading dose of 2 mg/kg followed by maintenance, e.g., 1.7 mg/kg q8h. Max. doses 0.4 g/d. Pediatric IM, IV: 2–2.5 mg/kg q8h **Mild to Moderate Infections:** IM, IV: 3 mg/kg/d in 3 doses. **Bacterial Endocarditis Prophylaxis:** PO: 1–2 g ampicillin plus 1.5 mg/kg gentamycin IV or IM ½ h prior to procedure; then 6 h after initial dose give 1.5 g ampicillin. Apply 1 to 4 times daily. Cover with sterile bandage as appropriate.	**Injection:** 2,10,40 mg/ml **Ointment:** 0.1%, 0.3% **Cream:** 0.1% **Solution:** 0.3%	ANTI-INFECTIOUS CHEMOTHERAPY (G) Aminoglycosides (SG) OPHTHALMIC AGENTS (G) Antibacterial (SG) **Cost:** Low
Geocillin	See INDANYL CARBENICILLIN		Lactam Antibiotic
Geopen	See CARBENICILLIN		Lactam Antibiotic
Gesterol 50	See PROGESTERONE		Progestin
Gesterol L.A. 250	See HYDROXYPROGESTERONE		Progestin
GLATIRAMER Copaxone	**Multiple Sclerosis (relapsing):** SC: 20 mg daily	**Ampoule:** 20 mg of Lyophilized Material	ANTI-INFLAMMATORY ETC (G) Immunomodulating (SG) **Cost:** Prohibitively expensive

GENERIC NAME Trade Name	INDICATIONS AND DOSAGES	DOSE FORMS	GROUP (G)/SUBGROUP (SG) Relative Cost within Group
GLIMEPIRIDE Amaryl	**Non-Insulin Dependent Diabetes:** Initially 1–2 mg/d increasing at 1–2 week intervals to, usually, 4 mg/d.	**Tablets:** 1, 2, 4 mg	ENDOCRINE AGENTS (G) Oral Antidiabetic Agents (SG) Sulfonylurea (SSG)
GLIPIZIDE Generic, Glucotrol	**Diabetes:** PO: 5 mg with breakfast initially. Increase dose 5 mg/d every three months if glycosylated Hgb control is inadequate. No benefit established above 10 mg. Selected patients may benefit up to 20 mg.	**Tablet:** 5, 10 mg **Tablet:** (Ext'd release) 5, 10 mg	ENDOCRINE AGENTS (G) Oral Antidiabetic Agents (SG) Sulfonylurea (SSG) **Cost:** Medium
GLUCAGON INJECTION	**Hypoglycemia, Stomach and small bowel imaging:** 0.25–0.5 mg IV for rapid, brief effect; 1–2 mg IM or IV for longer duration.	**Powder for injection:** 1, 10 mg/vial	ENDOCRINE AGENTS (G) Miscellaneous (SG)
Glucocerebrosidase-β-glucosidase	See ALGLUCERASE		Enzyme
Glucophage	See METFORMIN		Oral Antidiabetic Agent
Glucotrol	See GLIPIZIDE		Oral antidiabetic
GLUTETHIMIDE Generic, Doriden	**Hypnotic:** PO: 250–500 mg hs.	**Tablet:** 250, 500 mg	CNS SEDATIVE-HYPNOTICS (G) Short Acting Hypnotics (SG) **Cost:** Low
GLYBURIDE Generic, DiaBeta, Micronase, Glynase PresTab	**Diabetes:** PO (DiaBeta, Micronase): 1.25–5 mg/d at breakfast to start, then maintenance of 1.25–20 mg/d. Increase daily dose in increments of 2.5 mg at weekly intervals while monitoring response (max. dose 20 mg/d). PO (Glynase PresTab): 1.5–3 mg/d at breakfast to start, then maintenance of 0.75–12 mg/d (max. dose 12 mg/d). Increase daily dose in increments of 1.5 mg at weekly intervals while monitoring response. Give dose q12h if > 6 mg/d.	**Tablet** (DiaBeta, Micronase): 1.25, 2.5, 5 mg **Tablet** (Glynase PresTab): 1.5, 3, 6 mg	ENDOCRINE AGENTS (G) Oral Antidiabetic Agents (SG) Sulfonylurea (SSG) **Cost:** Medium
GLYCERIN Generic, Osmoglyn	**Edematous Cornea:** Apply 1–2 drops to cornea after local anesthetic. **Lower IOP in Glaucoma, Cataract Surgery (Pre-op):** PO: 1–2 g/kg 1–1.5 h prior to surgery. Off label use IV to lower intracranial pressure.	**Solution:** topical (Ophthalgan) **Solution:** 50%, oral (0.6 g glycerin/ml)	RENAL AGENTS (G) Osmotic Diuretics (SG) **Cost:** High
Glyceryl Trinitrate	See NITROGLYCERIN		Vasodilator
GLYCOPYRROLATE Generic, Robinul	**Peptic Ulcer:** PO: 1–2 mg bid-tid, maintenance 1 mg bid. IV, IV: 0.1–0.2 mg tid or QID. **Pre-anesthetic:** IM: 0.004 mg/kg given 30–60 minutes prior to procedure.	**Tablet:** 1, 2 mg **Injection:** 0.2 mg/ml	AUTONOMIC NS AGENTS (G) Parasympatholytics (SG) Quaternary Amines (SSG) **Cost:** PO: Medium IV, IM: High

GENERIC NAME Trade Name	INDICATIONS AND DOSAGES	DOSE FORMS	GROUP (G)/SUBGROUP (SG) Relative Cost within Group
GOLD SODIUM THIOMALATE Myochrysine, Aurolate	**Rheumatoid Arthritis (initial therapy):** IM: 50 mg/week to a total of 1.0 gram (if some response by 700 mg then longer intervals) (if no improvement after 1 gram total dose is reached, may increase dose by steps of 10 mg every 1–4 weeks—not to exceed 100 mg in any single dose). **Rheumatoid Arthritis (maintenance therapy):** IM: 25–50 mg every other week for 2–20 weeks; then 25–50 mg every third or fourth week may be given for indefinite maintenance.	**Injection:** 50 mg/ml (2 & 10 ml vials)	ANTIINFLAMMATORY ETC AGENTS (G) Gold Compounds and Antirheumatic (SG) **Cost:** High
GoLYTELY	See POLYETHYLENE GLYCOL-ELECTROLYTE SOLUTIONS		Bowel Cleanser
GOSERELIN Zoladex	**Endometriosis, Prostatic Carcinoma:** SC: 3.6 mg q28d.	**Implant:** 3.6 mg	ENDOCRINE AGENTS (G) Hypothalamic Releasing Factor Antagonist (SG)
GRANISETRON Kytril	**Chemotherapy Emesis Prophylaxis:** IV: 10 mg/kg (given SLOWLY over 5 minutes), give dose 30 minutes prior to chemotherapy. Pediatric IV (2 to 16 yrs): 10 mcg/kg kg (given SLOWLY over 5 minutes), give dose 30 minutes prior to chemotherapy.	**Injection:** 1 mg/ml	GASTROINTESTINAL AGENTS (G) ANTIEMETICS (SG) Serotonin Antagonists (SG) **Cost:** High
Granulocyte Colony-Stimulating Factor	See FILGRASTIM		Repair neutropenia
Grifulvin	See GRISEOFULVIN		Antifungal
Gris-PEG	See GRISEOFULVIN		Antifungal
Grisactin	See GRISEOFULVIN		Antifungal
GRISEOFULVIN Generic, Fulvicin U/F, Grifulvin, Grisactin, Gris-PEG	**Tinea (corporis, cruris, capitis):** PO: 0.5 g/d microsize crystals OR 330–375 mg/d ultramicrosize in 1–2 doses. **Tinea (pedis, unguium):** PO: 0.75–1.0 g/d microsize crystals OR 660–750 mg/d ultramicrosize in 1–2 doses. **Fungal Infections:** Pediatric PO (> 23 kg): 250–500 mg/d microsize OR 165–330 mg/d ultramicrosize in 1–2 doses. Pediatric PO (13.5–23 kg): 125–250 mg/d microsize OR 82.5–165 mg/d ultramicrosize in 1–2 doses.	**Capsule:** 125, 250 mg **Tablet:** 250, 500 mg **Oral Suspension:** 125 mg/5 ml Ultramicrosize **Tablet:** 125, 165, 250, 330 mg	ANTI-INFECTIOUS AGENTS (G) Systemic Antifungal Agents (SG) **Cost:** Low

GENERIC NAME Trade Name	INDICATIONS AND DOSAGES	DOSE FORMS	GROUP (G)/SUBGROUP (SG) Relative Cost within Group
GUAIFENESIN Generic, OTC,	PO: (Adults and children > 12 yrs): 100–400 mg q4h (max. dose 2.4 g/day). Pediatric PO: (6 to 12 yrs): 100–200 mg q4h (max. dose 1.2 g/day). Pediatric PO: (2 to 6 yrs): 50–100 mg q4h (max. dose 600 mg/day).	**Tablet:** 100, 200 mg **Tablet:** (ER) 600 mg **Liquid:** 100 mg/5 ml, 200 mg/5 ml **Capsule:** 200 mg **Capsule:** (ER) 300 mg **Syrup:** 100 mg/5 ml	RESPIRATORY AGENTS (G) Expectorants and Mucolytic Agents (SG) **Cost:** Low
GUANABENZ Wytensin	**Hypertension:** PO: 4 mg bid initially, increment by 4–8 mg per day q1–2 weeks, maintenance dose 8–64 mg/d in 2 divided doses.	**Tablet:** 4, 8 mg	AUTONOMIC NS AGENTS (G) Sympathoplegics (SG) Centrally-Acting Sympathoplegics (SSG) **Cost:** Medium
GUANADREL Hylorel	**Hypertension:** PO: 10 mg/d initially; 20–75 mg/d maintenance as 2–4 doses/d.	**Tablet:** 10, 25 mg	AUTONOMIC NS AGENTS(G) Sympathoplegics (G) Adrenergic Neuron (Postganglionic) Blockers (SG) **Cost:** High
GUANETHIDINE Ismelin	**Hypertension:** PO (outpatient): 10 mg/d initially; 20–50 mg/d maintenance as single dose. PO (inpatient): 25–50 mg/d initially, increase by 25–50 mg/d or qod as indicated.	**Tablet:** 10, 25 mg	AUTONOMIC NS AGENTS(G) Sympathoplegics (G) Adrenergic Neuron (Postganglionic) Blockers (SG)
GUANFACINE Tenex	**Hypertension:** PO: 1 mg qhs; if needed, in 3–4 weeks increase to 2 mg qhs; and later to 3 mg qhs.	**Tablet:** 1 mg	AUTONOMIC AGENTS (G) Sympathoplegics (SG) Centrally-Acting Sympathoplegics (SG) **Cost:** Medium
HALAZEPAM Paxipam	**Sedation:** PO: 20–40 mg tid or QID to start; maintenance 80–160 mg/d in 3–4 doses.	**Tablet:** 20, 40 mg	CNS AGENTS (G) Sedative-Hypnotics (SG) Intermediate-Acting (SG)
HALCINONIDE Halog	Apply to affected area 1–3 times a day.	**Ointment:** 0.1%. **Cream:** 0.025%, 0.1%. **Solution:** 0.01%. **Cream (Halog-E):** 0.1%	DERMATOLOGIC AGENTS (G) Anti-Inflammatory Steroids, Topical (SG) **Cost:** High
Halcion	See TRIAZOLAM		Hypnotic, ultra-short
Haldol	See HALOPERIDOL		Antipsychotic
Halog	See HALCINONIDE		Corticosteroid, topical

GENERIC NAME Trade Name	INDICATIONS AND DOSAGES	DOSE FORMS	GROUP (G)/SUBGROUP (SG) Relative Cost within Group
HALOPERIDOL Generic, Haldol	**Psychotic Disorders:** PO: 0.5–2 mg bid or tid to start (3–5 mg if symptoms severe); max. dose 100 mg/d. Pediatric (3–12 yrs or 15–40 kg) PO: 0.5 mg/d to start, increase by 0.5 mg/d q1week; maintenance 0.05–0.15 mg/kg/d in 2–3 doses (max. dose 6 mg/d). **IM Depot (Decanoate):** Give deep IM injection q 4 weeks, may start with 10–15 times daily oral dose (do not exceed 100 mg q 4 wks). **Severe Agitation:** IM (lactate): 2–5 mg q60 min–8h, then PO maintenance dosing. **Tourette's Syndrome:** Pediatric PO: 0.05–0.075 mg/kg/d in 2–3 doses (max. dose 6 mg/d).	**Tablet:** 0.5, 1, 2, 5, 10, 20 mg **Liquid:** 2 mg/ml **Injection:** 5 mg/ml (as lactate), 50 mg (as 70.5 mg decanoate)/ml, 100 mg (as 141.04 mg decanoate/ml)	CNS AGENTS (G) Antipsychotics (G) Prominent Extrapyramidal Effects (SG) **Cost:** Low
HALOPROGIN Halotex	**Tinea pedis, cruris, corporis, manuum:** Topical: Apply to affected area bid for 2–3 weeks.	**Cream:** 1% **Solution:** 1%	DERMATOLOGIC AGENTS (G) Topical Fungicides (SG) **Cost:** High
Halotestin	See FLUOXYMESTERONE		Androgen
Halotex	See HALOPROGIN		Fungicide, Topical
Harmonyl	See DESERPIDINE		Hypotensive
HCTZ	See HYDROCHLOROTHIAZIDE		Sodium Diuretic
Healon	See HYALURONATE		Viscoelastic filler
Hemabate	See CARBOPROST		Oxytocic PG
Hemofil	See ANTIHEMOPHILIC FACTOR VIII (Non-recombinant)		Hematopoietic Hormone
HEPARIN Generic, Heparin Injection, Liquaemin Sodium	Note: Doses are recommendations for initiating therapy. Adjust dosage so that APTT is 1.5–2 times control value or when WBCT is 2.5–3 times control value. **Full-Dose Anticoagulation:** IV: 10,000 units initially, then 5,000–10,000 units q4–6h. IV infusion: Initially 5,000 unit loading dose, then 20,000–40,000 units/d in 1000 ml isotonic saline (continuous). SC: 10,000–20,000 units to start, then 8,000–10,000 units q8h. (Alternatively, follow initial dose with 15,000–20,000 units q12h.) **Low-Dose Thromboembolism Prophylaxis:** SC: 5000 units q8–12h (treat for 7 days postoperatively; give initial dose 2 h prior to surgery). Discontinue and begin protamine sulfate therapy if bleeding continues postoperatively.	**Injection:** 1,000, 2,500, 5,000, 10,000, 20,000, 40,000 units/ml in vials	METABOLIC AGENTS (G) Anticoagulants And Coagulants (SG) Heparin and Related Agents (SSG) **Cost:** Low
Heparin Injection	See HEPARIN		Anticoagulant
Herplex	See IDOXURIDINE		Antiviral
Hexadrol	See DEXAMETHASONE		Corticosteroid
Hexalen	See ALTRETAMINE		Cancer Chemotherapy

GENERIC NAME Trade Name	INDICATIONS AND DOSAGES	DOSE FORMS	GROUP (G)/SUBGROUP (SG) Relative Cost within Group
Hexamethylmelamine	See ALTRETAMINE		Cancer Chemotherapy
HEXOCYCLIUM Tral	**Peptic Ulcer:** PO: 25 mg QID (with meals and hs).	**Tablet:** 25 mg	AUTONOMIC NS AGENTS (G) Parasympatholytics (G) Quaternary Amines (SG) **Cost:** High
Hiprex	See METHENAMINE		Antibacterial, Urinary
Hismanal	See ASTEMIZOLE		Antihistamine
Hivid	See ZALCITABINE		Antiviral
HMS	See MEDRYSONE		Corticosteroid, Ocular
HN_2	**See MECHLORETHAMINE**		
HOMATROPINE Generic, Isopto Homatropine, AK-Homatropine, Homatropine HBr	**Refraction:** Instill 1–2 drops immediately before procedure, repeat in 5–10 min PRN. **Uveitis:** Solution: Instill 1–2 drops up to q3–4h.	**Solution:** 2, 5%.	OPHTHALMIC AGENTS (G) Mydriatics (SG) Cycloplegic Mydriatics (SG) **Cost:** Medium
Homatropine HBr	See HOMATROPINE		Anticholinergic
HUMAN CHORIONIC GONADOTROPIN (FSH) Profasi, Pregnyl	**Prepubertal cryptorchidism:** IM: 4000 USP units, 3 times/week, treat for 3 weeks. Alternate regimen: 5000 USP units qod for 4 injections (many other regimens are advocated). **Male hypogonadotropic hypogonadism (selected cases):** IM: 500 to 1000 USP units, 3 times/week, treat for 3 weeks; followed with 500 to 1,000 USP units, 2 times/week, for 3 additional weeks (other regimens are advocated). Alternate regimen: 4000 USP units 3 times/week, treat for 6 to 9 months; followed with 2000 USP units 3 times/week for an additional 3 months. **Use with menotropins to stimulate spermatogenesis:** IM: 5000 IU, 3 times/week for 4 to 6 months as pretreatment before using menotropins; once menotropins started, give concurrent HCG 2000 IU 2 times/week. **Use with menotropins to induce ovulation:** IM: 5000–10,000 IU as single dose following menotropin pretreatment. Profasi	**Injection:** (powder) 5,000 U,10,000 U per 10 ml vial	ENDOCRINE AGENTS (G) Anterior Pituitary Hormones (SG) **Cost:** High
Humate	See ANTIHEMOPHILIC FACTOR VIII (Non-recombinant)		Hemostatic
Humatin	See PAROMOMYCIN		Aminoglycoside
Humatrope	See SOMATOTROPIN		Growth Hormone
Humulin R, N, 70/30,50/50, L,U	See INSULINS		
Hy-Gestrone	See HYDROXYPROGESTERONE		Progestin

GENERIC NAME Trade Name	INDICATIONS AND DOSAGES	DOSE FORMS	GROUP (G)/SUBGROUP (SG) Relative Cost within Group
HYALURONATE Generic, Healon, Amvisc	Viscoelastic filler. May also be used to coat instruments.	**Injection:** 10, 12, 14, 16, 30 mg/ml	OPHTHALMIC AGENTS (G) Adjuncts To Surgery (SG)
HYALURONIDASE Wydase	**Increase Dispersion and Absorption of Injected Drugs Or Fluids**	**Injection:** Solution 150 U/ml **Injection: Powder:** 150.1500 U/vial	METABOLIC AGENTS (G) Enzyme (SG)
Hycamtin	See TOPOTECAN		Cancer Chemotherapy
Hycodan	See HYDROCODONE See PART III for many additional mixtures		Narcotic
Hycomine	See HYDROCODONE See PART III for many additional mixtures		Narcotic
HYDRALAZINE Generic, Apresoline	**Hypertension:** PO: 10 mg QID initially; 40–300 mg/d maintenance given in 4 divided doses. **Hypertensive Crisis:** IM, IV: 20–40 mg PRN (Onset 10–80 min). Change to PO therapy w/in 1–2 days.	**Tablet:** 10, 25, 50, 100 mg **Injection:** 20 mg/ml	ANS AGENTS (G) Sympathomimetics (SG) Beta 1 and 2 Effect (SSG) **Cost:** Low
HYDRALAZINE-HCTZ COMBINATION Generic Apresazide	**Hypertension:** PO: Capsules: Combination in fixed proportion of hydralazine/hydrochlorothiazide 100/50, 25/25, 50/50 mg		
Hydrea	See HYDROXYUREA		Cancer Chemotherapy
Hydro-Z-50	See HYDROCHLOROTHIAZIDE		Sodium Diuretic
Hydrochlor	See HYDROCHLOROTHIAZIDE		Sodium Diuretic
HYDROCHLOROTHIAZIDE Generic, HCTZ, Esidrix, Hydrodiuril, Oretic, Hydromal, Thiuretic, Diaqua, Hydrochlor,, Dydrozide-50, Hyperetic, Lexer	**Hypertension:** PO: First Dose 25 mg; Maintenance 25–50 mg/d given in 1 or 2 divided doses. **Edema:** PO: First Dose 25–200 mg qd; Maintenance 25–200 mg/d.	**Tablet:** 25, 50, 100 mg **Solution:** 50 mg/5 ml **Intensol Solution:** 100 mg/ml	RENAL AGENTS (G) Sodium Diuretics (G) Thiazide Diuretics (SG) **Cost:** Low
HYDROCODONE	**See Tables**		CNS AGENTS (G) Narcotic Analgesics (G) Lowest Potency (SG) **Cost:** Low
HYDROCORTISONE Generic, Cortisol, Cortef, Hydrocortisone Acetate, Solu-Cortef,	**Addison's:** PO: 10–30 mg/d with fludrocortisone. PO: 20–240 mg/d. IV/IM (succinate): 100–500 mg and may repeat q2–6 hrs. IV/IM/SC (phosphate): ⅓ to ½ the oral dose for maintenance. **Intraarticular** (acetate): 10–37.5 mg/injection. **Tendonitis** (acetate): 5–25 mg/injection.**Tablet:** 5, 10, 20 mg	**Oral suspension:** 10 mg/5 ml. **Injection:** Phosphate: 20 mg/ml in 2, 10 ml vials. Succinate: 100, 250, 500, 1g. Acetate: 25 & 50 mg/ml.	ENDOCRINE AGENTS (G) Anti-Inflammatory Steroids (SG) **Cost:** Low

GENERIC NAME Trade Name	INDICATIONS AND DOSAGES	DOSE FORMS	GROUP (G)/SUBGROUP (SG) Relative Cost within Group
Hydrodiuril	See HYDROCHLOROTHIAZIDE		Sodium Diuretic
HYDRO-FLUMETHIAZIDE Generic, Saluron, Diucardin	**Hypertension:** PO: Initially 50 mg bid; Maintenance 50–100 mg/d (max. dose 200 mg/d). **Edema:** PO: Initially 50 mg qd or bid; Maintenance 25–200 mg/d.	**Tablet:** 50 mg	RENAL AGENTS (G) Sodium Diuretics (SG) Thiazide Diuretics (SSG) **Cost:** Medium
Hydromal	See HYDROCHLOROTHIAZIDE		Sodium Diuretic
HYDROMOR-PHONE Generic, Dilaudid, Dihydromorphone	**Pain Management:** IV: 1–1.5 mg (administer at rate > 1 mg/min) q4–6h. PO: 2–4 mg q4–6h. IV, SC: 1–2 mg q4–6h (max. dose 4 mg q4–6h PRN).	**Tablet:** 1, 2, 3, 4 mg **Suppositories:** 3 mg **Injection:** 1, 2, 3, 4, 10 mg/ml	CNS AGENTS (G) Narcotic Analgesics (SG) Greatest Potency (SSG) **Cost:** High
Hydromox	See QUINETHAZONE		Sodium Diuretic
HYDROPRES 25, 50	**Hypertension:** PO:1 tablet bid.	**Tablet:** Combination of hydrochlorothiazide (25, 50 mg)and reserpine (0.125 mg)	CV AGENTS (G) Sodium Diuretic (SG) and Central Sympathoplegic (SG)
HYDROQUINONE Generic, Melanex, Solaquin	**Skin Bleaching:** Topical: Apply twice daily.	**Cream:** 1.5%, 2%, 4% **Solution:** 3% **Gel:** 4%	DERMATOLOGIC AGENTS (G) Miscellaneous (SG) **Cost:** High
HYDROXYCHLO-ROQUINE Plaquenil	**Rheumatoid arthritis:** PO: 400 mg/d initially (usually 4–12 weeks); after response give maintenance of 200 mg/d (discontinue if no improvement seen after 6 months of treatment). **Systemic lupus erythematosus:** PO: 400 qd or bid initially (usually several weeks or months), then maintenance of 200–400 mg/d. **Malaria chemoprophylaxis:** PO: 400 mg once/wk. Begin 1–2 weeks before exposure. **Acute Malaria:** PO: 800 mg to start; then 400 mg at 6 hours; then 400 mg/day for 2 days.	**Tablets:** 200 mg (equivalent to 155 mg base)	ANTI-INFLAMMATORY AGENTS (G) Cytotoxic Immunosuppressants (SG)
HYDROXYPRO-GESTERONE Generic. Hydroxyprogesterone caproate in oil, many names.	**Primary/Secondary Amenorrhea, Abnormal Uterine Bleeding:** IM: 375 mg (single dose). Test for Continuous Estrogen Production: IM: 125–250 mg given on day 10 of cycle, repeat q week until no further suppression desired.	**Injection:** 125, 250 mg/ml	ENDOCRINE AGENTS (G) Progestins (SSG) **Cost:** High
Hydroxyprogesterone caproate in oil	See HYDROXYPROGESTERONE		Progestin
HYDROXYUREA Hydrea	CANCER CHEMOTHERAPY (G) React With DNA (SG) Other Miscellaneous (SSG)		

GENERIC NAME Trade Name	INDICATIONS AND DOSAGES	DOSE FORMS	GROUP (G)/SUBGROUP (SG) Relative Cost within Group
HYDROXYZINE Generic, Atarax, Vistaril	**Pruritus:** PO: 25 mg tid or QID. Pediatric (> 6 yrs) PO: 50–100 mg/d in divided doses. Pediatric (< 6 yrs) PO: 50 mg/d in divided doses. **Nausea and Vomiting:** IM: 25–100 mg per dose. Pediatric IM: 1.1 mg/kg per dose. **Anxiety:** PO: adults 50–100 mg QID. Pediatric (> 6 yrs) PO: 50–100 mg/d in divided doses. Pediatric (< 6 yrs) PO: 50 mg/d in divided doses. IV: 50–100 mg initially, repeat q4–6h as needed.	**Tablet:** 10, 25, 50, 100 mg **Syrup:** 10 mg/5 ml **Capsule:** 25, 50, 100 mg **Oral Suspension:** 25 mg/5 ml **Injection:** 25, 50 mg/ml	ANTI-INFLAMMATORY ETC AGENTS (G) Antihistamines (H1) (SG) Miscellaneous (SSG)
Hygroton	See CHLORTHALIDONE		Sodium Diuretic
Hylorel	See GUANADREL		Alpha Adrenergic Blocker
Hylutin	See HYDROXYPROGESTERONE		Progestin
Hyoscine	See SCOPOLAMINE		Parasympatholytic
HYOSCYAMINE Generic, Levsin, l-atropine	**Antispasmodic:** PO Adults 0.125–0.25 mg tid or QID. PO (ext'd release): 0.375–0.75 mg q12 hours. SC, IM or IV 0.25–0.5 mg 2–4 times daily, PRN.	**Tablet:** 0.125, 0.15 mg **Tablet:** (sublingual) 0.125 mg **Capsule:** (Ext'd release) 0.375 mg **Solution:** 0.125 mg/ml **Elixir:** 0.125 mg/5 ml **Drops:** 0.125 mg/ml **Injection:** 0.5 mg/ml	ANS/CNS AGENTS (G) Antiparkinsonian Agents (SG) Anticholinergics (SSG) **Cost:** High
Hyperetic	See HYDROCHLOROTHIAZIDE		Sodium Diuretic
Hyperstat	See DIAZOXIDE		Vasodilator
HypRho-D	See RHo(D)IMMUNE GLOBULIN		Anti Rh antibody
Hyprogest 250	See HYDROXYPROGESTERONE		Progestin
Hyproval P.A.	See HYDROXYPROGESTERONE		Progestin
Hyproxon	See HYDROXYPROGESTERONE		Progestin
Hytakerol	See DIHYDROTACHYSTEROL		D Vitamin Equivalent
Hytrin	See TERAZOSIN		Alpha Adrenergic Blocker
IBUPROFEN OTC, Generic, Motrin, Advil, Susprin	**Arthritic Conditions:** PO: 300–600 mg q6–8h (max. dose 3200 mg/d). **Dysmenorrhea:** PO: 400 mg q4h PRN. **Pain:** PO: 200–600 mg q4–6h.	**Tablet:** 200, 300, 400, 600, 800 mg **Suspension:** 100 mg/5 ml	ANTI-INFLAMMATORY ETC AGENTS (G) Non-Narcotic Analgesics (SG) Aspirin and Related (SSG) **Cost:** Low
IBUTILIDE Corvert	**Conversion of Atrial Fibrillation or Flutter:** IV: 1 mg infused over 10 min	**Ampoule:** 0.1 mg/ml in 10 ml	CARDIOVASCULAR AGENTS (G) Antiarrhythmic (SG) **Cost:**

GENERIC NAME Trade Name	INDICATIONS AND DOSAGES	DOSE FORMS	GROUP (G)/SUBGROUP (SG) Relative Cost within Group
Idamycin	See IDARUBICIN		
IDARUBICIN Idamycin	CANCER CHEMOTHERAPY (G) React With DNA (SG) Antibiotics (SSG)		
IDOXURIDINE Dendrid, Herplex, Stoxil	Solution: Instill 1–2 drops q1h (daytime) and q2h (night-time) to start, with improvement may decrease to 1 drop q2h (daytime) and q4h (night-time). Continue rx for 3–7 days after full resolution. Alternate regimen: 1 drop q minute for 5 minutes, repeat q4h around the clock.	**Solution:** 0.1%	OPHTHALMIC AGENTS (G) Antiviral Agents (SG) **Cost:** Low
Ifex	See IFOSFAMIDE		
IFOSFAMIDE Ifex	CANCER CHEMOTHERAPY (G) Alkylating Agents (SG) Nitrogen Mustards (SSG)		
Iletin I,II,II U-500	See INSULINS		
Ilosone	See ERYTHROMYCIN		Macrolide Antibiotic
INDINAVIR Crixivan	**Aids:** 800 mg tid reverse transcriptase inhibitor.	**Capsules:** 200, 400 mg	ANTI-INFECTIOUS AGENTS (G) Antiviral Agents (G) Protease Inhibitor (SSG)
Imdur	See ISOSORBIDE MONONITRATE		Vasodilator
IMIPENEM WITH CILASTATIN Primaxin, IV,IM.	**Infections:** IV: 250–750 mg of each q6h by IV infusion over 20–30 minutes IM: 500–750 mg of each q12h	**Injection:** Mixture of powders: Imipenem/ cilastatin: 250 mg, 500 mg or 750 mg of each.	ANTI-INFECTIOUS AGENTS (G) A carbapenem (similar to lactam antibiotic) given with agent to protect from inactivation. **Cost:** Very High
IMIPRAMINE Generic, Tofranil, Pramine, Presamine, Janimine	**Endogenous Depression:** PO: 75 mg/d to start (single dose); maintenance 50–150 mg/d (max. dose 200 mg/d). Geriatric/adolescent PO: 30–40 mg/d to start; maintenance 30–100 mg/d. IV: 100 mg/d max. dose, give in divided doses.	**Tablet:** 10, 25, 50 mg **Capsule:** 75, 100, 125, 150 mg **Injection:** 12.5 mg/ml	CNS AGENTS (G) Tricyclic Antidepressants (SG) **Cost:** Low
Imitrex	See SUMATRIPTAN		Vasoconstrictor (migraine)
Imodium	See LOPERAMIDE		Antidiarrheal Narcotic
Imuran	See AZATHIOPRINE		Immunosuppressant
INDANYL CARBENICILLIN Geocillin	**Urinary Tract Infections:** PO: 382–764 mg q6h. **Prostatitis:** PO: 764 mg QID.	**Tablet:** equivalent to 382 mg carbenicillin	ANTI-INFECTIOUS AGENT (G) Non-Sulfonamide for UTI (SG) **Cost:** Low
INDAPAMIDE Generic, Lozol	**Hypertension:** PO: 1.25 mg qAM, maintenance 1.25–5 mg qd (adjust dose q4 weeks). **Edema:** PO: 2.5 mg qAM, maintenance 2.5–5 mg qAM.	**Tablet:** 1.25, 2.5 mg	RENAL AGENTS (G) Sodium Diuretics (G) Thiazide Diuretics (SG) **Cost:** High
Inderal	See PROPRANOLOL		Beta Adrenergic Blocker

GENERIC NAME Trade Name	INDICATIONS AND DOSAGES	DOSE FORMS	GROUP (G)/SUBGROUP (SG) Relative Cost within Group
INDERIDE	See BETA-BLOCKER-HCTZ COMBINATION		
INDINAVIR Crixivan	**Aids:** 800 mg tid with AZT or other reverse transcriptase inhibitor.		ANTI-INFECTIOUS AGENTS (G) Antiviral Agents (SG) Protease Inhibitor
Indocin	See INDOMETHACIN		Non-Narcotic Analgesic
INDOMETHACIN Generic, Indocin	**Arthritic Conditions:** PO: 25 mg q8–12h to start, increase 25–50 mg/d; (max. dose 200 mg/d in 3 or 4 divided doses). PO (Ext'd release): 75 mg/d to start, increase to 75 mg bid. **Acute Gouty Arthritis:** 50 mg tid until pain subsides (do not use sustained release).	**Capsule:** 25, 50 mg **Capsule:** (Ext'd release) 75 mg **Oral Suspension:** 25 mg/5 ml **Suppositories:** 50 mg	ANTI-INFLAMMATORY ETC AGENTS (G) Non-Narcotic Analgesics (SG) Aspirin and Related (SSG) **Cost:** Low
InFeD	See IRON DEXTRAN INJECTION		Injectable Iron
INH	See ISONIAZID		Tuberculostatic
INJECTION POSTERIOR PITUITARY, Pituitrin	**Post op Ileus:** PO: 10 units SC or IM	**Injection:** 20 units/1 ml vial	ENDOCRINE AGENTS (G) Posterior Pituitary Hormones (Antidiuretic) (SG)
Innovar	See CONSCIOUS SEDATION, Part I		Narcotic-Antipsychotic Combination
Inocor	See AMRINONE		Antiarrhythmic
INSULIN INJECTION Generic, Regular Insulin, Humulin R, Novolin R, Novolin R PenFil, Clear Insulin, Iletin I, Iletin II, Velosulin Human	**Diabetes Mellitus:** Dosage individualized. Regular insulin generally required in IDDM. In NIDD longer acting form and lower requirement if diet and oral antidiabetics inadequate. Prescribe with control of amount and distribution of Calories. Children and adults: 0.5 to 1 U/kg/day. Adolescents (during growth spurt): 0.8 to 1.2 U/kg/day.	**Vials and Cartridges:** 100 units/ml "R" indicates recombinant origin. Iletin I indicates beef and pork origin. Iletin II indicates pork origin. Semisynthetic: Velosulin, human	ENDOCRINE AGENTS (G) Insulins (SG) Insulins, Rapidly Acting (SSG) **Cost:** Low
INSULIN INJECTION CONCENTRATED Concentrated Regular Iletin II U-500	**Insulin Resistant Patients: SC:**	**Injection:** 500 units/ml. Preparation is purified pork.	ENDOCRINE AGENTS (G) Insulins (SG) Insulins, Intermediate Acting (SSG)
INSULIN,LISPRO Humalog	**Diabetes SC:** More rapid onset (15 min), peak effect (40 min)	**Injection:** 100 units /ml	Insulin, Very Rapidly Acting, (SSG)
INSULIN, PROMPT INSULIN ZINC SUSPENSION Semilente.	Used in preparation of lente insulin		ENDOCRINE AGENTS (G) Insulins (SG) Insulins, Rapidly Acting (SSG)

GENERIC NAME Trade Name	INDICATIONS AND DOSAGES	DOSE FORMS	GROUP (G)/SUBGROUP (SG) Relative Cost within Group
INSULIN, ISOPHANE Generic NPH Insulin NPH Isletin I NPH Isletin II (Pork) Humulin N Novolin N	**Diabetes:**	**Injection and Cartridges:** 100 units/ml. "N" suffix indicates brand of isophane insulin. NPH is old name for mixture with no excess of protamine as is present in PZI (Protamine Zinc Insulin).	ENDOCRINE AGENTS (G) Insulins (SG) Insulins, Intermediate Acting (SSG) **Cost:** Low
INSULIN, REGULAR-ISOPHANE MIXTURE Humulin 70/30 Novolin 70/30 Humulin 50/50	**Diabetes:**	**Injection and Cartridges:** 100 units/ml. All of recombinant origin.	ENDOCRINE AGENTS (G) Insulins (SG) Insulins, Intermediate Acting (SSG) **Cost:** Low
INSULIN ZINC SUSPENSION Lente Insulin, Lente Iletin I, Lente Iletin II, Lente L Humulin L, Novolin L	**Diabetes:**	**Injection:** 100 units/ml Mixture of 70% ultralente and 30% semilente."L" Indicates Brand of Lente Insulin	ENDOCRINE AGENTS (G) Insulins (SG) Insulins, Mixed Duration Combinations (SSG) **Cost:** Low
INSULIN, EXTENDED ZINC SUSPENSION Ultralente Ultralente U Humulin U	**Diabetes:** See Insulin, Regular	**Injection:** 100 units/ml "U" Indicates Brand of Ultralente Insulin	ENDOCRINE AGENTS (G) Insulins (SG) Insulins, Long Acting (SSG) **Cost:** Low
Intal	See CROMOLYN		Mast Cell Stabilizer
INTERFERON ALFA-2A(r) Roferon-A	**Hairy Cell Leukemia, AIDS-Related Kaposi's Sarcoma:**		ANTI-INFLAMMATORY, ETC AGENTS (G) Cytokines, Other Immunomodulators (SG)
INTERFERON ALFA-2B Intron	**Hairy Cell Leukemia, AIDS-Related Kaposi's Sarcoma, Malignant Melanoma, Chronic Hepatitis:**		ANTI-INFLAMMATORY, ETC AGENTS (G) Cytokines, Other Immunomodulators (SG)
INTERFERON ALFA-N3 Alferon N	**Condylomata Accuminata:** Intralesional injection into refractory lesions		ANTI-INFLAMMATORY, ETC AGENTS (G) Cytokines, Other Immunomodulators (SG)
INTERFERON BETA-1A Avonex	**Multiple Sclerosis (relapsing):** SC: 0.25 mg (8 mIU) qod.	**Powder for injection/ reconstitution:** 0.3 mg (9.6 mIU).	ANTI-INFLAMMATORY, ETC AGENTS (G) Cytokines, Other Immunomodulators (SG)
INTERFERON BETA-1B Betaseron, rIFN-B	**Multiple Sclerosis (relapsing):** SC: 0.25 mg (8 mIU) qod.	**Powder for injection/ reconstitution:** 0.3 mg (9.6 mIU).	ANTI-INFLAMMATORY, ETC AGENTS (G) Cytokines, Other Immunomodulators (SG)

GENERIC NAME Trade Name	INDICATIONS AND DOSAGES	DOSE FORMS	GROUP (G)/SUBGROUP (SG) Relative Cost within Group
INTERFERON GAMMA-1B Actimmune	**Chronic Granulomatous Disease, (Anti-Infectious):**		ANTI-INFLAMMATORY, ETC AGENTS (G) Cytokines, Other Immunomodulators (SG)
Interleukin-2	See ALDESLEUKIN		Immunostimulant
Intron	See INTERFERON ALFA-2B		Cytokine
Intropin	See DOPAMINE		Sympathomimetic
Inversine	See MECAMYLAMINE		Hypotensive
Invirase	See SAQUINAVIR		Reverse Transcriptase Inhibitor
IODIDE IODINE SOLUTION (STRONG) Generic, Lugol's Solution **POTASSIUM IODIDE** Generic	**Preparation for Thyroid Surgery:** PO: 2–6 qtt tid, treat for 10 days prior to surgery. **Thyroid Blocking in Radiation Exposure:** PO (adults and children > 1 yr.): 130 mg (1 tablet) q day for 10 days. PO (children < 1 yr.): 65 mg q day (½ tablet, crushed) for 10 days.	**Solution:** 5% iodine and 10% potassium iodide. **Tablets:** 130 mg potassium iodide.	ENDOCRINE AGENTS (G) Antithyroid Agents and Related (SG) **Cost:** Low
IODOQUINOL Diiodohydroxy-quin, Mobequin, Yodoxin	**Parasitic Infections:** PO: 650 mg q8h after meals for 20 days. Pediatric PO: 10–13 mg/kg q8h for 20 days (max single dose 650 mg/dose).	**Tablet:** 210, 650 mg **Powder:** in 25 g	ANTI-INFECTIOUS AGENTS (G) Antiparasitic Agents (SG)
Ionamin	See PHENTERMINE		Diet Pill
IPRATROPIUM Atrovent	**COPD or asthma associated bronchospasm:** Inhalation: 2 puffs (36 mcg) QID (do not exceed 12 puffs/day). **Allergic Rhinitis, Common Cold:**	**Aerosol:** approx. 18 mcg is delivered each puff. **Nasal Spray:** 0.03, 0.06%	RESPIRATORY AGENTS (G) Parasympatholytic for Deep Inhalation (SG) **Cost:** Low **Cost:** Higher and less effective compared to corticosteroids
IRON DEXTRAN INJECTION In FeD	**Iron Deficiency:** IM: calculate dose (in mg) as follows: 0.3 × (Weight in pounds) × (100—[(6.75) × (hemoglobin [in gm/d]/ 14.8)]); divide dose such that no more than 100 mg/d (2.0 ml) is given.	**Injection:** 50 mg iron per ml (as dextran).	METABOLIC AGENTS (G) Specific Ions (SG)
Ismelin	See GUANETHIDINE		Hypotensive
Ismo	See ISOSORBIDE MONONITRATE		Vasodilator
Ismotic	See ISOSORBIDE		Vasodilator
Isorbid	See ISOSORBIDE DINITRATE		Vasodilator
ISOETHARINE Generic, Bronkosol	**Asthma, Bronchospasm:** Inhalation: Solutions of graded strength are diluted and aerosolized by oxygen stream or IPPB.	**Aerosol:** Metered nebulizer gives 340 mcg/puff **Solution:** 0.062%, 0.08%, 0.01%, 0.125%, 0.167%, 0.17%, 0.2%, 0.25%, 1%	RESPIRATORY AGENTS (G) Beta Adrenergic Agonist (SG) for Inhalation (SG)

GENERIC NAME Trade Name	INDICATIONS AND DOSAGES	DOSE FORMS	GROUP (G)/SUBGROUP (SG) Relative Cost within Group
ISONIAZID Generic, INH, Laniazid, Niconyl, Nydrazid	**Tuberculosis (Initial Therapy, given in combination):** Adults (single dose/day): 5–10 mg/kg/d (max. dose 300 mg/d). Adults (two doses/week): 15 mg/kg twice per week (max. dose 900 mg/week). Pediatric (single dose/day): 10–20 mg/kg/d (max. dose 300 mg/d). Pediatric (two doses/week): 20–40 mg/kg/week (max. dose 900 mg/week). **Tuberculosis Prevention:** Adults PO: 300 mg/d in a single dose. Pediatric PO: 10 mg/kg/d (max. dose 300 mg/d).	**Tablet:** 50, 100, 300 mg **Injection: 100 mg/ml** **Syrup:** 50 mg/5 ml	ANTI-INFECTIOUS AGENTS (G) Antituberculous Agents of First Choice (SG) **Cost:** Low
Isophan	See MAGALDRATE		Antacid
ISOPROTERENOL Generic, Isuprel	**Chronic Obstructive Pulmonary Disease:** IPPB: 0.5 ml of 0.5% (in 2–2.5 ml of saline) over 15–20 min (max. dose 5 times/d). Metered Aerosol: 1–2 puffs q3–4h. **Bradycardia:** IV: 2 mcg/min initially; then titrate upward until satisfactory heart rate (usually not more than 10 mcg/min) is reached.	**Tablet:** (sublingual) 10, 15 mg **Solution:** (for inhalation) 0.25%, 0.5%, 1% **Injection:** 0.2 mg/ml **Aerosol:** 0.25% **Aerosol:** delivers 80 mcg, 131 mcg per dose	AUTONOMIC NS AGENTS (G) Sympathomimetics (SG) Beta 1 and 2 Agonists (SSG) **Cost:** Low
Isoptin	See VERAPAMIL		Calcium Channel Blocker
Isoptocarbachol	See CARBACHOL		Cholinergic
Isordil	See ISOSORBIDE DINITRATE		Vasodilator
ISOSORBIDE Ismotic	**IOP Reduction:** PO: 1.5 g/kg, initial dose; dose range, 1–3 g/kg bid-QID PRN	**Solution:** 45%	RENAL AGENTS (G) Osmotic Diuretics (SG)
ISOSORBIDE DINITRATE Generic, Isordil, Sorate, Sorbitrate, Dilatrate, Isorbid, Isotrate, Sorbide-TD	**Angina Prophylaxis:** Sublingual: 5–10 mg q2–3h (take 3 or more minutes prior to situations likely to provoke anginal attacks). PO: (chewable tablets) 5–10 mg q2–3h. PO: initially 5–20 mg, maintenance 10–40 mg q6h. PO: (Ext'd release) initially 40 mg, maintenance 40–80 mg q8–12h. Acute Angina (in NTG intolerant Patients): Sublingual: starting dose 2.5–5 mg. PO: (chewable tablets) 5 mg.	**Tablet:** (sublingual) 2.5, 5, 10 mg **Tablet:** 5, 10, 20, 30, 40 mg **Tablet:** (Ext'd release) 40 mg **Tablet:** (chewable) 5, 10 mg **Capsule:** (Ext'd release, Imdur) 40 mg	CV AGENTS (G) Vasodilators (SG) Post-Arteriolar (Antianginal) (SSG) **Cost:** Low
ISOSORBIDE MONONITRATE Ismo, Monoket, Imdur	**Prevention of angina:** PO: 20 mg bid, with doses 7 hours apart. PO (Ext'd release): Initially 30–60 mg qAM, after several days increase to 120 mg qAM PRN (max dose: 240 mg/d).	**Tablet:** 10, 20 mg **Tablet:** (Ext'd release, Imdur) 60 mg	CV AGENTS (G) Vasodilators (SG) Post-Arteriolar (Antianginal and Related Agents) (SSG) **Cost:** Medium
Isotrate	See ISOSORBIDE DINITRATE		Vasodilator

GENERIC NAME Trade Name	INDICATIONS AND DOSAGES	DOSE FORMS	GROUP (G)/SUBGROUP (SG) Relative Cost within Group
ISOTRETINOIN Accutane, 13-cis-Retinoic Acid	**Severe Cystic Acne:** PO: 0.5–1 mg/kg/d (max. dose 2 mg/kg/d) divided q12h for 15–20 weeks. For persistent acne may repeat after 2 month intermission.	**Capsule:** 10, 20, 40 mg	DERMATOLOGIC AGENTS (G) Keratolytic-plastic Agents (SG) Acne and Psoriasis (SSG) **Cost:** Very High
ISOXSUPRINE Generic, Vasodilan, Vasoprin, Voxsuprine	**Vascular Disease:** PO: 10–20 mg q6–8h.	**Tablet:** 10, 20 mg	ANS AGENTS (G) Sympathomimetics (SG) Beta 1 and 2 Agonists (SSG) **Cost:** Low
ISRADIPINE DynaCirc	**Hypertension:** See discussion, Part 1		CV AGENTS (G) Vasodilators (SG) Calcium Channel Blockers (SSG) **Cost:** Medium
Isuprel	See ISOPROTERENOL		Beta Adrenergic Agonist
ITRACONAZOLE Sporanox	**Blastomycosis/Histoplasmosis:** PO: 200 mg qd, if needed increase in 100-mg increments to a max. dose of 400 mg daily (if dose > 200 mg/d give in 2 divided doses). **Aspergillosis:** PO: 200–400 mg/d. **Serious Fungal Infections:** PO: 200 mg tid loading dose for 3 days, then 200 mg/d for a minimum of 3 months. **Onychomycosis:** PO: 200 mg/d for 12 weeks	**Capsule:** 100 mg	ANTI-INFECTIOUS AGENTS (G) Systemic Antifungal Agents (SG) **Cost:** Low
Janimine	See IMIPRAMINE		Antidepressant
JENEST-28	**Contraception:** PO: 28-day regimen.		**Tablet:** ethinyl estradiol (35 mcg), norethindrone (0.5 mg) in 28-Day Cyclic Tablet Dispensers
JOK	See DOCUSATE		Stool Softener
K-Dur	See POTASSIUM CHLORIDE		
K-lor	See POTASSIUM CHLORIDE		
K-Pek	See KAOLIN + PECTIN		Antidiarrheal
K1-Vitamin	See PHYTONADIONE (K1)		Coagulant
Kabikinase	See STREPTOKINASE		Thrombolytic
KANAMYCIN Generic, Kantrex	**Serious Infection:** IM, IV: 15 mg/kg/d given in 2–4 divided doses (IM) or 2–3 divided doses (IV), may start with an initial loading dose of 10 mg/kg followed by lower maintenance doses, e.g., 7.5 mg/kg q12h (max. dose 1.5 g/d; desirable peak serum levels 15–30 mcg/ml, trough levels should not exceed 10 mcg/ml). **Suppression of Intestinal Bacteria:** PO: 1 g q4h to start, then 1 g q6h for 36–72 hours. **Hepatic Coma:** PO: 8–12 g/d in divided doses. Aerosol Treatment: Aerosol: 250 mg bid-QID by nebulizer (250 mg in 3 ml normal saline to nebulize)	**Capsule:** 500 mg. **Injection:** 500 mg, 1g **Injection:** (pediatric) 75 mg	ANTI-INFECTIOUS AGENTS (G) Aminoglycosides (SG) **Cost:** Medium

GENERIC NAME Trade Name	INDICATIONS AND DOSAGES	DOSE FORMS	GROUP (G)/SUBGROUP (SG) Relative Cost within Group
Kantrex	See KANAMYCIN		Aminoglycoside Antibiotic
KAOLIN + PECTIN Kaopectate, K-Pek	PO: 60–120 ml/dose (give after each bowel movement). Pediatric PO (6–12 yrs): 30–60 ml/dose. Pediatric PO (3–6 yrs): 15–30 ml/dose.	**Suspension:** 90 g kaolin, 2 g pectin/ 30ml	GI AGENTS (G) Anti-Diarrheal Agents (SG) **Cost:** Low
Kaopectate	See KAOLIN + PECTIN		Antidiarrheal
Keflet	See CEPHALEXIN		Lactam Antibiotic
Keflex	See CEPHALEXIN		Lactam Antibiotic
Keflin	See CEPHALOTHIN		Lactam Antibiotic
Kefros	See CEPHALEXIN		Lactam Antibiotic
Kefurox	See CEFUROXIME		Lactam Antibiotic
Kefzol	See CEFAZOLIN		Lactam Antibiotic
Kemadrin	See PROCYCLIDINE		Anticholinergic
Kenacort	See TRIAMCINOLONE		Corticosteroid
Kenalog	See TRIAMCINOLONE ACETONIDE		Corticosteroid
Kerlone	See BETAXOLOL		Beta Adrenergic Blocker
Ketalar	See KETAMINE		Incomplete Anesthetic
KETAMINE Ketalar	IV: 1–4.5 mg/kg (give SLOWLY over 60 or more seconds) IM: 6.5–13 mg/kg.	**Injection:** 10, 50, 100 mg/ml	GENERAL ANESTHETICS (G) Conscious Sedation (SG) **Cost:** High
KETOCONAZOLE Nizoral	**Cutaneous candidiasis; tinea corporis, cruris and versicolor (pityriasis):** Topical: apply once daily to cover the affected and immediate surrounding area (treat versicolor for 2 weeks; pedis for 6 weeks) **Seborrheic dermatitis:** Topical: apply to the affected area twice daily for 4 weeks or until clinical clearing. Shampoo: twice a week for 4 weeks with at least 3 days between each reshampooing (at each shampoo apply for 1 minute, rinse hair, reapply for 3 minutes, rinse).	**Cream:** 2% **Shampoo:** 2%	DERMATOLOGIC AGENTS (G) Topical Fungicides (SG) **Cost:** Moderate
KETOPROFEN Generic, OTC, Actron, Orudis	**Minor Pain Including Arthritic and Dysmenorrhea:** PO: starting dose 75 mg tid. PO: Daily dose 150 to 300 mg divided into 3 or 4 doses. (Max. dose 300 mg/d).	**Capsule:** 25, 50, 75 mg **Capsule:** (Ext'd release) 200 mg	ANTI-INFLAMMATORY ETC (G) Aspirin And Other NSAIDs(SG) **Cost:** High
KETOROLAC Toradol	**Pain:** IM: 30–60 mg loading dose, then 15–30 mg q6h PRN (discontinue after 5 days). PO: 10 mg q4–6h (max. dose 40 mg/d give only after IM dose) (discontinue after 5 days).	**Tablet:** 10 mg **Injection:** 15, 30, 60 mg/ml	ANTI-INFLAMMATORY ETC (G) Aspirin And Other NSAIDs (SG) **Cost:** Medium
Kidrolase	See ASPARAGINASE		
Klavikordal	See NITROGLYCERIN		Vasodilator

GENERIC NAME Trade Name	INDICATIONS AND DOSAGES	DOSE FORMS	GROUP (G)/SUBGROUP (SG) Relative Cost within Group
Klonopin	See CLONAZEPAM		Ultrashort-Acting Hypnotic
Klor-Con	See POTASSIUM CHLORIDE		
Klorvess	See POTASSIUM CHLORIDE		
Koate	See ANTIHEMOPHILIC FACTOR VIII Non-Recombinant		Hemostatic
KoGENate	See ANTIHEMOPHILIC FACTOR VIII RECOMBINANT		Hemostatic
Konyne 80	See COAGULANT FACTOR IX		Hemostatic
Kwell	See LINDANE		Ectoparasiticide
Kytril	See GRANISETRON		Antiemetic
l-atropine	See HYOSCYAMINE		Parasympatholytic
L-Deprenyl	See SELEGILINE		MAO Inhibitor, Type B
L-DESOXYEPHEDRINE (Inhaler) OTC, Vicks Inhaler	**Nasal Congestion:** Intranasal: 1–2 inhalations, each nostril q 2 hours or more (do not use for more than 7 days).	**Inhaler:** 50 mg	RESPIRATORY AGENTS (G) Nasal (Topical) Decongestants (SG) **Cost:** Low
L-Dopa	See LEVODOPA		Dopamine Precursor
L-HYOSCYAMINE Generic, Levsin	PO, SL: 0.125–0.25 mg q6–8h. PO: (ext'd release) 0.375–0.75 q12h. SC, IM, IV: 0.25–0.5 mg bid-QID.	**Tablet:** 0.125, 0.15 mg. **Tablet:** (sublingual) 0.125 mg. **Capsule:** (ext'd release) 0.375 mg. **Solution, Drops:** 0.125 mg/ml. **Elixir:** 0.125 mg/5 ml. **Injection:** 0.5 mg/ml	ANS AGENTS (G) Parasympatholytics (SG) Tertiary Amines (SSG) **Cost:** Medium
LAM	See LEVOMETHADYL		Narcotic Analgesic
LABETALOL Normodyne, Trandate	**Hypertension:** PO: 100 mg bid initially; 200–1200 mg/d maintenance in 2–3 doses (max. dose 2400 mg/d). Increase doses in 100 mg bid increments at 2–3 day intervals (as needed). IV: 20 mg initially, add 40–80 mg q10min (max. dose: 300 mg). Each injection must be given over a 2-min period.	**Tablet:** 100, 200, 300 mg **Injection:** 5 mg/ml	ANS AGENTS (G) Sympathoplegics (SG) Alpha And Beta Blocker (SSG) **Cost:** Medium
Lactaid	See LACTASE		Enzyme

GENERIC NAME Trade Name	INDICATIONS AND DOSAGES	DOSE FORMS	GROUP (G)/SUBGROUP (SG) Relative Cost within Group
LACTASE OTC, Generic Lactaid, Surelac	**Lactose Intolerance:** PO (Liquid): 5 to 15 drops per quart of milk. PO (Tablets): 1 to 3 tablets when commence eating dairy product (max single meal dose: 6 tablets). PO (Capsules): 1 or 2 capsules taken with milk or dairy products (more if severely intolerant of lactose).	**Liquid:** 1250 neutral lactase units per 5 drop dosage. **Tablet:** 3000 FCC lactase units of beta-D-galactosidase. **Capsule:** 250 mg standardized lactase. **Tablet:** (chewable) 3000, 3300 FCC lactase units.	GI AGENTS (G) Enzymes (SG)
LACTULOSE Duphalac, Chronulac, Constilac, Cholac, Enulose	**Encephalopathy of Hepatic Failure:** PO: 20–30 gm lactulose (= 30–45 ml) tid or QID. (May initiate therapy with 20–30 gm lactulose qh until desired laxative effect (ie., 2–3 soft stools per day) is seen, then reduce to maintain desired effect. **Constipation:** PO: 10–20 g lactulose (15–30 ml) per day (max. dose 40 ml/day).	**Syrup:** 10 gm lactulose/15 ml with added sugars.	MISCELLANEOUS GI AGENTS (G) Hyperosmolar Solution (SG) **Cost:** High
Lamisil	See TERBINAFINE		Antifungal, Topical
LAMIVUDINE Epivir	**HIV Infection:** PO: 150 mg bid with a protease inhibitor Pediatric 4 mg/kg to 150 mg bid	**Tablets:** 150mg **Oral Sol'n:** 10 mg/kg	ANTI-INFECTIOUS AGENTS (G) Antiviral Agents (SG) Transcriptase Inhibitor (SSG) **Cost:** High
Laniazid	See ISONIAZID		Tuberculostatic
Lanoxicaps	See DIGOXIN		Cardiac Glycoside
Lanoxin	See DIGOXIN		Cardiac Glycoside
LANSOPRAZOLE Prevacid	**Peptic Ulcer:** PO: 15–30 qd	**Capsule:** ER: 15, 30 mg	GASTROINTESTINAL AGENTS (G) Inhibit Gastric Acid Secretion (SG) Inhibit H ion Transport (SSG)
Lariam	See MEFLOQUINE		Antimalarial
Larodopa	See LEVODOPA		Dopamine Precursor
Larotid	See AMOXICILLIN		Lactam Antibiotic
Lasix	See FUROSEMIDE		Sodium Diuretic
LATANOPROST Xalatan Isopropyl-PGF_{2a}	**Lower IOP:** One drop in the affected eye(s) no oftener than once daily in the evening.	**Ophthalmic Solution:** 0.005%,	OPHTHALMIC AGENTS (G) Lower IOP (SG) Prostaglandin Prodrug (SSG) **COST:** Expensive
Lasan	See ANTHRALIN		Keratoplastic (Tar)
Lente Iletin I	See INSULIN ZINC SUSPENSION		
Lente Insulin	See INSULIN ZINC SUSPENSION		
Lente L	See INSULIN ZINC SUSPENSION		
Lente Iletin II	See INSULIN ZINC SUSPENSION		
Lescol	See FLUVASTATIN		Lipid Lowering Agent

GENERIC NAME Trade Name	INDICATIONS AND DOSAGES	DOSE FORMS	GROUP (G)/SUBGROUP (SG) Relative Cost within Group
LEUCOVORIN Generic, Folinic Acid, Citrovorum Factor	**Rescue:** Oral: 15 mg q6hrs × 10 doses from 24h after start of methotrexate IV, IM: Same as PO: **(Note:** this is dose when MTX elimination is normal.)	**Tabs:** 5, 15, 25 mg. **Powder for Injection:** 50, 100, 350 mg/ vial **Amps:** 3 mg/ml	ANTIDOTE OR USED IN POISONING (G)
Leukeran	See CHLORAMBUCIL		
Leukine	See SARGRAMOSTIM		Stimulate Granulocyte Recovery
LEUPROLIDE Lupron, Lupron Depot, Lupron Depot-Ped	**Advanced Prostate Cancer:** SC: 1 mg qd. IV (depot form): 7.5 mg q28 to q33 days. **Precocious Puberty (central):** SC: 50 mcg/kg/day to start (single dose), increase daily dose by 10 mcg/ kg if needed for proper suppression. (depot form): 0.3 mg/kg given q4 weeks to start (minimum: 7.5 mg for weight < 25 kg; intermediate 11.25 mg for weight between 25 and 37 kg; maximum 15 mg for weight > 37 kg as a single IM injection, increase monthly dose by 3.75 mg/kg if needed for proper suppression. **Endometriosis:** IM (depot form only): 3.75 mg q month (safety of treatment beyond 6 months has not been established)	**Injection:** 5 mg. **Powder for Injection (depot forms):** 3.75 & 7.5 mg ([6]Lupron Depot); 11.25 & 15 mg([6]Lupron Depot-Ped).	ENDOCRINE AGENTS (G) Hypothalamic Releasing Factor Antagonist (SG)
Leustatin	See CLADRIBINE		
LEVAMISOLE Ergamisol	**Colon Cancer (Adjuvant given with 5-FU treatment):** PO. 50 mg q8h, give for 3 days initially (start 7–30 days post-surgery); maintenance is 50 mg q8h for a 3 day period then repeat q2 weeks.	**Tablet:** 50 mg levamisole base	CANCER CHEMOTHERAPY (G) Immunomodulators (SG)
Levaquin	See LEVOFLOXACIN		Quinolone Antibacterial
Levarterenol	See NOREPINEPHRINE		Sympathomimetic
Levatol	See PENBUTOLOL		Beta Adrenergic Blocker
LEVLEN	**Oral Contraception:** PO: 21- or 28-day regimen.	**Tablet:** ethinyl estradiol (30 mcg), levonorgestrel (0.15 mg) in 21-Day and 28-Day Slidecases	
Levo-Dromoran	See LEVORPHANOL		Narcotic Analgetic
LEVOBUNOLOL Generic, Betagan	**Elevated IOP:** Instill 1 drop 1–2 times/d.	**Solution:** 0.25%, 0.5%	OPHTHALMIC AGENTS (G) Used in The Treatment of Glaucoma (SG) Beta-Adrenergic Receptor Blockers (SSG) **Cost:** Low

GENERIC NAME Trade Name	INDICATIONS AND DOSAGES	DOSE FORMS	GROUP (G)/SUBGROUP (SG) Relative Cost within Group
LEVOCABASTINE Livostin	**Allergic Conjunctivitis:** Into conjunctival sac (suspension): 1 drop QID (use up to 2 weeks).	**Suspension:** 0.05%	OPHTHALMIC AGENTS (G) Ocular Anti-Inflammatory Agents (SG) Antihistamines (SSG)
LEVODOPA Generic, L-Dopa, Dopar, Larodopa	**Parkinsonism:** PO: 250–500 mg bid to start; increase 100–750 mg/d q3–7d; (max. dose 8 g/d).	**Tablet:** 100, 250, 500 mg **Capsule:** 100, 250, 500 mg	ANTIPARKINSONIAN AGENTS (G) Dopamine Related Agents (SG) **Cost:** Low
LEVODOPA AND CARBIDOPA (MIXTURE) Generic, Sinemet	**Parkinsonism:** Levodopa and Carbidopa are combined in standard preparations in two ratios: 4:1 and 10:1 (Max. dose of carbidopa: approx. 200 mg/d). PO: (Patients not currently receiving levodopa): One tab of 100 mg/10 mg or 100 mg/25 mg (levodopa/carbidopa) tid to start; increase 1 tab qd or qod; maintenance 6 tab's/d. If additional levodopa required: substitute 250 mg/25 mg, 1 tab tid-QID; increase by 1 tab qd or qod (max. dose: 8 tab/d). PO: (Patients currently receiving levodopa): Start more than 8 hours since patient last received levodopa. Choose levodopa/carbidopa dose that will provide 25% of previous levodopa daily dosage.	**Tablet:** Levodopa/carbidopa:100 mg/10 mg,100 mg/25 mg,250 mg/25 mg **Tablet:** (Ext'd release) Levodopa/carbidopa: 100 mg/25 mg,200 mg/50 mg	CNS AGENTS (G) Antiparkinsonian Agents(SG) Dopamine Precursor (SSG) **Cost:** Medium
LEVOFLOXACIN Levaquin	**Infections:** PO, IV: 500 mg each day	**Tablets:** 250, 500 mg **IV Solution** 25 mg/ml	ANTI-INFECTIOUS AGENTS (G) Quinolone Antibacterial (SG)
Levomepro-mazine	See METHOTRIMEPRAZINE		Phenothiazine Analgetic
LEVOMETHADYL L-alpha-acetyl-methadyl, Orlaam, LAM, Long Acting Methadone	**Methadone Maintenance:** Labeled for use in maintenance treatment of heroin abuse in appropriate programs. **Pain Management:** Initial dose 5–10 mg, with severe pain use 80–120 mg as tolerance develops.	**Solution:** 10 mg/ml	NARCOTIC ANALGESICS (G) Greatest Potency (SG)
LEVONORGES-TREL Norplant System	**Subdermal:** Implant 6 Silastic capsules (total 216 mg) in mid portion of upper arm during the first 7 days of the onset of menses.	**Kit:** 6 implant capsules, each containing 36 mg levonorgestrel	ENDOCRINE AGENTS (G) Progestins (SG) Progestin Only Contraceptive (SSG)
Levophed	See NOREPINEPHRINE		Sympathomimetic
Levoprome	See METHOTRIMEPRAZINE		Phenothiazine Analgetic
LEVORPHANOL Levo-Dromoran	**Pain Management:** PO, SC: 2 mg (max. dose 3 mg).	**Tablet:** 2 mg **Injection:** 2 mg/ml	CNS AGENTS (G) Narcotic Analgesics (SG) Of Greatest Potency (SSG) **Cost:** Low
Levothroid	See LEVOTHYROXINE(T4)		Thyroid Replacement

GENERIC NAME Trade Name	INDICATIONS AND DOSAGES	DOSE FORMS	GROUP (G)/SUBGROUP (SG) Relative Cost within Group
LEVOTHYROXINE (T4) Generic, Levothroid, Synthroid, Levoxine	**Hypothyroidism:** PO: 0.05–0.2 mg/d, increase by 0.025 mg q2–3 weeks PRN. Maintenance dose up to 0.2 mg/d (in debilitated, aged or long-standing hypothyroid conditions: 0.025 mg/d to start, increase by <0.025 mg/d q3–4 wks PRN). **Congenital Hypothyroidism (Guidelines):** Pediatric PO: At 0–6 months use 8–10 mcg/kg/d increasing with age. **Thyroid Suppression:** PO: 2.6 mcg/kg/d, treat for 7–10 days. **Severe Hypothyroidism or Cretinism:** Pediatric PO: 0.025–0.5 mg/d to start, increase by 0.05–0.1 mg/d q7d PRN (max. dose 0.3–0.4 mg/d). **Hypothyroidism with Myxedema Coma or Obtundation:** IM, IV: 0.4 mg given as starting dose (lower if cardiac debility), then 0.1–0.2 mg IV; maintenance dose of 0.05–0.1 mg/day can maintain euthyroid state; convert to PO as soon as clinically feasible.	**Tablet:** 0.025, 0.05, 0.075, 0.088, 0.1, 0.112, 0.125, 0.15, 0.175, 0.2, 0.3 mg **Injection:** (powder) 200, 500 microg/vial (6 & 10 ml)	ENDOCRINE AGENTS (G) Thyroid Replacements (SG) **Cost:** Medium
Levoxine	See LEVOTHYROXINE (T4)		Thyroid Hormone
Levsin	See L-HYOSCYAMINE		Belladonna Alkaloid
Lexer	See HYDROCHLOROTHIAZIDE		Sodium Diuretic
Librax	See CLIDINIUM AND CHLORDIAZEPOXIDE		Sedative and Cholinergic Combination
Librium	See CHLORDIAZEPOXIDE		Sedative, Long Acting
Lidex	See FLUOCINONIDE		Corticosteroid, Topical
LIDOCAINE Generic, Xylocaine, Anestacon	**Acute Ventricular Arrhythmias:** IV: Loading dose 1 mg/kg/dose given q5–10 minutes (do not exceed a rate 25–50 mg/min, monitor EKG during administration) until desired effect or total dose of 5 mg/kg is reached; maintenance infusion 1–4 mg/min (20–50 mcg/kg/min); change to oral antiarrhythmic as soon as practical (max. dose 300 mg total during a 1 hour period). IV: 300 mg, may repeat once in 60–90 minutes PRN.	**Injection:** 300 mg/3 ml **Injection:** 0.2%, 0.4%, 0.8%, 1%, 2%, 4%, 10%, 20%	CV AGENTS (G) Group I Antiarrhythmic Agents (SG) **Cost:** Medium
LIG	See ANTI-THYMOCYTE GLOBULIN		Immunomodulator
LIMBITROL	See CHLORDIAZEPOXIDE AND AMITRIPTYLINE		Sedative and TCA Combination
Lincocin	See LINCOMYCIN		Macrolide Antibiotic

GENERIC NAME Trade Name	INDICATIONS AND DOSAGES	DOSE FORMS	GROUP (G)/SUBGROUP (SG) Relative Cost within Group
LINCOMYCIN Lincocin, Lincorex	**Bacterial Infections:** PO: 500 mg q8h (max. dose 500 mg q6h). Pediatric PO: 30 mg/kg/d in 3–4 doses. IV: 600 mg q24h (max. dose 600 mg q12h). IV: 600–1000 mg q8–12h (max. dose 8 g/d); (administer doses SLOWLY over 60 or more minutes).	**Capsule:** 250, 500 mg **Injection:** 300 mg/ml	ANTI-INFECTIOUS AGENTS (G) Macrolide Antibiotics (SG) **Cost:** Medium
Lincorex	See LINCOMYCIN		Macrolide Antibiotic
LINDANE Generic, Kwell, G-well, Scabene	**Scabies:** Lotion: Apply 2 oz. to entire skin surface, leave on for 8–12 hours; remove by thorough washing. Repeat after 7 days if needed. Pediculosis pubis and Pediculosis capitis: Lotion and cream: Rub into skin and hair, leave on for 8–12 hours; remove by thorough washing. Repeat after 7 days if necessary. Treat sexual contacts at same time. Shampoo: Apply 1–2 oz, massage thoroughly into hair, leave for 4 min; remove by rinsing thoroughly. Use fine-tooth comb or tweezers to remove remaining nits.	**Cream:** 1% **Lotion:** 1% **Shampoo:** 1%	TOPICAL ANTI-INFECTIOUS AGENTS (G) Ectoparasiticidal Agents (SG) **Cost:** Low
Lioresal	See BACLOFEN		Muscle Relaxant
LIOTHYRONINE (T3) Generic, Cytomel, Triostat, Triiodothyronine	**Hypothyroidism:** PO: 25 mcg/d to start, increase by 12.5–25 mcg/d q1–2 wks; maintenance 25–75 mcg/d. **Myxedema:** PO: 5 mcg/d to start, increase by 5–10 mcg/d q1–2 wk until 25 mcg/d dose is attained, then can increase by 12.5–25 mcg/d q1–2 wk; maintenance dose is 50–100 mcg/d. Note: In elderly, use 5 mcg/d to start, increase 5 mcg q1–2 wks PRN. **Myxedema Coma:** IV: 25–50 mcg initially such that >65 mcg/d is given; give doses 4 h apart (10–20 mcg initial dose if cardiac concerns exist but are not too severe to preclude use). **Congenital Hypothyroidism (Guidelines):** Pediatric PO (1–3 years): 5 mcg/d to start, increase by 5 mcg/d q3–4d PRN, maintenance 50 mcg/d. Pediatric PO (6–12 months): 5 mcg/d to start, increase by 5 mcg/d q3–4d PRN, maintenance 20 mcg/d. **Nontoxic Goiter:** PO: 5 mcg/d to start, increase by 5–10 mcg/d q1–2 wks, until 25 mcg/d dose is attained, then can increase by 12.5–25 mcg/d q1–2 wk; maintenance 25–75 mcg/d. **T3 Suppression Test:** PO: 75–100 mcg/d for 7 days, then repeat thyroid uptake test (>49% suppression rules out autonomous thyroid function).	**Tablet: 5,** 25, 50 mcg **Injection:** 10 mcg/ml	ENDOCRINE AGENTS (G) Thyroid Replacements (SG) **Cost:** Medium

GENERIC NAME Trade Name	INDICATIONS AND DOSAGES	DOSE FORMS	GROUP (G)/SUBGROUP (SG) Relative Cost within Group
LIOTRIX Euthroid, Thyrolar	**Untreated Hypothyroidism:** PO: 15–30 mg/d to start, increase by 15 mg q2–3 wks; maintenance dosage usually 60–120 mg/d.	**Tablet:** Tablet strength in grains (thyroid equivalent in mgs): ¼ (15), ½ (30), 1 (60), 2 (120), 3 (180)	THYROID REPLACEMENTS (SG) **Cost:** Low
Lipitor	See ATORVASTATIN		Hypocholesterolemic
Lipoxide	See CHLORDIAZEPOXIDE		Sedative, Long Acting
Liquaemin Sodium	See HEPARIN		Anticoagulant
LiquidPred	See PREDNISOLONE		Corticosteroid
LISINOPRIL Zestril, Prinivil	**Hypertension:** PO: 10 mg qd to start; 20–40 mg qd maintenance. PO (patient on diuretics): 5 mg qd to start, observe till BP stable. **Congestive Heart Failure:** PO: 5 mg qd to start; 10–20 mg qd maintenance (2.5 mg qd to start in hypotensive or hyponatremic patients), observe till BP stable, give with digoxin and diuretics.	**Tablet:** 2.5, 5, 10, 20, 40 mg	CV AGENTS (G) Vasodilators (SG) ACE Inhibitors (SSG) **Cost:** Low
LITHIUM Lithium carbonate, generic, Eskalith, Lithium citrate, generic, Cibalith	**Acute Mania:** Dosage must be controlled with blood levels PO: 600 mg tid. PO (Ext'd release): 900 mg bid. Long term use 300 mg tid or QID.	**Tablet:** 300 mg **Tablet:** (Ext'd release) 300, 450 mg **Capsule:** 150, 300, 600 mg **Syrup:** 8 mEq lithium (as citrate equivalent to 300 mg lithium carbonate) per 5 ml	CNS AGENTS (G) Antimanic Agents (SG) **Cost:** Medium
Lithium carbonate	See LITHIUM		Antimanic
Lithium citrate	See LITHIUM		Antimanic
Livostin	See LEVOCABASTINE		Mast Cell Stabilizer
LO/OVRAL	**Oral Contraception:** PO: 21-Day regimen or 28-Day regimen.	**Tablet:** ethinyl estradiol (30 mcg), norgestrel (0.3 mg) in 21-Day and 28-Day Pilpaks	
LOCARBEF Lorabid	**Respiratory & Other Infections:** PO: 200–400 mg q 12h. Cystitis (uncomplicated): PO: 400 mg/d.	**Tablet:** 200 mg **Powder (Sup):** 20 mg & 100 mg per ml	LACTAM ANTIBIOTICS (G) Benzyl Penicillins and First Generation Cephalosporins (SG)
Lodine	See ETODOLAC		Non-Narcotic Analgesic
Lodosyn	See CARBIDOPA		Adjunct to Levodopa
LODOXAMIDE Alomide	**Vernal Keratoconjunctivitis:** Adults and children (> 2 yrs): 1 to 2 drops in affected eye QID, use up to 3 months.	**Solution:** 0.1%	OPHTHALMIC AGENTS (G) Mast Cell Stabilizers (SG)

GENERIC NAME Trade Name	INDICATIONS AND DOSAGES	DOSE FORMS	GROUP (G)/SUBGROUP (SG) Relative Cost within Group
LOESTRIN Loestrin 21 Loestrin Fe	**Oral Contraception:** PO: Combination of norethindrone/ ethinyl estradiol: 1.5 mg/30 mcg in 21d package 1.0 mg/20 mcg in 21d package 1.5 mg/30 mcg in 28d package with added iron 1.0 mg/20 mcg in 28d package with added iron		
Logen	See DIPHENOXYLATE WITH ATROPINE		Antidiarrheal
Lognex	See TACRINE		Cholinesterase Inhibitor, Central
LOMEFLOXACIN Maxaquin	**Lower Respiratory Tract Or Urinary Tract Infections:** PO: 400 mg once daily for 10 days. **Prophylaxis:** PO: 400 mg dose 2–6 hours before surgery. **Gonococcal Infections:** PO: 400 mg as a single dose.	**Tablet:** 400 mg	ANTI-INFECTIOUS AGENTS (G) Quinolone Antibacterial (SG) **Cost:** High
LOMOTIL	See DIPHENOXYLATE with ATROPINE		Control Diarrhea
Loniten	See MINOXIDIL		Alpha Blocker
LOMUSTINE CCNU CEENU	CANCER CHEMOTHERAPY (G) Alkylating Agents (SG) Nitrosoureas (SSG)		
Lonox	See DIPHENOXYLATE WITH ATROPINE		Antidiarrheal
LOPERAMIDE Generic, OTC, Imodium	Diarrhea: PO: 4 mg to start, then 2 mg PRN after each stool (max. dose 16 mg/d). Pediatric PO (2–5 yrs): 1 mg q8h to start, then 0.1 mg kg PRN after each stool (max. dose 3 mg/d).	**Capsule:** 2 mg **Tablet:** 2 mg **Liquid:** 1 mg/5 ml, 1 mg/ml	GI AGENTS (G) Anti-Diarrheal Agents (SG) Weak Narcotic (SSG) **Cost:** Medium
Lopid	See GEMFIBROZIL		Alter Lipid Metabolism
Lopidine	See APRACLONIDINE		Lower IOP
Lopressor	See METOPROLOL		Beta Blocker
LOPRESSOR HCT 100/ 25,100/50,50/25	See Beta-Blocker-Diuretic Hypotensive Combination		
Loprox	See CICLOPIROX		Fungicide, Topical
Lopurin	See ALLOPURINOL		Inhibit Urate Synthesis
Lortab	See HYDROCODONE		Narcotic and Aspirin or Acetaminophen
Lorabid	See LORACARBEF		Lactam Antibiotic
LORACARBEF Lorabid	**Acute Bronchitis, Skin Infections:** PO: 200–400 mg q12h for 1 week. **Pyelonephritis, pneumonia, sinusitis,** PO: 400 mg q12h, treat for 2 weeks. **UTI** (uncomplicated): PO: 200 mg q d, treat for 1 week.	**Capsules:** 200 mg **Powder for Suspension:** 20 mg/5 ml, 100 mg/5 ml	LACTAM ANTIBIOTICS (G) Resistant to Staphylococcal Lactamase (SG)

GENERIC NAME Trade Name	INDICATIONS AND DOSAGES	DOSE FORMS	GROUP (G)/SUBGROUP (SG) Relative Cost within Group
LORATADINE Claritin	**Allergic (Type 1) Reactions:** PO (Adults and children >12 yrs): 10 mg qd ac.	**Tablet:** 10 mg	ANTI-INFLAMMATORY ETC (G) Antihistamines (H1) (SG) Non-Sedating (SSG) **Cost:** Very High
LORAZEPAM Generic, Ativan	**Sedation:** PO: 2–3 mg/d start; maintenance 1–10 mg/d in 2–3 doses (max. dose 4 mg). **Pre-Operative Sedation:** IM: 0.05 mg/kg, at least 2 hours before surgery. IV: 0.044–0.05 mg/kg, 15–20 min before surgery (max. dose: 2 mg total). **Hypnotic:** PO: 2–6 mg/d in 2–3 doses (largest at hs).	**Tablet:** 0.5, 1, 2 mg **Injection:** 2, 4 mg/ml	CNS AGENTS (G) Sedative-Hypnotics (SG) Ultrashort-Acting Hypnotics (SSG) **Cost:** Medium
Lorcet	See HYDROCODONE		Narcotic Analgesic Mixture
Lorelco	See PROBUCOL		Affects Lipids
LOSARTAN Cozaar	**Hypertension:** PO: 50 mg once daily then 25–100 mg in 1–2 doses daily	**Tablet:** 25, 50 mg	CV AGENTS (G) Vasodilator (SG) ACE Inhibitor (SSG) (Angiotensin II Receptor Blocker)
Lotensin	See BENAZEPRIL		ACE Inhibitor
Lotrimin	See CLOTRIMAZOLE		Fungicide
LOVASTATIN Mevacor	PO: 20 mg q PM initially, maintenance dose 20 to 80 mg/day in single or divided doses (max. dose 80 mg/d), make adjustments q 4 weeks. Use initial dose = 40 mg/d if serum cholesterol >300 mg/dl.	**Tablet:** 10, 20, 40 mg	METABOLIC AGENTS (G) Lipid Lowering Drugs (SG) HMG-CoA Reductase Inhibitors (SSG) **Cost:** Medium
Lovenox	See ENOXAPARIN		Anticoagulant
Low Molecular Weight Heparin	See ENOXAPARIN		Anticoagulant
LOXAPINE Generic, Loxitane	**Psychotic Disorders:** PO: 10 mg bid to start, maintenance 60–100 mg/d in 2–4 doses (max. dose 250 mg/d). IV: 12.5–50 mg q4–6h; then PO maintenance.	**Capsule:** 5, 10, 25, 50 mg **Liquid:** 25 mg/ml **Injection:** 50 mg/ml	CNS AGENTS (G) Antipsychotics (SG) Prominent Extrapyramidal Effects (SSG) **Cost:** High
Loxitane	See LOXAPINE		Antipsychotic
Lozol	See INDAPAMIDE		Sodium Diuretic
Ludiomil	See MAPROTILINE		TCA Antidepressant
Lufyllin	See DYPHYLLINE		Bronchodilator, Xanthine
Lugol's Solution	See IODINE SOLUTION (STRONG)		Inhibit Thyroid
Luminal	See PHENOBARBITAL		Sedative, Long Acting
Lupron	See LEUPROLIDE		LH-RH Antagonist
Luvox	See FLUVOXAMINE		Stimulant
Lymphocyte Immune Globulin	See ANTI-THYMOCYTE GLOBULIN		Immunomodulator
Lyphocin	See VANCOMYCIN		Lactamase Resistant Antibiotic

GENERIC NAME Trade Name	INDICATIONS AND DOSAGES	DOSE FORMS	GROUP (G)/SUBGROUP (SG) Relative Cost within Group
LYPRESSIN (8-Lysine Vasopressin) Diapid	**Diabetes Insipidus:** Nasal spray: 1–2 sprays q4–6h (maximum 10 sprays/nostril q3–4h).	**Nasal spray:** 0.185 mg lypressin (equiv. to 50 USP posterior pituitary pressor units)/ml	ENDOCRINE AGENTS (G) Posterior Pituitary Hormones (Antidiuretic) (SG)
M.S.	See MORPHINE		Morphine Sulfate
Maalox	See ALUMINUM HYDROXIDE-MAGNESIUM HYDROXIDE		Antacid
Macrodantin	See NITROFURANTOIN		Antibacterial
MAGALDRATE OTC, Generic, Riopan, Isophan	**Gastric hyperacidity:** PO: 10–15 ml between meals and at bedtime.	**Suspension:** 540 mg/5 ml)	GI AGENTS (G) Antacids (SG) **Cost:** Low
MAGNESIA (MILK of) Generic, OTC, Magnesium Hydroxide	PO: 30–60 ml of standard formulation.	**Liquid:** (magnesium hydroxide 7–8.5%; approx. 80 mEq of magnesium/30 ml)	GI AGENTS (G) Bulk and Saline Laxatives (SG) Antacid (SG) **Cost:** Inexpensive
Magnesia Magma	See MAGNESIA (MILK of)		Laxative
MAGNESIUM SALICYLATE OTC, Generic, Magan, Mobidin,	PO: 650 mg q4h (max. dose 4800 mg/d in 3 or 4 divided doses)	**Caplet:** 325, 500 mg. **Tablet:** 545, 650 mg **Tablet:** (Enteric) 500 mg	GI AGENTS (G) Non-Narcotic Analgesics (SG) Aspirin and related NSAIDs (SG) **Cost:** Low
MAGNESIUM SULFATE Generic	**Severe Hypomagnesemia:** IV: 5 g (approx. 40 mEq/L) diluted in 1000 ml D5W or NS; infuse Slowly over 3 hours. **Mild Magnesium Deficiency:** IM: 1 g (8.12 mEq) q6h for 4 doses; max. dose 32.5 mEq/d. **Eclampsia, Toxemia of Pregnancy, Nephritis:** IV: 1–4 g of 10–20% solution (rate NOT >1.5 ml/min for 10% solution; Not > 0.75 ml/min for 20% sln), DO not give in the 2h preceding delivery. IV: 1–5 g of a 50% sln q4–6h PRN, DO NOT give in the 2h preceding delivery.	**Injection:** 10, 12.5, 20, 50% slns (0.8, 1, 2, 4 mEq/ml)	METABOLIC AGENTS (G) Specific Ions (SG)
Magnesium Hydroxide	See MAGNESIA (MILK of)		Laxative
MALATHION	Withdrawn by manufacturer		
Maltsupex	See METHYLCELLULOSE		Laxative
Mandelamine	See METHENAMINE		Antibacterial
Mandol	See CEFAMANDOLE		Lactam Antibiotic

GENERIC NAME Trade Name	INDICATIONS AND DOSAGES	DOSE FORMS	GROUP (G)/SUBGROUP (SG) Relative Cost within Group
MANNITOL Generic, Resectisol, Osmitrol	**Test Dose:** IV: 0.2 g/kg over 3–5 min if urine flow does not increase, repeat once then reevaluate. **Oliguria:** IV: 50–100 g (of a 15–25% sln, give over 3–5 min). **Increased Intracranial (ICP) or Intraocular (IOP) Pressure:** IV: 1.5–2 g/kg (as a 15–20% sln) over 30–60 min. (Many other dosing schemes exist.)	**Injection:** 10, 15, 20, 25%	RENAL AGENTS (G) Osmotic Diuretics (SG) **Cost:** Low
MANTADIL	**Topical:** Apply bid—QID.	**Cream:** hydrocortisone acetate (0.5%), chlorcyclizine (2%)	ANTI-INFLAMMATORY STEROID (G) and ANTIHISTAMINE (G)
Maolate	See CHLORPHENESIN CARBAMATE		Muscle Relaxant
MAPROTILINE Generic, Ludiomil	**Endogenous Depression:** PO (>17 yrs): 75–150 mg/d to start in 1–3 doses; maintenance 75–150 mg/d (max. dose 225 mg/d). Geriatric PO: 25 mg/d to start; maintenance 50–75 mg/d.	**Tablet:** 25, 50, 75 mg	Tricyclic Antidepressants (G) **Cost:** Low
MARAX		**Tablet:** theophylline (130 mg), ephedrine sulfate (25 mg), hydroxyzine (10 mg)	
Marcaine	See BUPIVACAINE		Local Anesthetic
Marezine	See CYCLIZINE		Motion Sickness Preventive
Marinol	See DRONABINOL		Sedative
Matulane	See PROCARBAZINE		Cancer Chemotherapy
Mavik	See TRANDOLAPRIL		ACE Inhibitor
Maxaquin	See LOMEFLOXACIN		Quinolone Antibacterial
Maxiflor	See DIFLORASONE		Corticosteroid
MAXITROL	**Ophthalmic (suspension):** 1 or 2 qtt q 1 h in severe cases; in mild cases, 1–2 qtt 4 to 6 times/d. **Ophthalmic (ointment):** Apply 0.25–0.5 inch tid or QID.	**Ophthalmic Suspension (per cc):** polymyxin B sulfate (10,000 Units), neomycin sulfate (equal to 3.5 mg of neomycin base), dexamethasone (0.1%) **Ophthalmic Ointment (per g):** polymyxin B sulfate (10,000 Units), neomycin sulfate (equal to 3.5 mg of neomycin base), dexamethasone (0.1%)	

GENERIC NAME Trade Name	INDICATIONS AND DOSAGES	DOSE FORMS	GROUP (G)/SUBGROUP (SG) Relative Cost within Group
Maxolon	See METOCLOPRAMIDE		Antiemetic
MAXZIDE **MAXZIDE-25 MG**	**Edema:** PO: 1 tablet qd.	**Tablet:** triamterene (75 mg), hydrochlorothiazide (25 or 50 mg)	RENAL AGENT (G) K Sparing Diuretic (SG)
Mazanor	See MAZINDOL		Diet Pill
MAZINDOL Mazanor, Sanorex	**Exogenous Obesity:** PO: 1 mg tid or 2 mg qd.	**Tablet:** 1, 2 mg	SYMPATHOMIMETIC STIMULANTS (G) Other Schedule 3 Or 4 "Diet Pills" (SG) **Cost:** Very High
Mebaral	See MEPHOBARBITAL		Anticonvulsant
MEBENDAZOLE Vermox	**Trichuriasis, Ascariasis and Hookworm Infection:** PO (adults and pediatric): 100 mg bid for 3 days. **Enterobius vermicularis (pinworm):**PO (adults and pediatric): 100 mg as a single dose.	**Tablet:** (chewable) 100 mg	ANTI-INFECTIOUS AGENTS (G) Antiparasitic Agents (G) **Cost:** High
MECAMYL-AMINE Inversine	**Hypertension:** Start with 2.5 mg bid. Adjust dosage in increments of 2.5 mg at intervals > 2d. The average total daily dosage is 25 mg, usually in 3 divided doses.	**Tablet:** 2.5 mg	AUTONOMIC AGENTS (G) Sympathoplegics (SG) Ganglionic Blockers (SSG) **Cost:** Low
MECHLORETH-AMINE HN2 Mustargen	CANCER CHEMOTHERAPY (G) Alkylating Agents (SG) Nitrogen Mustards (SSG)		
MECLIZINE OTC, Generic, Antivert, Antivert-25, Bonine	**Motion Sickness:** PO: 25–50 mg 1 hour before departure; repeat qd as needed. Vertigo: PO: 25–100 mg/d in divided doses.	**Tablet:** 12.5, 25, 50 mg **Tablet:** (chewable) 25 mg **Capsule:** 25, 30 mg	ANTI-INFLAMMATORY AGENTS (G) Antihistamines (H1) (SG) Motion Sickness Prevention (SG) **Cost:** Low
MECLOFENA-MATE Generic, Meclomen	**Pain, Arthritic Conditions:** PO: 50–100 mg q4–6h (max. dose 400 mg/d).	**Capsule:** 50, 100 mg	ANTI-INFLAMMATORY ETC AGENTS (G) Non-Narcotic Analgesics (SG) Other NSAIDs (SSG) **Cost:** Medium
Meclomen	See MECLOFENAMATE	Non-Narcotic Analgetic	
Medrol	See METHYLPREDNISOLONE		Corticosteroid
MEDROXY-PROGESTERONE Generic, Provera, Amen, Curretab, Cycrin	**Secondary Amenorrhea:** PO: 5–10 mg/d for 5–10 days, expect withdrawal bleeding 3–7 days after last dose. **Menopause (Maintenance):** 2.5 mg/d with estrogen continuously. **Abnormal Uterine Bleeding:** PO: 5–10 mg/d for 5–10 days; start on day 16 or 21 of menstrual cycle; expect withdrawal bleeding 3–7 days after last dose; continue therapy for 2 cycles after bleeding is controlled.	**Tablet:** 2.5, 5, 10 mg	ENDOCRINE AGENTS (G) Progestins (SG) **Cost:** Low

GENERIC NAME Trade Name	INDICATIONS AND DOSAGES	DOSE FORMS	GROUP (G)/SUBGROUP (SG) Relative Cost within Group
MEDRYSONE HMS	**Solution, Suspension:** 1 or 2 drops into the conjunctival sac qh during the day and q2h during the night.	**Suspension:** 1%	OPHTHALMIC AGENTS(G) (G) Anti-Inflammatory Steroids (SG) **Cost:** High
MEFENAMIC ACID Ponstel	**Pain/Dysmenorrhea:** PO: 500 mg to start, then 250 mg q6h.	**Capsule:** 250 mg	NON-NARCOTIC ANALGESICS (G) Aspirin and Related NSAIDs (SG) Other NSAID's (SSG) **Cost:** Medium
MEFLOQUINE Lariam	**P. vivax or P. falciparum Malaria (treatment):** PO: give 1250 mg (5 tablets) as a single dose—give with at least 8 oz of water. (For P. vivax follow this treatment with an 8-aminoquinolone (primaquine) to eliminate hepatic phase parasites. **Malaria prophylaxis:** PO: 250 mg q week for 1st four weeks then 250 mg q other week. Start doses 1 week prior to travel to, and continue 4 weeks after return from malarious area. Pediatric PO: (weight >45 kg): 1 tab weekly. Pediatric PO: (weight 31–45 kg): 3/4 tab weekly. Pediatric PO: (weight 20–30 kg): tab weekly. Pediatric PO: (weight 15–19 kg): 1/4 tab weekly. Start all pediatric doses one week prior to travel to and continue weekly doses for 4 weeks after return from malarious area	**Tablet:** 250 mg	ANTI-INFECTIOUS AGENTS (G) Antiparasitic Agents (G) **Cost:** Medium
Mefoxin	See CEFOXITIN		Lactam Antibiotic
Megace	See MEGESTROL		Progestin
MEGESTROL Megace	Weight loss in AIDS, Palliation of CA of Breast or Endometrium: PO: 400–800 mg/d	PO: Suspension 40 mg/ml	ENDOCRINE AGENTS (G) Progestins (SG)
Melanex	See HYDROQUINONE		Skin Lightener
Mellaril	See THIORIDAZINE		Antipsychotic
MELPHALAN Alkeran Phenylalanine Mustard	CANCER CHEMOTHERAPY Alkylating Agents (SG) Nitrogen Mustards (SSG)		
Menest	See ESTERIFIED ESTROGENS		Estrogen

GENERIC NAME Trade Name	INDICATIONS AND DOSAGES	DOSE FORMS	GROUP (G)/SUBGROUP (SG) Relative Cost within Group
MENOTROPINS (FSH and LH) Pergonal	**Induction Of Ovulation In Anovulatory But Functional Ovaries:** IM: 75 IU-FSH/75 IU-LH per day initially, give for 9–12 days; follow w/ 10,000 U of HCG, one day after the last menotropins dose (observe for signs of excess ovarian stimulation [e.g., total estrogen secretion >100 mcg/d or estriol excretion >50 mcg/d] and/or ovarian enlargement—do NOT give HCG if evidence of excess ovarian stimulation. May repeat sequence at least twice with larger (double) menotropins dose if ovulation w/o pregnancy occurred. **Induction of Spermatogenesis In Primary or Secondary Pituitary Hypofunction:** IM: 75 IU-FSH/75 IU-LH 3 times/week, give concomitantly w/ HCG 2000 IU 2 times/week (may require 3–4 months of therapy to assess efficacy of treatment); prior to initiation of therapy give HCG alone (5000 IU 3 times a week) for approximately 4–6 months to achieve adequate masculinization.	**Injection:** (powder) 75 IU FSH activity and 75 IU LH activity per aml, 150 IU FSH activity and 150 IU LH activity per aml	ENDOCRINE AGENTS (G) Anterior Pituitary Hormones (SG)
MEPENZOLATE Cantil	PO: 25–50 mg QID (with meals and hs).	**Tablet:** 25 mg	AUTONOMIC AGENTS (G) Parasympatholytics (SG) Parasympatholytics, Quaternary Amines (SG) **Cost:** Very High
MEPERIDINE Generic, Demerol, Pethidine	**Pain Management:** PO, IM, SC: 50–150 mg q3–4h. Pediatric PO, IM, SC: 1–1.8 mg/kg q3–4h.	**Tablet:** 50, 100 mg **Syrup:** 50 mg/5 ml **Injection:** 10 mg/10 ml; 25, 50, 75, 100 mg/ml	**CNS AGENTS (G)** Narcotic Analgesics (SG) Intermediate Potency (SG) **Cost:** Medium
MEPHENYTOIN Mesantoin	**Seizure Disorders:** PO: 50–100 mg/d to start, increase by 50–100 mg/d q1week; maintenance 200–600 mg/d in 3 doses (max. dose 800 mg/d). Pediatric PO: 50–100 mg/d to start, increase by 50–100 mg/d q1week; maintenance 100–400 mg/d in 3 doses.	**Tablet:** 100 mg	CNS AGENTS (G) Anticonvulsants (SG) Hydantoins And Equivalent (SG) **Cost:** Medium
MEPHOBAR-BITAL Mebaral, Methyl-phenobarbital	**Sedative:** PO: 32–100 mg tid-QID Pediatric PO: 16–32 mg tid-QID **Anti-convulsant:** PO: 400–600 mg/d. Pediatric PO: (<5 yrs) 16–32 mg tid-QID. Pediatric PO: (>5 yrs) 32–64 mg tid-QID	**Tablet:** 32, 50, 100 mg	CNS AGENTS (G) Anticonvulsants (SG) Sedative-Hypnotics (SG) **Cost:** Medium
Mephyton	See PHYTONADIONE (K1)		K Vitamin (Coagulant)

GENERIC NAME Trade Name	INDICATIONS AND DOSAGES	DOSE FORMS	GROUP (G)/SUBGROUP (SG) Relative Cost within Group
MEPIVACAINE Generic, Carbocaine, Polocaine	**Infiltration:** 1% Peripheral Nerve Block: 1–2%	**Injection:** 1, 1.5, 2, 3%	LOCAL ANESTHETICS (G) Injectable or Topical (SG) **Cost:** Low
MEPROBAMATE Generic, Miltown, Equanil	**Sedation:** PO: 1200–1600 mg/d in 3–4 doses; max. dose 2,400 mg/d. PO (Ext'd release): 400–800 mg bid.	**Tablet:** 200, 400, 600 mg **Capsule (ER):** 200 mg, 400 mg	CNS AGENTS (G) Sedative-Hypnotics (SG) Intermediate-Acting (SG) **Cost:** Low
Mepyramine	See PYRILAMINE		Antihistamine
MERCAPTOPURINE Purinethol 6-MP	CANCER CHEMOTHERAPY (G) Antimetabolites (SG) Purine Analogues (SSG)		
MESALAMINE Pentasa, Asacol, Rowasa	**Chronic Inflammatory Bowel Disease:** PO (Tablet): 800 mg tid (total dose: 2.4 g/d for 6 weeks). PO (Capsule): 1 g QID (give for up to 8 weeks). Rectal (Suppository): 500 mg bid—retain for 1–3 hrs if possible (treat for 3–6 weeks). **Rectal (Suspension):** 4g (60 ml) once a day at hs—retain for up to 8h if possible (treat for 3–6 weeks).	**Tablet:** (Ext'd release) 400 mg **Capsule:** (Ext'd release) 250 mg **Suppositories:** 500 mg **Suspension:** (rectal) 4 g/60 ml	GI AGENTS (G) 5-Aminosalicylates (SG) **Cost:** Low
Mesantoin	See MEPHENYTOIN		Anticonvulsant
MESORIDAZINE Serentil	**Psychotic Disorders:** PO: 50 mg tid to start; 100–400 mg/d maintenance in 3 doses. IV: 25 mg; can repeat at 0.5–1 hour (max. dose 200 mg/d). **Alcohol Dependence:** PO: 25 mg bid to start (max. dose 50–200 mg/d).	**Tablet:** 10, 25, 50, 100 mg **Concentrate:** 25 mg/ml **Injection:** 25 mg/ml	CNS Agents(G) Antipsychotics (G) Moderate Extrapyramidal Effects (SG) **Cost:** Medium
Mestinon	See PYRIDOSTIGMINE		Cholinesterase Inhibitor
Metamucil	See PSYLLIUM		Bulk Laxative
Metaprel	See METAPROTERENOL		Beta Adrenergic Agonist
METAPROTERENOL Generic, Alupent, Metaprel	**Asthma, Bronchospasm:** Metered Inhaler: 2–3 inhalations tid-QID (max. dose 12 inhalations/d). **Nebulizer:** 10 (range 5–15) inhalations undiluted (0.5%) sln q4h. IPPB: Dilute 0.2–0.3 ml in 2.5 ml saline. PO: 20 mg tid-QID. Pediatric PO (<6 y.o.): 1.3–2.6 mg/kg/d in 3–4 doses. Pediatric PO (6–9 y.o.): 10 mg tid-QID.	**Syrup:** 10 mg/5 ml **Tablet:** 10, 20 mg	ANS AGENTS (G) Sympathomimetics (G) Beta 1 and 2 Effects (SG) **Cost:** Medium

GENERIC NAME Trade Name	INDICATIONS AND DOSAGES	DOSE FORMS	GROUP (G)/SUBGROUP (SG) Relative Cost within Group
METARAMINOL Generic, Aramine	**Hypotension:** IV: 0.5–5 mg initially; then mix a 0.025–0.2 mg/ml sln and adjust rate to establish blood pressure at desired level (eg., >90 mm Hg systolic). IV, SC: 2–10 mg initially; reassess blood pressure in 10 min and readminister PRN.	**Injection:** 10 mg/ml	ANS AGENTS (G) Sympathomimetics (SG) Predominantly Alpha Agonists (SG) **Cost:** High
METAXALONE Skelaxin	PO: 800 mg tid or QID (if older than 12 years).	**Tablet:** 400 mg	CNS AGENTS (G) Muscle Relaxants (SG) Sedative Hypnotics (SG) **Cost:** Medium
METFORMIN Glucophage	**Diabetes:** (II, NIDDM) PO: Initially 500 mg bid with meals. Increase daily dose by 500 or 850 mg q 1 or 2 weeks to 1500–2550 mg/d	**Tablet:** 500, 850 mg	ENDOCRINE AGENT (G) Oral Antidiabetic Agent (SG) Biguanide (SSG)
METHACHOLINE Provocholine	**Diagnosis Of Bronchial Airway Hyperactivity:** **Nebulizer:** Serial increases in nebulizer doses as follows—Dose 1–0.025 mg/ml Dose 2–0.25 mg/ml Dose 3–2.5 mg/ml Dose 4–10 mg/ml Dose 5–25 mg/ml. Measure FEV1 at 5 minutes after dose given. Target for positive challenge is 20% or greater reduction in FEV1 from baseline; stop test at this point. If reduction is 15 to 19% repeat challenge at same dose.	**Solution:** 100 mg/5ml	AUTONOMIC AGENTS (G) Cholinergic Agents (SG) Choline Esters (SG) **Cost:** Low
METHADYL (L-ALPHA-ACETYL)	See LEVOMETHADYL		Narcotic Analgesic
METHADONE Generic, Dolophine	**Pain Management:** PO, IM, SC: 2.5–10 mg q3–4h. **Detoxification treatment:** PO: 5–20 mg q6–8h. After 2–3 days dose should be gradually decreased.	**Tablet:** 5, 10mg **Oral Solution:** 5 mg/5ml, 10 mg/5ml, 10 mg/10ml **Oral Concentrate:** 10 mg/ml **Dispersible Tablet:** 40 mg **Injection:** 10 mg/ml	CNS AGENTS (G) Narcotic Analgesics (SG) Greatest Potency (SG)
METHAMPHETAMINE Generic, Desoxyn, Desoxyephedrine, Speed	**Exogenous Obesity:** PO: 2.5–5 mg bid or tid (given 30 min before meals). PO (Ext'd release): 10–15 mg qAM. **Attention Deficit:** Pediatric PO (>5 yrs): 5 mg, q12–24h to start; increase 5 mg/d q1week PRN; maintenance 20–25 mg/d.	**Tablet:** 5 mg **Tablet: (Ext'd release):** 5, 10, 15 mg	CNS AGENTS (G) Sympathomimetic Stimulants (SG) Schedule II Agents (SG) **Cost:** High
METHAZOLAMIDE Neptazane	**Glaucoma:** PO: 50–100 mg bid—tid.	**Tablet:** 25, 50 mg	OPHTHALMIC AGENTS (G) USED IN GLAUCOMA (SG) Carbonic Anhydrase Inhibitors (SG) **Cost:** Medium

GENERIC NAME Trade Name	INDICATIONS AND DOSAGES	DOSE FORMS	GROUP (G)/SUBGROUP (SG) Relative Cost within Group
METHENAMINE Mandelamine, Danazol, Uroqid, Hippurate: Hiprex, Urex	**Urinary Tract Infections—Mandelate:** PO: 1 g q6h, after meals and hs. Pediatric (6–12 y.o.) PO: 500 mg q6h. **Urinary Tract Infections—Hippurate:** PO: 1 g q12h. Pediatric (6–12 y.o.) PO: 0.5–1 g q12h.	**Mandelate:** **Tablet:** 0.5, 1 g **Tablet:** (Enteric) 0.25, 0.5, 1 g **Oral Suspension:** 0.25 g per 5 ml **Suspension Forte:** 0.5 g per 5 ml **Granules:** 1 g packets **Hippurate:** Tablet: 1 g	ANTI-INFECTIOUS AGENTS (G) Non-Sulfonamide For UTI (SG)
Methergine	See METHYLERGONOVINE		Vasoconstrictor
METHIMAZOLE Tapazole	**Mild Hyperthyroidism:** PO: 15 mg/d to start; maintenance 5–15 mg/d, give in 3 divided doses. Pediatric PO: 0.4 mg/kg/d to start; maintenance 0.2 mg/kg/d in 3 divided doses. **Moderate Hyperthyroidism:** PO: 30–40 mg/d to start; maintenance as above. **Severe Hyperthyroidism:** PO: 60 mg/d to start; maintenance as above.	**Tablet:** 5, 10 mg	ENDOCRINE AGENTS (G) Anti-Thyroid Agents and Related (SG) **Cost:** High
METHOCARBAMOL Generic, Robaxin	PO: 1500 mg QID initially, then maintenance 1000 mg QID.	**Tablet:** 500, 750 mg **Injection:** 100 mg/ml	CNS AGENTS (G) Muscle Relaxants (SG) Sedative Hypnotics (SG) **Cost:** Low
METHOHEXITAL Brevital	Administer IV in a concentration no higher than 1%. Induction 50–120 mg (adults 1–1.5 mg/kg). Maintenance: intermittent injection of 1% solution or by continuous IV drip of a 0.2% solution.	**Injection:** (powder) 500 mg, 2.5 g, 5g	GENERAL ANESTHETICS (G) Agents For Induction (SG)
METHOTREXATE Generic, Mexate, Amethopterin	**Antineoplastic:** **Rheumatoid Arthritis:** Initially 7,5 mg weekly or 2,5 mg tid one day each week. **Abortifacient:** with misoprostol CANCER CHEMOTHERAPY (G) Antimetabolites (SG) Folate Analogue (SSG)		
METHOTRIMEPRAZINE Levomepromazine, Levoprome	**Pain:** IM: 10–20 mg q4–6h to start; maintenance 5–40 mg q1–24h. **Preoperative:** IM: 2–20 mg 45–180 min prior to procedure (decrease if concurrent atropine or scopolamine is being used).	**Injection:** 20 mg/ml	ANTI-INFLAMMATORY AGENTS (G) Non-Narcotic Analgesics (SG) Other Nonnarcotic Analgesics (SG) **Cost:** Very High

GENERIC NAME Trade Name	INDICATIONS AND DOSAGES	DOSE FORMS	GROUP (G)/SUBGROUP (SG) Relative Cost within Group
METHOXAMINE Vasoxyl	**Hypotension:** IM: 5–15 mg, depending on degree of decrease; repeat PRN. IV: 3–5 mg if systolic pressure <60 mm; may be given with 10–15 mg IM for prolonged effect or an infusion may be given with an initial dose of 5 mcg/min. (Give IV SLOWLY). **Paroxysmal Supraventricular Tachycardia:** IV: 10 mg SLOWLY (over 3–5 min).	**Injection:** 20 mg/ml	ANS AGENTS (G) Sympathomimetics (SG) Predominantly Alpha Agonists (SG) **Cost:** High
METHOXSALEN Generic, Oxsoralen, 8-MOP	**Vitiligo:** PO: 20 mg daily, take dose 2 to 4 hours before UV exposure.	**Capsule:** 10 mg	DERMATOLOGIC AGENTS (G) Miscellaneous (SG)
METHSCOPOL-AMINE Dura-Vent,	PO: 2.5 mg, take 30 minutes ac, and 2.5–5 mg at hs.	**Tablet:** 2.5 mg	ANS AGENTS (G) Parasympatholytics (SG) Quaternary Amines (SG)
METHSUXIMIDE Celontin	**Seizure Disorders:** PO: 300 mg/d for 1 week, each wk add 300 mg/d (max. dose 1200 mg/d).	**Capsule:** 150, 300 mg	CNS AGENTS (G) Anticonvulsants (SG) Succinimides (SG)
METHYCLOTHIA-ZIDE Generic, Aquatensen, Enduron	**Hypertension:** PO: 2.5–5 mg qd. **Edema:** PO: Initially 2.5–10 mg qd.	**Tablet:** 2.5, 5 mg	RENAL AGENTS (G) Sodium Diuretics (G) Thiazide Diuretics (SG) **Cost:** Low
METHYL TESTOSTERONE Generic, Virilon, Testred	**Androgen Deficiency in Males:** PO: 10–50 mg/d.	**Capsule:** 10 mg	ENDOCRINE AGENTS (G) Androgenic/Anabolic Steroids (SG) **Cost:** Low
METHYLCELLU-LOSE Generic, OTC, Citrucel, Maltsupex, others	PO: 1 heaping tbsp in 8 oz cold water 1–3 times daily. Children (6–12 yrs): ½ heaping tbsp in 4 oz cold water, 1–3 times daily. PO: 1–2 tbsp qd or bid (mix in liquid).	**Citrucel:** Powder; 2g methylcellulose/heaping tbsp	LAXATIVES AND BOWEL CLEANSERS (G) Bulk Laxatives(SG) **Cost:** Medium
METHYLDOPA Generic, Aldomet, Aldoril	**Hypertension:** PO: 250 mg bid or tid initially; 500–3000 mg/d maintenance in 2–4 doses. IV: 250–500 mg q6h (max dose: 1000 mg q6h).	**Tablet:** 125, 250, 500 mg **Oral Suspension:** 250 mg/5 ml **Injection:** 250 mg/5 ml	ANS AGENTS (G) Sympathoplegics (G) Centrally-Acting Adrenergic Inhibitors (SG) **Cost:** Low
METHYLDOPA-DIURETIC COMBINATION Generic, Aldoril	**Hypertension:**	**Tablet:** Methyldopa/hydrochlorothiazide in following doses: 15/250 mg, 25/250 mg, 30/500 mg, 50/500 mg	CENTRAL SYMPATHOPLEGIC (G) AND DIURETIC
METHYLENE BLUE Generic	**Methemoglobinemia:** 1–2 mg/kg IV over several minutes.	**Injection:** 10 mg/ml	ANTIDOTES AND USED IN POISONINGS (G)

GENERIC NAME Trade Name	INDICATIONS AND DOSAGES	DOSE FORMS	GROUP (G)/SUBGROUP (SG) Relative Cost within Group
METHYLERGO-NOVINE Methergine	**Prevent Post-Partum Bleeding:** PO: 0.2 mg q6–8h for a max. duration of 1 week. IV, IV: 0.2 mg after placenta delivered; repeat q2–4h PRN. (Infuse IV dose SLOWLY over 1 min with careful BP monitoring.)	**Tablet:** 0.2 mg **Injection:** 0.2 mg/ml (1 ml)	CV AGENTS (G) Vasoconstrictors And Oxytocics (G)
METHYLPHENI-DATE Generic, Ritalin	**Attention Deficit:** Pediatric (>5 yrs) PO: 5 mg bid; increase 5–10 mg/d q1week; maintenance 10–60 mg/d.	**Tablet:** 5, 10, 20 mg **Tablet:** (Ext'd release) 20 mg	SYMPATHOMIMETIC STIMULANTS (G) Schedule II Agents (SG) **Cost:** Medium
Methylphenobar-bital	See MEPHOBARBITAL		Anticonvulsant
METHYLPRED-NISOLONE Generic, Medrol, Solu-Medrol, Depo-Medrol, Depoject	PO: 4–48 mg/d. IV (succinate): 10–40 mg. IV (acetate): 40–120 mg weekly. Intraarticular (acetate): 4–80 mg.	**Tablet:** 2, 4, 8, 16, 24, 32 mg	ENDOCRINE AGENTS (G) Anti-Inflammatory Steroids (SG) **Cost:** Low
METHYPRYLON Noludar	**Hypnotic:** PO: 200–400 mg hs. Pediatric PO (>12 yrs. only): 50–200 mg hs.	**Tablet:** 200 mg **Capsule:** 300 mg	CNS AGENTS (G) Sedative-Hypnotics (SG) Short-Acting Hypnotics (SG) **Cost:** Low
METHYSERGIDE Sansert	**Prevention of Migraine Attacks:** PO: 4–8 mg/d (discontinue after 3 wks if no benefit). Discontinue drug for 3–4 weeks q6months.	**Tablet:** 2 mg	CV AGENTS (G) Vasoconstrictors and Oxytocics (SG) **Cost:** Low
Meticorten	See PREDNISOLONE		Corticosteroid
METIMYD	**Ophthalmic (suspension):** 2–3 qtt q 1–2 h during the day and hs. **Ophthalmic (ointment):** Apply 0.25–0.5 inch tid or QID and hs.	**Ophthalmic Suspension:** sulfacetamide sodium (10%), prednisolone acetate (0.5%) **Ophthalmic Ointment:** sulfacetamide sodium (10%), prednisolone acetate (0.5%)	
METIPRANOL OptiPranolol	**Elevated IOP:** Instill 1 drop bid.	**Solution:** 0.3%	OPHTHALMIC PREPARATIONS (G) Used In Glaucoma (G) Beta-Adrenergic Receptor Blockers (SG) **Cost:** Low

GENERIC NAME Trade Name	INDICATIONS AND DOSAGES	DOSE FORMS	GROUP (G)/SUBGROUP (SG) Relative Cost within Group
METOCLO-PRAMIDE Reglan, Maxolon	**Diabetic Gastroparesis:** PO, IV: 10 mg 30 min ac and hs, for 2–8 weeks (infuse IV over 2 or more minutes, convert to PO as soon as feasible). **Post-Op Nausea & Vomiting:** IM: 10–20 mg near end of procedure. **Chemotherapy Emesis Prophylaxis:** IV: 1–2 mg/kg (give slowly over 15–30 min) repeat q2h for 2 doses, then give q3h for 3 doses. **Gastroesophageal Reflux:** PO: 10–15 mg 30 min ac and hs (max. dose: 45 mg/d).	**Tablet:** 5, 10 mg **Syrup:** 5 mg/5 ml **Injection:** 5 mg/ml **Concentrated Solution:** 10 mg/ml	GI AGENTS (G) Antiemetics (Minor) (SG) **Cost:** Medium
METOCURINE Metubine	**Surgery:** IV: 0.2–0.4 mg/kg to start, then 0.5–1 mg PRN. **Electroconvulsive Therapy:** IV: 1.75–5.5 mg; administer SLOWLY, until head-drop is produced (average dose range 2–3 mg).	**Injection:** 2 mg/ml	GENERAL ANESTHETICS AND ADJUNCTS (G) Neuromuscular Blocking Agents (SG) Non-Depolarizing Agents (SSG) **Cost:** Medium
METOLAZONE Zaroxolyn, Mykrox	**Hypertension:** PO: 2.5–5 mg qd (Zaroxolyn). PO: initially 0.5 mg qd, maintenance 0.5–1.0 mg qd (Mykrox). **Edema:** PO: 5–20 mg qd (Zaroxolyn only).	**Tablet:** 2.5, 5, 10 mg Zaroxolyn, slow onset **Tablet:** 0.5 mg Mykrox, rapid onset	RENAL AGENTS (G) Thiazide Diuretics (SG) **Cost:** Medium
METOPROLOL Generic, Lopressor, Toprol	**Hypertension:** PO: 100 mg/d initially given as 1 or 2 doses; 100–450 mg/d maintenance in 1–3 doses (smaller doses may require > once a day dosing). PO (Ext'd release): 50–100 mg qd initially; 100–400 mg qd maintenance. **Angina:** PO: 50 mg bid initially; 100–400 mg/d maintenance. When discontinuing, taper dose over two or more weeks. PO (Ext'd release): 100 mg qd initially; 100–400 mg qd maintenance. Reassess at weekly (or longer) intervals and increase if needed. **Acute MI:** IV: 1–3 mg SLOWLY (not > 1 mg/min), initially; repeat after 2 minutes to a total dose of 0.1 mg/kg. Oral therapy (180–320 mg/d) thereafter.	**Tablet:** 50, 100 mg **Tablet:** (ER) 50,100 mg **Injection:** 1 mg/ml	ANS AGENT(G) Sympathoplegics (SG) Cardioselective, Beta 1 Blocker (SG) **Cost:** Medium
Metremia	See TRIMETHOPRIM		Antibacterial
Metrodin	See UROFOLLITROPIN (FSH)		Fertility Agent

GENERIC NAME Trade Name	INDICATIONS AND DOSAGES	DOSE FORMS	GROUP (G)/SUBGROUP (SG) Relative Cost within Group
METRONIDA-ZOLE Generic, Flagyl, Protostat	**Anaerobic Bacterial Infections:** PO: 7.5 mg/kg q6h; max. dose 4 g/d. IV: 15 mg/kg to start, then 7.5 mg/kg q6h for 7–10 days—bone, heart, pulmonary and joint infections may take longer (max. dose 4 g/d). Infuse doses over 1 hour. **Prophylaxis for Surgery:** IV: 15 mg/kg given SLOWLY (over 30–60 min) 1 hour prior to surgery; then 7.5 mg/kg at 6 hours and 12 hours after first dose. **Bacterial Vaginosis:** PO: 500 mg bid for 7 days (alternate regimen 2 g given as a single dose). **Giardiasis (quinacrine alternate):** PO: 250 mg tid for 7 days. **Acute Amebiasis (dysentery):** PO: 750 mg tid for 5–10 days. Pediatric PO: 30–50 mg/kg/d in 3 divided doses for 10 days (max. single dose 750 mg/dose). **Amebic Liver Abscess:** PO: 500–750 mg tid for 5–10 days. **Trichomoniasis:** PO (single dose): 2 g in one day given as 1 or 2 doses. PO (7 day): 250 mg tid for 7 days. **Acne Rosacea:** Apply gel bid.	**Tablet:** 250, 500 mg **Injection:** 500 mg/100 ml **Injection:** (powder) 500 mg (as HCL) ANTI-INFECTIOUS AGENTS (G)	Miscellaneous Antibacterials (SG) **Cost:** Low (PO) Medium (IV)
Metubine	See METOCURINE		Curariform
Mevacor	See LOVASTATIN		HMG-CoA Reductase Inhibitors
Mexate	See METHOTREXATE		Cancer Chemotherapy
MEXILETINE Mexitil	**Ventricular Arrhythmias** **(Not recommended):** PO: 200 mg q 8h; may increase up to 400 mg q 8h (max. dose 1200 mg/d).	**Capsule:** 150, 200, 250 mg	CV AGENTS (G) Antiarrhythmic Agents (SG) Group I (SG) **Cost:** High
Mexitil	See MEXILETINE		Antiarrhythmic
Mezlin	See MEZLOCILLIN		Lactam Antibiotic
MEZLOCILLIN Mezlin	IM dose should not exceed 2 g/injection. **General Infection:** IV, IM: 3 g q4h (18 g/d) or 4 g q6h (16 g/d). **Serious Infection:** IV, IM: 200–350 mg/kg/d given in 4–6 divided doses (max. dose 24 g/d). **Uncomplicated Gonorrhea:** IM, IV: 1–2 g (single dose); plus 1 g probenecid PO 30 min prior to injection. **Surgical Prophylaxis:** IV: 4 g 30–90 minutes prior to surgery, repeat at 6 and 12 hours. Lower Respiratory Tract, Skin, Intra-abdominal **Infection:** IV: 4 g q6h or 3 g q4h.	**Injection:** (powder) 1, 2, 3, 4, 20 g	LACTAM ANTIBIOTICS (G) Wider Gram Negative Coverage (SG) No/Marginal Effectiveness In Meningitis and vs. P. aeruginosa (SSG) **Cost:** Low
Miacalcin	See CALCITONIN		Inhibit Osteoclastic Activity

GENERIC NAME Trade Name	INDICATIONS AND DOSAGES	DOSE FORMS	GROUP (G)/SUBGROUP (SG) Relative Cost within Group
MIBEFRADIL Posicor	**Hypertension, Angina:** PO: 50–100 once daily	**Tablet:** 50 mg	CV AGENTS (G) Vasodilators, Post-Arteriolar (SG) Calcium Channel Blockers (SSG)
Micatin	See MICONAZOLE		Fungicide
MICONAZOLE Generic, OTC, Micatin, Monistat, Zeasorb	**Tinea, Cutaneous Candidiasis:** (Topical): apply to affected and surrounding skin areas bid (treat pedis for four weeks, others for two weeks).	**Cream:** 2% **Powder:** 2% **Spray:** 2% **Solution:** 2%	TOPICAL ANTI-INFECTIOUS AGENTS (G) Topical Fungicides (SG) **Cost:** Low as generics
Micro-K	See POTASSIUM CHLORIDE		Supplementary K Ion
Micronase	See GLYBURIDE		Oral Antidiabetic Agent
Midamor	See AMILORIDE		K Sparing Diuretic
MIDAZOLAM Versed	**Conscious Sedation:** IV: 1–2.5 mg (administered over >2 minutes. May repeat after evaluation of effect in 2–4 minutes (max. dose usually not >5 mg to produce desired effect). Lower dose in elderly, debilitated or if other CNS depressants acting or given simultaneously.	**Injection:** 1, 5 mg/ml	GENERAL ANESTHETICS AND ADJUNCTS (G) Preprocedural Agents (Conscious Sedation) (SG) **Cost:** High
MIDODRINE ProAmatine	**Orthostatic Hypotension:** PO: 10mg tid	**Tablets: 2.5, 5 mg**	ANS AGENT (G) Sympathomimetic, Pure Alpha Agonist (SG)
MIDRIN	**Tension Headache:** PO: 1–2 capsules q 4 h, up to 8 capsules qd. **Migraine Headache:** PO: 2 capsules stat, then 1 capsule q h until relieved, up to 5 capsules within a 12-hour period.	**Capsule:** isometheptene mucate (65 mg), dichloral-phenazone (100 mg), acetaminophen (325 mg)	
MIFEPRISTONE RU486	**Abortifacient (investigational drug):** PO: 600 mg as a single dose followed in 48 h by a prostaglandin agonist intravaginally.	Availability pending.	ENDOCRINE AGENTS (G) Antiprogestins (SG)
Milkinol	See MINERAL OIL		Stool Softener
Milontin	See PHENSUXIMIDE		Anticonvulsant
Milophene	See CLOMIPHENE		Fertility Agent
MILRINONE Primacor	**CHF:** IV: Loading dose 50 mcg/kg given over 10 minutes, infuse maintenance dose at 0.375–0.75 mcg/kg/min (max. dose 1.13 mg/kg).	**Injection:** 1 mg/ml	CV AGENT (G) Xanthine (SG) **Cost:** Very High
Miltown	See MEPROBAMATE		Sedative-Hypnotic
MINERAL OIL Agoral Plain, Milkinol, Neo-Cultol	PO: 5–45 ml. Pediatric PO: 5–20 ml.	**Liquid:** heavy mineral oil **Emulsion:** 1.4 g mineral oil/ 5 ml **Jelly:** refined mineral oil	GI AGENTS (G) Fecal Softener Laxatives (SG) **Cost:** Medium
Minipress	See PRAZOSIN		Alpha Adrenergic Receptor Blockers

GENERIC NAME Trade Name	INDICATIONS AND DOSAGES	DOSE FORMS	GROUP (G)/SUBGROUP (SG) Relative Cost within Group
Minizide 1, 2, 5	See PRAZOSIN-DIURETIC COMBINATION		Hypotensive-Diuretic Combination
Minocin	See MINOCYCLINE		Tetracycline Antibiotic
MINOCYCLINE Generic, Minocin, Dynacin	**Bacterial Infections:** PO, IV: 200 mg to start; then 100 mg bid (max. IV dose 400 mg/d). Pediatric (> 8 yrs) PO: IV: 4 mg/kg to start; then 2 mg/kg bid. **Syphilis:** PO: 200 mg to start; then 100 mg bid for 10–15 days. **Chlamydia trachomatis or U. urealyticum (mycoplasmas):** PO: 100 mg bid for 7 days. **Gonorrhea (Penicillin-Sensitive Patients):** PO: 200 mg to start; then 100 mg bid for 4 days or longer. **Meningococcal-Carrier State:** PO: 100 mg bid for 5 days. **Mycobacterium marinum Infections:** PO: 100 mg bid for 6–8 weeks.	**Capsule:** 50, 100 mg **Injection:** (powder) 100 mg **Oral Suspension:** 50 mg per 5 ml	TETRACYCLINES (G) **Cost:** Medium
MINOXIDIL Generic, Loniten, Rogaine	**Hypertension:** PO: 5 mg/d to start; 5–40 mg/d maintenance in 1–2 doses (max. dose 100 mg/d). **Alopecia (includes Male Pattern Baldness):** Topical (2% sln.): 1 ml to scalp bid.	**Tablet:** 2.5, 10 mg	CV AGENTS (G) Vasodilators (SG) Arteriolar Dilators (SG) **Cost:** Low (PO) Very High (topical)
Mintezol	See THIABENDAZOLE		Parasiticide
Miostat	See CARBACHOL		Cholinergic
MIRTAZAPINE Remeron	**Depression:** PO: Initially 15 mg, then 15–45 mg.	**Tablet:** 15,30 mg	CNS AGENTS (G) TCA Antidepressants (SG)
MISOPROSTOL Cytotec	**NSAID Induced Ulcer Prophylaxis:** PO: 100–200 mcg QID as tolerated (take with food).	**Tablet:** 100, 200 mcg	ANTACIDS (G) Surface and Mixed Activity (SG) **Cost:** Medium
Mithracin	See PLICAMYCIN		
MITOMYCIN Mitomycin-C	CANCER CHEMOTHERAPY (G) React With DNA (SG) Antibiotics (SSG)		
Mitomycin-C	See MITOMYCIN		
MITOXANTRONE Novantrone	CANCER CHEMOTHERAPY (G) React With DNA (SG) Antibiotics (SSG)		
Mivacron	See MIVACURIUM		Curariform
MIVACURIUM Mivacron	**Endotracheal Intubation:** 0.15 mg/kg given over 5–15 seconds (effective neuromuscular block duration 15–20 minutes AVE).	**Injection:** 0.5, 2 mg/ml	GENERAL ANESTHETICS AND ADJUNCTS (G) Neuromuscular Blocking Agents (SG) Non-Depolarizing (SSG) **Cost:** High
Moban	See MOLINDONE		Antipsychotic
Mobequin	See IODOQUINOL		Parasiticide

GENERIC NAME Trade Name	INDICATIONS AND DOSAGES	DOSE FORMS	GROUP (G)/SUBGROUP (SG) Relative Cost within Group
Mobidin	See MAGNESIUM SALICYLATE		Non-Narcotic Analgetic
Moctanin	See MONOCTANOIN		Gall Stone Dissolution
Modicon	PO: 21-Day regimen or 28-Day regimen.	**Tablet:** ethinyl estradiol (35 mcg), norethindrone (0.5 mg) in 21-Day and 28-Day packs	
Moduretic	PO: Initially 1 tablet/d. Dosage may be raised to 2 tabs/d as a single dose or in divided doses.	**Tablet:** amiloride HCl (5 mg), hydro-chlorothiazide (50 mg)	
MOEXIPRIL Univasc	**Hypertension:** PO: Initially 7.5 mg qd ac, maintenance of 7.5–30 mg/d in 1–2 doses ac	**Tablet:** 7.5, 15 mg	CV AGENTS (G) Vasodilator (SG) ACE Inhibitor (SSG)
MOLINDONE Moban	**Psychotic Disorders:** PO: 50–75 mg/d to start; maintenance 5–25 mg tid-QID (max. dose 225 mg/d).	**Tablet:** 5, 10, 25, 50, 100 mg **Concentrate:** 20 mg/ ml	CNS AGENTS (G) Antipsychotics (SG) Prominent Extrapyramidal Effects (SG) **Cost:** Medium
MONOBENZONE Benoquin	**Depigmentation After Vitiligo:** Topical: rub into the pigmented areas to be treated 2 to 3 times daily (effects seen in 1–4 months, discontinue after 4 months if no improvement).	**Cream:** 20%	DERMATOLOGIC AGENTS (G) Miscellaneous (SG) **Cost:** Medium
Monocid	See CEFONICID		Lactam Antibiotic
MONOCTANOIN Moctanin	**Dissolution of Post-OP Radiolucent Gallbladder Stone :** Intra-biliary-tree Infusion: 3–5 ml/hour of diluted solution. (Discontinue if no effect after 72h. Usual treatment lasts 2–10 days.)	**Infusion:** 120 ml bottles	MISCELLANEOUS GI AGENTS (G) Gallstone Dissolving Agents (SG)
Monodox	See DOXYCYCLINE		Tetracycline
Monoket	See ISOSORBIDE MONONITRATE		Vasodilator
Mononine	See COAGULANT FACTOR IX		Hemostatic
Monopril	See FOSINOPRIL		ACE Inhibitor
MORICIZINE Ethmozine	**Arrhythmias:** PO: 200–300 mg q 8 h (within range increase PRN by 150 mg/d every three days). (q12h dosing may also be effective in some patients.)	**Tablet:** 200, 250, 300 mg	CV AGENTS (G) Antiarrhythmic Agents (SG) Group I (SG)

GENERIC NAME Trade Name	INDICATIONS AND DOSAGES	DOSE FORMS	GROUP (G)/SUBGROUP (SG) Relative Cost within Group
MORPHINE Generic, Morphine, M.S., MS Contin, Oramorph	**Pain Management:** Initial doses: IV: 2.5–15 mg q3–4h SC: 5–20 mg q4h. Rectal: 10–20 mg q4h. PO: 10–30 mg q4h. PO: (Ext'd release) 30 mg q8–12h.	**Tablet:** 15, 30 mg **Tablet:** (ER) 15, 30, 60, 100 mg **Soluble Tablet:** 10, 15, 30 mg **Solution:** 10, 20,100 mg/5 ml **Suppositories:** 5, 10, 20, 30 mg **Injection:** 0.5, 1, 2, 3, 4, 5, 8, 10, 15, 25, 50 mg/ml	CNS AGENTS (G) Narcotic Analgesics (G) Of Greatest Potency (SG) **Cost:** High
Motofen	See DIFENOXIN WITH ATROPINE		Antidiarrheal
Motrin	See IBUPROFEN		Non-Narcotic Analgesics
Mucomyst	See ACETYLCYSTEINE		Mucolytic
Mucosil-20	See ACETYLCYSTEINE		Mucolytic
Muse	See ALPROSTADIL		Vasodilator
Mustargen	See MECHLORETHAMINE		Cancer Chemotherapy
Myambutol	See ETHAMBUTOL		Tuberculostatic
Mycelex	See CLOTRIMAZOLE		Fungicide
Mycifradin	See NEOMYCIN		Aminoglycoside
MYCITRACIN TRIPLE ANTIBIOTIC	Topical: Apply 1–3 times/d.	**Ointment (per g):** polymyxin B sulfate (5000 Units), neomycin sulfate (3.5 mg), bacitracin (500 Units)	
MYCOLOG-II	Topical: Apply bid in the AM and PM.	**Cream and Ointment (per g):** triamcinolone acetonide (1.0 mg), nystatin (100,000 Units)	
Mycostatin	See NYSTATIN		Fungicide
Mydriacyl	See TROPICAMIDE		Local Anesthetic
Mykrox	See METOLAZONE		Sodium Diuretic
Mylanta	See ALUMINUM HYDROXIDE with MAGNESIUM HYDROXIDE		Antacid
Myleran	See BUSULFAN		Cancer Chemotherapy
Myochrysine	See GOLD SODIUM THIOMALATE		Antirheumatic
Myolin	See ORPHENADRINE		Anticholinergic
Mysoline	See PRIMIDONE		Anticonvulsants

GENERIC NAME Trade Name	INDICATIONS AND DOSAGES	DOSE FORMS	GROUP (G)/SUBGROUP (SG) Relative Cost within Group
NABUMETONE Relafen	**Arthritic Condition:** 1000 mg qd or bid	**Tablet:** 500, 750 mg	ANTI-INFLAMMATORY (G) Non-Narcotic Analgesics (SG) Aspirin and Related NSAIDs (SG) **Cost:** High
NADOLOL Generic, Corgard	**Hypertension:** PO: 40 mg/d initially; 40–320 mg/d maintenance as 1 dose (max dose: 320 mg/d). Assess and change dose if needed q3–7d. **Angina:** PO: 40 mg/d initially; 40–240 mg/d maintenance given as 1 dose (max dose: 240 mg/d). Assess and change dose if needed q3–7d.	**Tablet:** 20, 40, 80, 120, 160 mg	ANS AGENTS (G) Sympathoplegics (SG) Beta Adrenergic Blockers (SSG) Non-Selective (Beta 1 and 2) Blockers (SSG) **Cost:** Medium
NAFARELIN Synarel	**Endometriosis:** Nasal Spray: 400 mcg/d given in two divided doses as single spray, in one nostril qAM & qPM; (max. dose: 800 mcg/d; safety of treatment beyond 6 mo. has not been established). **Central precocious puberty**	Nasal Spray: 1600 mcg/d, given in two divided doses as two sprays (400 mcg ea. spray) into each nostril qAM & qPM for a total of 8 sprays per day (max. dose: 1800 mcg/d).	ENDOCRINE AGENTS (G) Hypothalamic Releasing Factor Antagonist (SG)
NAFCILLIN Generic, Unipen	**Infections:** PO: 250 mg-1 g q4–6h. IV: 500 mg q4–6h. IV: 3000–6000 mg/d in 4 divided doses. **Pediatric Infections:** Pediatric PO: 50–100 mg/kg/d in 4 doses. Pediatric IM: 150 mg/kg/d in 4 doses. Pediatric IV: 150–200 mg/kg/d in 4–6 doses. **Streptococcal Pharyngitis (when Pen V not used):** Pediatric PO: 250 mg tid for 10 days.	**Capsule:** 250 mg **Tablet:** 500 mg **Injection:** (powder) 500 mg, 1, 2, 10 g	ANTI-INFLAMMATORY AGENTS (G) Lactam antibiotics (SG) Penicillins: Resistant to Staphylococcal Lactamase (SSG) **Cost:** Low
NAFTIFINE Naftin	**Tinea pedis, cruris, corporis:** Topical: massage into affected areas qd with the cream (bid with the gel).	**Cream:** 1% **Gel:** 1%	ANTI-INFECTIOUS AGENTS (G) Topical Fungicides (SG) **Cost:** Medium
Naftin	See NAFTIFINE		Fungicide, Topical
NALBUPHINE Generic, Nubain	**Pain Management:** IV, IM, SC: 10–20 mg q3–6h. (max. dose: 160 mg/d IV, IM, SC).	**Injection:** 10, 20 mg/ml	CNS AGENTS (G) Narcotic Analgesics And Related Agents (SG) Mixed Agonist-Antagonist Effects (SSG) **Cost:** Medium
Nalfon	See FENOPROFEN		Non-Narcotic Analgetic
NALIDIXIC ACID Generic, NegGram	**Urinary Tract Infections:** PO: initial 1–2 weeks give 1 g QID; may reduce to 2 g/d for time greater than 2 weeks.	**Tablet:** 250 mg, 500 mg, 1 g **Suspension:** 250 mg per 5 ml	ANTI-INFECTIOUS AGENT (G) Quinolone (SG) **Cost:** High

GENERIC NAME Trade Name	INDICATIONS AND DOSAGES	DOSE FORMS	GROUP (G)/SUBGROUP (SG) Relative Cost within Group
NALMEFENE Revex	**Reverse Effects of Narcotics: Intra- and post-operative:** 0.25 mcg/kg q 2–5 min prn to 1 mcg /kg.**Overdose:** 50 mcg (0.5 mg) q 2–5 to max of 1.5 mg. Repeat only after 4 h.	**Injection:** 100 mcg/ml and 1 mg/ml	CNS AGENTS(G) Narcotic Antagonist (SG) **Cost:** Low
NALOXONE Generic, Narcan	**Post-Operative Narcotic Reversal:** IV: 0.1–0.2 mg q2–3 min until desired state of reversal obtained. Pediatric IV: 0.005–0.01 mg q2–3 minutes until desired state of reversal obtained. **Opiate Overdose Reversal:** IV: 0.4–2.0 mg q2–3 min prn to 10 mg. Pediatric IV**:** 0.01 mg/kg to start; if not effective, then administer an additional dose of 0.1 mg/kg**.** **Naloxone Challenge:** Patient should be opioid free for at least 7d and not be manifesting withdrawal symptoms.) **IV: Step 1—put 0.8 mg (2 ml) naloxone in a syringe;** **Step 2**—inject IV 0.2 mg initially and observe for evidence of withdrawal for 30 sec (don't remove syringe); **Step 3—**if no withdrawal, give the remaining 0.6 mg and observe for s/sx withdrawal for 20 minutes more; If there is doubt about s/sx, a confirmatory rechallenge of 1.6 mg (4 ml) may be administered. **SC:** Inject SC 0.8 mg (2 ml) and observe for evidence of withdrawal for 45 minutes; if no s/sx of withdrawal are noted, challenge is considered negative and naltrexone may be started.	**Injection:** 0.4, 1 mg/ml **Injection:** (neonatal) 0.02 mg/ml	CNS AGENTS (G) Narcotic Analgesics And Related Agents (SG) Narcotic Antagonists (SSG) **Cost:** Very High
NALTREXONE ReVia, Trexan	**Opiate Blockade (Treatment):** PO: 50 mg/d (start slowly and only if opioid-free and if naloxone iv challenge is negative). **Chronic Alcoholism:** Limited Experience	**Tablet:** 50 mg	CNS AGENTS (G) Narcotic Analgesics And Related Agents (SG) Narcotic Antagonists (SSG) **Cost:** High
NANDROLONE Generic, Durabolin, Deca-Durabolin	**Anemia Of Renal Disease:** IM: (men) 100–200 mg per week. IV: (women) 50–100 mg per week. **Breast Cancer Palliation:** IM (phenylpropionate): 50–100 mg per week.	**Injection:** (in oil) 25, 50, 100, 200 mg/ml	ENDOCRINE AGENTS (G) Androgenic/Anabolic Steroids (SG) **Cost:** Medium
NAPHAZOLINE OTC, Privine	**Nasal Decongestion:** Intranasal (adults and children >12 yrs): 1–2 drops or sprays in each nostril q6h.	**Solution:** 0.05%	SYMPATHOMIMETICS (G) Incomplete Sympathomimetics (SG) **Cost:** Medium
Naphcon-A		**Ophthalmic Solution:** naphazoline HCl (0.025%), pheniramine maleate (0.3%)	
Naprosyn	See NAPROXEN		Non-Narcotic Analgetic

GENERIC NAME Trade Name	INDICATIONS AND DOSAGES	DOSE FORMS	GROUP (G)/SUBGROUP (SG) Relative Cost within Group
NAPROXEN OTC, Generic, Naprosyn, Anaprox, Aleve	**Arthritic Conditions:** PO: 250–500 mg naproxen q12h; max. dose 1250 mg/d. PO: 275 mg qAM, 550 mg qPM N-sodium; max. dose 1375 mg/d. **Acute Gout:** PO: 750 mg naproxen to start, then 250 mg q8h. PO: 825 mg N-sodium to start, then 275 mg q8h. **Pain/Dysmenorrhea:** PO: 500 mg naproxen to start, then 250 mg q6–8h; max. dose 1250 mg/d. PO: 550 mg N-sodium to start; then 275 mg q6–8h; max. dose 1375 mg/d.	**Tablet:** 200 mg (220 mg naproxen sodium), 250 mg (275 mg naproxen sodium), 500 mg (550 mg naproxen sodium), 250 mg, 375 mg, 500 mg **Oral Suspension:** 125 mg/5 ml	ANTI-INFLAMMATORY AGENTS (G) Non-Narcotic Analgesics (SG) Aspirin And Related (SSG) **Cost:** Medium
Naqua	See TRICHLORMETHIAZIDE		Sodium Diuretic
Narcan	See NALOXONE		Narcotic Antagonist
Nardil	See PHENELZINE		MAO Inhibitor
Nasalcrom	See CROMOLYN		Mast Cell Stabilizer
Nasalide	See FLUNISOLIDE		Corticosteroid
Natacyn	See NATAMYCIN		Antifungal, Ocular
NATAMYCIN Natacyn	**Fungal keratitis:** **Suspension:** 1 drop q1–2h into conjunctival sac to start, then decrease frequency to q3–4h after 3–4 d (treat for ave. 14–21 d). **Fungal conjunctivitis, blepharitis:** **Suspension:** 1 drop q4–6h times/d into conjunctival sac.	**Suspension:** 5%	OPHTHALMIC AGENTS (G) Anti-Fungal Agent (SG)
Naturetin	See BENDROFLUMETHIAZIDE		Sodium Diuretic
Navane	See THIOTHIXENE		Antipsychotic
Navelbine	See VINORELBINE		Cancer Chemotherapy
NebuPent	See PENTAMIDINE		Antiparasitic
NEDOCROMIL Tilade	**Bronchial Asthma:** Inhalation (adults and children >12 yrs): 2 puffs QID (use at regular intervals) to provide 14 mg/d.	**Aerosol:** 1.75 mg per puff	RESPIRATORY AGENTS (G) Antiallergic Agents, Non-Steroidal (SG)
NEFAZODONE Serzone	**Endogenous Depression:** PO: 100 mg bid increased at intervals of 1 week to 150 to 300 mg bid (less in older patients).	**Tablet:** 100 mg	CNS AGENTS (G) Tricyclic Antidepressants (SG)
NegGram	See NALIDIXIC ACID		Quinolone Antibacterial
NELFINAVIR Viracept	**HIV Infection:** PO; In combination with nucleoside analogue.	**Tablet: 250 mg**	ANTI-INFECTIOUS AGENT (G) Antiretroviral (SG) Protease Inhibitor (SSG) **Cost:** Very High

GENERIC NAME Trade Name	INDICATIONS AND DOSAGES	DOSE FORMS	GROUP (G)/SUBGROUP (SG) Relative Cost within Group
NELOVA 0.5/ 35E, 1/35E, 1/ 50E	**Oral Contraceptive:** PO: 1 tab/d. 28-Day regimen.	**Tablet:** norethindrone (0.5 or 1.0 mg), ethinyl estradiol (35 or 50 mcg) in 28-Day packs	
NELOVA 10/11	**Oral Contraception:** PO: 1 tab qd. 28-Day regimen.	**Tablets:** triphasic dosage	
Nembutal	See PENTOBARBITAL		Hypnotic
NEO-CORTEF		**Cream and Ointment:** neomycin sulfate (0.5%), hydro-cortisone (1 %)	
Neo-Cultol	See MINERAL OIL		Stool Softener
NEO-DECADRON Many Equivalent Mixtures	**Ophthalmic (solution):** 1–2 qtt q1h during the day and q 2 h at night; may reduce to 1 qtt q4h with clinical improvement. **Ophthalmic (ointment):** Apply 0.25–.05 inch ribbon tid—QID. May reduce to bid doses with clinical improvement **Topical:** Apply tid—QID.	**Ophthalmic Solution:** neomycin sulfate (equal to 0.35% of neomycin base), dexamethasone sodium phosphate (0.1%) **Ophthalmic Ointment:** neomycin sulfate (equal to 0.35% of neomycin base), dexamethasone sodium phosphate (0.05%) **Topical Cream:** neomycin sulfate (0.5%), dexamethasone sodium phosphate (0.1 %)	
NEO-MEDROL	**Topical:** Apply bid—tid.	**Topical:** neomy-cin sulfate (0.5%), methyl-prednisolone acetate (0.25%)	
NEO-SYNALAR	**Topical:** Apply bid—QID.	**Cream:** neomycin sulfate (0.5%), fluocinolone acetonide (0.025%)	
Neo-Synephrine	See PHENYLEPHRINE		Sympathomimetic
Neobiotic	See NEOMYCIN		Aminoglycoside
Neoloid	See CASTOR OIL		Irritant Laxative

GENERIC NAME Trade Name	INDICATIONS AND DOSAGES	DOSE FORMS	GROUP (G)/SUBGROUP (SG) Relative Cost within Group
NEOMYCIN Generic, Mycifradin, Neobiotic	**Hepatic Coma:** PO: 4–12 g/d (in divided doses) for 5–6 days. Pediatric PO: 50–100 mg/kg/d (in divided doses) for 5–6 days. **Preoperative Gut Sterilization:** PO: (Give on day before surgery, i.e., 3rd day of bowel prep.) 1 g in the afternoon, then 1 g in 1 hour, then 1 g hs (erythromycin given concurrently with each dose of neomycin).	**Tablet:** 500 mg **Oral Solution:** 125 mg/5 ml	ANTI-INFLAMMATORY AGENTS (G) Aminoglycosides (G) **Cost:** Low
Neoral	See CYCLOSPORINE		Immunosuppressant
NEOSPORIN PLUS Many Equivalent Mixtures	Topical: Apply 1–3 times/d.	**Cream (per g):** polymyxin B sulfate (10,000 Units), neomycin sulfate (equal to 3.5 mg of neomycin base), lidocaine (40 mg) **Ointment (per g):** polymyxin B sulfate (10,000 Units), neomycin sulfate (equal to 3.5 mg of neomycin base), bacitracin zinc (500 Units), lidocaine (40 mg)	
NEOSPORIN	**Ophthalmic (solution):** 1–2 qtt bid—QID for 7–10 days. **Ophthalmic (ointment):** Apply 0.25–0.5 inch ribbon q 3–4 h for 7–10 days. **Topical:** Apply 1–3 times/d.	**Ophthalmic Solution (per cc):** polymyxin B sulfate (10,000 Units), neomycin sulfate (equal to 1.75 mg of neomycin base), gramicidin (0.025 mg) **Ophthalmic Ointment (per g):** polymyxin B sulfate (10,000 Units), neomycin sulfate (equal to 3.5 mg of neomycin base), bacitracin zinc (400 Units) **Topical Ointment (per g):** polymyxin B sulfate (5,000 Units), neomycin sulfate (equal to 3.5 mg of neomycin base), bacitracin zinc (400 Units)	

GENERIC NAME Trade Name	INDICATIONS AND DOSAGES	DOSE FORMS	GROUP (G)/SUBGROUP (SG) Relative Cost within Group
NEOSTIGMINE Generic, Prostigmin	**Reversal of Non-Depolarizing Neuromuscular Blockade:** IV: 0.5–2 mg SLOWLY (max. dose 5 mg) + atropine; observe closely. **Myasthenia Gravis Symptoms:** PO: 15 mg q8h initially; increase gradually until maximal response, maintenance doses range 15–375 mg/d. IV, IV, SC: 0.5–2.0 mg PRN (give IV slowly). **Myasthenia Gravis Diagnosis:** IM: 0.022 mg/kg as a single dose. **Postoperative Ileus or Urinary Retention:** SC or IM: 0.25–0.5 mg q 4–6 h.	**Tablet:** 15 mg **Injection:** 1:1000, 1:2000, 1:4000 (0.25 mg/ml)	ANS AGENTS (G) Cholinergic Agents (Parasympathomimetics) (SG) Cholinesterase Inhibitors, Reversible (SSG) **Cost:** Low
Neothylline	See DYPHYLLINE		Bronchodilator
Neptazane	See METHAZOLAMIDE		Carbonic Anhydrase Inhibitor
Nesacaine	See CHLOROPROCAINE		Local Anesthetic
NETILMICIN Netromycin	**UTI (complicated):** IM, IV: 1.5–2 mg/kg q 12h (+ 3–4 mg/kg/d). **Systemic Infection:** IM, IV: 1.3–2.2 mg/kg q8h (= 4–6.5 mg/kg/d); (alternate regimen = 2–3.25 mg/kg q 12h).	**Injection:** 100 mg/ml	ANTI-INFLAMMATORY AGENTS (G) Aminoglycosides (SG) **Cost:** High
Netromycin	See NETILMICIN		Aminoglycoside Antibiotic
Neupogen	See FILGRASTIM		Granulocyte Repair
Neurontin	See GABAPENTIN		Anticonvulsant
Noutrexin	See TRIMETREXATE		Pneumocystis pneumonia
NEVIRAPINE Viramune	**HIV Infection:** PO: With another transcriptase inhibitor. Initially 200 mg daily then 200 mg bid	**Tablet:** 200 mg	ANTI-INFECTIOUS AGENTS(G) Antiviral, Systemic (SG) HIV Reverse Transcriptase Inhibitor (SSG) **Cost:** Under special program
NIACIN OTC, Generic, B3, Nicolar, Nicotinic Acid	**Hyperlipidemia:** PO: 1–2 g tid (max. dose: 6–8 g/d), maximum effect seen in 3–5 weeks. May pretreat with 325 mg ASA given 30 min. prior to niacin to minimize flushing and headaches. **Pellagra:** PO: Up to 500 mg/d.	**Tablet:** 25, 50, 100, 250, 500 mg **Tablet:** (Ext'd release) 250, 500, 750 mg **Capsule:** (Ext'd release) 125, 250, 300, 400, 500 mg **Elixir:** 50 mg/5 ml (pint, gal) **Injection:** 100 mg/ml	LIPID LOWERING DRUGS Other Lipid Lowering Agents (SG) **Cost:** Low
NICARDIPINE Cardene	**Chronic Stable Angina, Hypertension:** See discussion, Part 1	**Capsule:** **Capsule:** (Ext'd release) 30, 45, 60 mg **Injection:**	CV AGENTS (G) Vasodilators (SG) Calcium Channel Blockers (SSG) **Cost:** Low
Nicoderm	See NICOTINE		Transdermal Dose Form
Nicolar	See NIACIN		Lipid Lowering Agent
Niconyl	See ISONIAZID		Tuberculostatic
Nicorette	See NICOTINE		Transdermal Dose Form

GENERIC NAME Trade Name	INDICATIONS AND DOSAGES	DOSE FORMS	GROUP (G)/SUBGROUP (SG) Relative Cost within Group
NICOTINE Habitrol Nicoderm Nicorette OTC, Nicotrol OTC	**Adjunct to Smoking Cessation Efforts:** Chewing Gum: (4 mg size—more dependent patient) 9–12 pieces per day, (max. dose 20 pc/d). (2 mg size—less dependent patient) 9–12 pieces per day, (max. dose 30 pc/d). Decrease number of pieces per day by 1 or more every 4–7 days. Decrease chewing time from 30 minutes to 10–15 minutes for 4–7 days, then decrease the number of pieces. Substitute some doses of regular sugarless gum for nicotine gum as tolerated. Do not use gum for more than 6 months. **Transdermal:** 1 patch q24h, rotate sites; **Habitrol and Nicoderm Systems:** 21 mg/d (largest size) patch qd for 6 weeks, 14 mg/d (medium size) patch qd for 2 weeks, 7 mg/d (smallest size) patch qd for 2 weeks. **ProStep System:** 22 mg/d (large size) patch qd for 4–8 weeks, 11 mg/d (small size) patch qd for 2–4 weeks. **Nicotrol System:** 15 mg/d (largest size) patch qd for 12 weeks, 10 mg/d (medium size) patch qd for 2 weeks, 5 mg/d (smallest size) patch qd for 2 weeks.		ANS AGENTS (G) Cholinergic Agents (SG) Choline Esters and Equivalent (SSG) **Cost:** Very High
Nicotinic Acid	See NIACIN		Lipid Lowering Agent
NIFEDIPINE Generic, Procardia, Adalat	**Chronic Stable and Vasospastic Angina:** See discussion, Part 1 **Hypertension:** See discussion, Part 1	**Capsule:** **Tablet:** (Ext'd release) 30, 60, 90 mg	CV AGENTS (G) Vasodilators (SG) Calcium Channel Blockers (SSG) **Cost:** Medium
Nilandron	See NILUTAMIDE		Antiestrogen
Nilstat	See NYSTATIN		Fungicide
NILUTAMIDE Nilandron	**Prostatic Cancer:** PO: 300 mg qd for 30 days then 150 mg/d	**Tablet:** 50 mg	ENDOCRINE AGENT (G) Antiestrogen (SG)
NIMODIPINE Nimotop	**Subarachnoid Hemorrhage (Vasospasm):** PO: 60 mg q4h, treat for 3 weeks. (start therapy within 96 hours of event).	**Capsule:** 30 mg	CV AGENTS (G) Vasodilators (SG) Calcium Channel Blockers (SSG) **Cost:** High
Nimotop	See NIMODIPINE		Calcium Channel Blocker
Niong	See NITROGLYCERIN		Vasodilator
Nipent	See PENTOSTATIN		Cancer Chemotherapy
Nisaval	See PYRILAMINE		Antihistamine
NISOLDIPINE Sular	**Hypertension:** See discussion, Part 1	**Tablet:**	CV AGENTS (G) Vasodilators (SG) Calcium Channel Blockers (SSG) **Cost:** Medium

GENERIC NAME Trade Name	INDICATIONS AND DOSAGES	DOSE FORMS	GROUP (G)/SUBGROUP (SG) Relative Cost within Group
Nitorlex-D	See NITROGLYCERIN		Antianginal
Nitrek	See NITROFURANTOIN		Antibacterial
Nitro-bid	See NITROGLYCERIN		Antianginal
Nitro-Dur	See NITROGLYCERIN		Antianginal
Nitrocaps	See NITROGLYCERIN		Antianginal
Nitrocels	See NITROGLYCERIN		Antianginal
Nitrocot	See NITROGLYCERIN		Antianginal
Nitrodisc	See NITROGLYCERIN		Antianginal
Nitrodan	See NITROFURANTOIN		Antibacterial
NIDRAFUR-ANTOIN Furadantin, Cyantin, Macrodantin, Nitrek, Trantoin, Furadantin, Nitrodan	**Urinary Tract Infections:** PO: 50–100 mg with meals and at hs; max. dose 400 mg/d. Pediatric PO: 5–7 mg/kg/d in 4 divided doses. **Long-Term Suppressive Therapy:** PO: 50–100 mg at hs.	**Tablet:** 50, 100 mg **Capsule:** 25, 50, 100, 250, 500 mg **Oral Suspension:** 25 mg/5 ml	ANTI-INFECTIOUS AGENTS (G) Non-Sulfonamide Urinary Tract Agents (SG) **Cost:** Low
NITROGLYCERIN Generic	Glyceryl Trinitrate, Nitroglycerol, Sublingual: Nitrostat, Topical Ointment: Nitro-bid, Nitrong, Nitrol, Patches: Nitrodisc, Transderm, Transderm-Nitro, Nitro-Dur, IV: Nitro-bid IV, Nitrol, Tridil, Oral Extended Release: Angiospan, Cardabid, Niong, Nitrocels, Nitro-bid plateau caps, Diaceles, Klavikordal, Nitrocol, Nitroglyn, Nitorlex-D, Nitrolin, Nitronet, Nitrospan, Nitrostat-SR, N-G-C, Nitrocaps **Angina Prophylaxis:** Buccal (Ext'd release): 1 mg tid to start; 3–12 mg/d maintenance as 3–12 doses. Sublingual: 0.3–0.6 before stress. PO (Ext'd release): 2.5–2.6 mg tid-QID to start; maintenance doses up to 26 mg QID have been given. Topical ointment: 0.5 inch q8h to start; increase by 0.5 inch with each application (max. dose 4–5 inches q4h). NTG Patches: 1 patch/d to start; 1–2 patches/d maintenance (lowest effective strength). Patch application q12h (on 12h, off 12h) may be necessary for sustained 24 hour effect (many different patch strengths). Spray: 1–2 metered sprays under tongue (max. dose: 3 sprays in 15 min). **Acute Angina:** Sublingual: 0.4 mg (range: 0.3–0.6 mg) q5min, (maximum 3 doses). **Hypertension Control:** IV: 5 mcg/min; increase by 5 mcg/min q3–5min to 20 mcg/min; then increase by 10–20 mcg/min increases. Max. dose determined by tolerance & response. With PVC tubing, increase 1st dose.	**Tablet:** (Ext'd release) 1, 2, 3 mg (Buccal) **Tablet:** (Ext'd release) 2.6, 6.5, 9.0 mg **Tablet:** (sublingual) 0.15, 0.3, 0.4, 0.6 mg **Spray:** 0.4 mg per metered dose **Capsule:** (Ext'd release) 2.5, 6.5, 9, 13 mg **Ointment:** 2% **Patches:** Order dose as mg/d NTG. **Total NTG content/patch ranges as follows (mg):** 9 (3.3 sq cm), 12.5, 16, 18, 20, 24, 25, 32, 36, 50, 54, 60, 62.5, 75, 80, 120, 125, 187.5, (32 sq cm)	CV AGENTS (G) Vasodilators (SG) Post-Arteriolar (Antianginal and related agents) (SG) **Cost** Low (Oral, Sublingual) High (Transdermal)

GENERIC NAME Trade Name	INDICATIONS AND DOSAGES	DOSE FORMS	GROUP (G)/SUBGROUP (SG) Relative Cost within Group
Nitroglycerol	See NITROGLYCERIN		
Nitroglyn	See NITROGLYCERIN		Antianginal
Nitrol	See NITROGLYCERIN		Antianginal
Nitrolin	See NITROGLYCERIN		Antianginal
Nitronet	See NITROGLYCERIN		Antianginal
Nitrong	See NITROGLYCERIN		Antianginal
Nitrospan	See NITROGLYCERIN		Antianginal
Nitrostat	See NITROGLYCERIN		Antianginal
Nivaquine	See CHLOROQUINE		Parasiticide (Malaria)
Nix	See PERMETHRIN		Ectoparasitide
NIZATIDINE Axid	**Active duodenal ulcer, benign gastric ulcer:** PO: 300 mg qhs (or 150 mg bid). **Maintenance of healed duodenal ulcer:** 150 mg qhs.	**Capsule:** 150, 300 mg	GI AGENTS (G) Inhibitors Of Gastric Acid Secretion (SG) H2 Antagonist (SSG) **Cost:** Low
Nizoral	See KETOCONAZOLE		Antifungal
Noctec	See CHLORAL HYDRATE		Hypnotic, ultra short
Nolahist	See PHENINDAMINE		Antihistamine
Noludar	See METHYPRYLON		Hypnotic
Nolvadex	See TAMOXIFEN		Antiestrogen
Norcuron	See VECURONIUM		Curariform
NORDETTE	**Oral Contraceptive:** PO: 1 tab/d. 21- or 28-day regimen.	**Tablet:** ethinyl estradiol (30 mcg), levonorgestrel (0.15 mg) In 21-Day and 28-Day Pilpaks	
NOREPINEPH-RINE Generic, Levart-erenol, Lev-ophed	**Hypotension:** IV: 0.5–1.0 mcg/min of norepinephrine base initially; adjust rate to establish blood pressure >80–100 mm Hg systolic, average maintenance dose 2–12 mcg per minute up to 30 mcg/min.	**Injection:** 1 mg/ml	ANS AGENTS (G) Sympathomimetics (SG) Predominantly Alpha Agonists (SSG) **Cost:** High
NORETHIN 1/35E	**Contraception:** PO: 1 tab/d. 21- or 28-day regimen.	**Tablet:** ethinyl estradiol (35 mcg), norethindrone (1 mg) in 21-Day and 28-Day packs	
NORETHIN 1/50 M	**Contraception:** PO: 1 tab/d. 21- or 28-day regimen.	**Tablet:** mestranol (50 mcg), norethindrone (1 mg) in 21-Day and 28-Day packs	
Norflex	See ORPHENADRINE		Muscle Relaxant

GENERIC NAME Trade Name	INDICATIONS AND DOSAGES	DOSE FORMS	GROUP (G)/SUBGROUP (SG) Relative Cost within Group
NORFLOXACIN Noroxin, Chibroxin	**UTI:** PO: 400 mg q 12h for three days or longer prn. **Gonorrhea:** 800 mg as single dose **Conjunctivitis or Corneal Ulcer:** Apply 1–2 drops QID for up to 1 week.	**Tablet:** 400 mg **Solution:** 3.0 mg/ml	ANTI-INFECTIVE AGENTS (G) Quinolone Antibacterial (SG) Ophthalmic Anti-Infective (SG) **Cost:** High
NORGESIC	PO: 1–2 tablet tid or QID.	**Tablet:** orphenadrine citrate [25, 50 (forte) mg], aspirin (385 mg) caffeine (30 mg)	
NORGESTREL Ovrette	**Contraception:** PO: Progestin only contraceptive: 1 tab every day beginning on first day of menses.	**Tablet:** 0.075 mg	ENDOCRINE AGENTS (G) Progestins (SG)
NORINYL	**Contraception:** PO: 1 tab/d. 21- or 28-day regimen	**Tablet: Norinyl 1 + 35:** Norethindrone (1 mg) and ethinyl estradiol (35 mcg) in 21-Day and 28-Day packs **Norinyl 1 + 50:** Norethindrone (1 mg) and mestranol (50 mcg) in 21-Day and 28-Day packs	
Normodyne	See LABETALOL		Alpha/Beta Blocker
Noroxin	See NORFLOXACIN		Quinolone Antibacterial
Norpace	See DISOPYRAMIDE		Antiarrhythmic
Norplant System	See LEVONORGESTREL		Progestin
Norpramin	See DESIPRAMINE		TCA Antidepressant
NORTRIPTYLINE Aventyl, Pamelor	**Endogenous Depression:** PO: 75–100 mg/d to start in 3–4 doses; maintenance 75–100 mg/d. Geriatric PO: 30–50 mg/d in 3–4 doses.	**Capsule:** 10, 25, 50, 75 mg **Liquid:** 2 mg/ml	CNS AGENTS (G) Tricyclic Antidepressants (SG) **Cost:** High
Norvasc	See AMLODIPINE		Calcium Channel Blocker
Norvin	See RITONAVIR		Protease Inhibitor
Norzine	See THIETHYLPERAZINE		Antiemetic
Novantrone	See MITOXANTRONE		Cancer Chemotherapy
NOVOBIOCIN Albamycin	**Infections Due To S. aureus:** PO: 250 mg q6h; or 500 mg q12h (max. dose 500 mg q6h; or 1 g q12h).	**Capsule:** 250 mg	ANTI-INFECTIOUS AGENTS (G) Lactam Antibiotics (SG) Others Resistant to Staphylococcal Lactamase (SSG) **Cost:** Medium

GENERIC NAME Trade Name	INDICATIONS AND DOSAGES	DOSE FORMS	GROUP (G)/SUBGROUP (SG) Relative Cost within Group
Novocain	See PROCAINE		Local Anesthetic
Novolin L, N, R, 70/30	See INSULINS		
NPH INSULIN	See INSULINS		
Nubain	See NALBUPHINE		Narcotic Agonist-Antagonist
NuLYTELY	See POLYETHYLENE GLYCOL SOLUTIONS		Bowel cleanser
Numorphan	See OXYMORPHONE		Narcotic Analgetic
Nupercaine	See DIBUCAINE		Local Anesthetic
Nutropin	See SOMATOTROPIN (GH)		Growth Hormone
Nydrazid	See ISONIAZID		Tuberculostatic
NYLIDRIN Generic, Arlidin	**Peripheral Vascular Disease:** PO: 3–12 mg tid or QID.	**Tablet:** 6, 12 mg	ANS AGENTS (G) Sympathomimetics (SG) Unselective Beta 1 and 2 Agonists (SSG) **Cost:** Low
NYSTATIN Generic, Mycostatin, Nilstat	**Topical:** Apply 2–3 times/d until lesions resolved and continue for 1 week afterward. **Vaginal:** 1 tablet qd for 14 days.	**Cream:** 100,000 units/g **Ointment:** 100,000 units/g **Lotion:** 100,000 units/g **Powder:** 100,000 units/g **Vaginal tablets:** 100,000 & 500,000 units	DERMATOLOGIC AGENTS (G) Topical Fungicides (SG) **Cost:** Medium
Ocusert Pilo	See PILOCARPINE HCL		Cholinergic
OCTREOTIDE Sandostatin	**Acromegaly:** SC: 50 mcg tid initially, then increase as indicated to 100 mcg tid (max. dose 1500 mg/day); goal is to achieve growth hormone levels <5 ng/ml or IGF-I levels < 1.9 U/mL in males and <2.2 U/mL in females. **Carcinoid Tumors:** SC: 100–600 mcg/d given QID or bid in divided doses (doses as low as 50 mcg/d and up to 1500 mg/d have been given in some cases) **Vasoactive Interstitial Peptide Tumors (VIPomas):** SC: 150–450 mcg/d given in 2–4 divided doses (max. dose 750 mcg/d).	**Injection:** 0.05 mg, 0.1 mg, 0.5 mg	ENDOCRINE AGENTS (G) Inhibits Release of Growth Hormone and Many Other Substances
Ocuflox	See OFLOXACIN		Quinolone Antibacterial
Ocupress	See CARTEOLOL		Beta Adrenergic Blocker

GENERIC NAME Trade Name	INDICATIONS AND DOSAGES	DOSE FORMS	GROUP (G)/SUBGROUP (SG) Relative Cost within Group
OFLOXACIN Floxin,Ocuflox	**Pneumonia, Bronchitis:** PO, IV: 400 mg q12h 10 days **Chlamydia, Cervicitis, Urethritis:** PO, IV: 300 mg q12h for 7 days. **Gonorrhea (uncomplicated):** PO, IV: 400 mg single dose, follow by doxycycline. **Cystitis:** PO, IV: 200 mg q 12h for 7 days (give IV dose over 60 minutes). **Prostatitis:** PO, IV: 300 mg q 12h for 6 weeks. **PID (outpatient):** PO: 400 mg bid for 14 days (given with clindamycin or metronidazole). **Epididymitis:** PO: 300 mg bid for 10 days. **Intraocular:** Apply 1–2 drops q2–4h for 2 days, then q 6h for up to 1 week total.	**Injection:** 200, 400 mg **Tablet:** 200, 300, 400 mg **Solution:** 3 mg/ml	ANTI-INFECTIVE AGENTS (G) Quinolone Antibacterial (SG) Ophthalmic Antibacterial (SG) **Cost:** High
Ogen	See ESTROPIPATE		Estrogens
OLANZAPINE Zyprexa	**Schizophrenia;** 5–15 mg/d	**Tablets:** 5,7.5, 10 mg	CNS AGENTS (G) Antipsychotics (SG) Atypical Antipsychotics (SSG) **Cost:** Very high
OLSALAZINE Dipentum	**Ulcerative Colitis (maintenance of remission):** PO: 1 g per day given in 2 divided doses .	**Capsule:** 250 mg	GASTROINTESTINAL AGENTS (G) 5-Aminosalicylates (SG) **COST:** High
OMEPRAZOLE Prilosec	**Peptic Ulcer:** PO: 20–40 mg daily	**Capsules, ER:** 20 mg	GASTROINTESTINAL AGENTS (G) Inhibit Acid Secretion (SG) Inhibit H ion Transport (SSG)
Omnipen	See AMPICILLIN		Lactam Antibiotic
Oncaspar	See PEGASPARGASE		Cancer Chemotherapy
Oncovin	See VINCRISTINE		Cancer Chemotherapy
ONDANSETRON Zofran	**Chemotherapy Emesis Prophylaxis:** PO: 8 mg bid. IV: Three slow infusions of 0.15 mg/kg given 30 min before and 4 and 8 hours after treatment or a single 32 mg infusion. (Give infusions over 15 min.)	**Tablets:** 4, 8 mg **Injection:** 2 mg/ml	GI AGENTS (G) Antiemetics (SG) Antiemetics (Serotonin ($5HT_3$) Antagonists) (SG) **Cost:** Medium
OnY-ClearNail	See TRIACETIN		Fungicide
Ophthaine	See PROPARACAINE		Local Anesthetic
Ophthetic	See PROPARACAINE		Local Anesthetic
OPHTHOCORT	**Ophthalmic:** Place 0.25–0.5 inch ribbon q3h, or more frequently if necessary.	**Ophthalmic Ointment (per g):** chloramphenicol (10 mg), polymyxin B sulfate (10,000 Units), hydrocortisone acetate (5 mg)	

GENERIC NAME Trade Name	INDICATIONS AND DOSAGES	DOSE FORMS	GROUP (G)/SUBGROUP (SG) Relative Cost within Group
OPIUM ALKALOIDS (TOTAL) Generic, Pantopon	**Pain:** IM, SC: 5–20 mg q4–5h.	**Injection:** 20 mg/ml (equivalent to 15 mg/ml of morphine).	NARCOTIC ANALGESICS AND RELATED AGENTS (G) Narcotic Analgesics of Greatest Potency (SG)
OPIUM TINCTURE-STRONG Generic	**Diarrhea, Analgesia:** PO: 0.6 ml QID	**Liquid:** 10% opium	CNS AGENTS (G) Narcotic Analgesics And Related Agents (SG) Narcotic Analgesics of Greatest Potency (SSG) **Cost:** High
Optimine	See AZATADINE		Antihistamine
OptiPranolol	See METIPRANOL		Beta Adrenergic Blocker
Or-Tyl	See DICYCLOMINE		Local Anesthetic
Oralet	See FENTANYL		Fentanyl Lozenge
Oramide	See TOLBUTAMIDE		Oral Antidiabetic Agent
Oramorph	See MORPHINE		Morphine, ER
Orap	See PIMOZIDE		Antipsychotic
Orasone	See PREDNISONE		Corticosteroid
Oretic	See HYDROCHLOROTHIAZIDE		Sodium Diuretic
Orinase	See TOLBUTAMIDE		Oral Antidiabetic Agent
Orlaam	See LEVOMETHADYL		Narcotic Analgetic
Ornidyl	See EFLORNITHINE		Fungicide, Systemic
ORPHENADRINE Generic, Norflex, Banflex, Myolin, Flexon	**Analgesia:** PO: 100 mg bid. IV or IM: 60 mg q12h.	**Tablet:** 100 mg **Tablet:** (Ext'd release) 100 mg **Injection:** 30 mg/ml	CNS AGENTS (G) Muscle Relaxants (SG) Other, Negligible Compounds (SG) **Cost:** Medium
ORTHO TRI-CYCLEN	**Oral Contraception:** PO: 1 tablet qd. 21- or 28-day regimen.	**Tablet:** PO: 21 day pack: Each tab with ethinyl estradiol (35 mcg), Norgestimate 0.18 mg in first 7 tabs, norgestimate 0.215 mg in next 7, norgestimate 0.25 mg final 7d. Also available with 7 inert tabs in 28-packs.	
ORTHO-CEPT	**Oral Contraceptive:** PO: 1 tab qd. 21- or 28-day regimen.	**Tablet:** PO: Ethinyl estradiol 30 mcg, desogestrel 0.15 mg in 21-day and 28-day Dialpaks	

GENERIC NAME Trade Name	INDICATIONS AND DOSAGES	DOSE FORMS	GROUP (G)/SUBGROUP (SG) Relative Cost within Group
ORTHO-CYCLEN	**Oral Contraceptive:** PO: 1 tab qd. 21- or 28-day regimen.	**Tablet:** Ethinyl estradiol 35 mcg, norgestimate (0.25 mg) in 21-Day and 28-Day packs	
Ortho-Est	See ESTROPIPATE		Estrogen
ORTHO-NOVUM 1/35 **ORTHO-NOVUM 1/50**	**Oral Contraceptive:** PO (1/35, 1/50): 1 tablet qd. 21- or 28-day regimen.	**Tablet (1/35):** ethinyl estradiol (35 mcg), norethindrone (1 mg) in 21- and 28-Day packs **Tablet (1/50):** mestranol (50 mcg), norethindrone (1 mg) in 21- and 28-Day packs	
ORTHO-NOVUM 10/11	**Oral Contraceptive:** PO: 1 tablet qd. 21- or 28-day regimen.	**Tablets:** PO: 10 tabs: ethinyl estradiol 35 mcg, norethindrone 0.5 mg; 11 tabs: ethinyl estradiol (35 mcg), norethindrone (1 mg) in 21-Day packs. aAlso available with 7 inert tabs in 28-Day packs	
ORTHO-NOVUM 7/7/7	**Oral Contraception:** PO: 1 tablet qd. 21- or 28-day regimen.	**Tablets:** PO: All 21 tabs contain ethinyl estradiol 35 mcg. Norethindrone 0.5 mg, 0.75, 1 mg in next 7–7-7 tablets. Also available with 7 inert tabs in 28-Day packs	
Orudis	See KETOPROFEN		Non-Narcotic Analgesics
Osmitrol	See MANNITOL		Osmotic Agent
Osmoglyn	See GLYCERIN		Osmotic Agent
OTOBIOTIC	**External Otitis:** External auditory canal: 4 qtt into ear(s) tid or QID.	**Otic Solution (per cc):** polymyxin B sulfate (10,000 Units), hydrocortisone (0.5%)	

GENERIC NAME Trade Name	INDICATIONS AND DOSAGES	DOSE FORMS	GROUP (G)/SUBGROUP (SG) Relative Cost within Group
Otrivin	See XYLOMETAZOLINE		Sodium Diuretic
Ovide	See MALATHION		Ectoparasiticide
Ovrette	See NORGESTREL		Progestin Only Contraceptive
OXACILLIN Generic, Bactocill, Prostaphlin	**Infections:** PO: 500–1000 mg q4–6h for a minimum of 5 days. IV, IV: 250–1000 mg q4–6h (max. dose 12g/d). Pediatric (<40 kg) Infections: Pediatric (<40 kg) PO: 50–100 mg/kg/d in 4 doses. Pediatric (<40 kg) IM, IV: 50–100 mg/kg/d in 4–6 doses (max. dose 100–300 mg/kg/d).	**Injection:** (powder) 0.25, 0.5, 1, 2, 4, 10 g	LACTAM ANTIBIOTICS (G) Penicillins: Resistant to Staphylococcal Lactamase(SG) **Cost:** Medium
Oxandrin	See OXANDROLONE		Androgen
OXANDROLONE Oxandrin	**Adjunct to foster weight gain:** PO: 2.5 mg 2–4 times a day (max. dose 20 mg/d); treat for 2–4 weeks.	**Tablet:** 2.5 mg	ENDOCRINE AGENTS (G) Androgenic/Anabolic Steroids (SG) **Cost:** High
OXAPROZIN Daypro	**Arthritic Condition:** 600–1200 mg qd (max. dose 1800 mg/d or 26 mg/kg: whichever is lower: in divided doses).	**Tablet:** 600 mg	CNS AGENTS (G) Non-Narcotic Analgesics (G) Aspirin and Related NSAIDs (SG) **Cost:** High
OXAZEPAM Generic, Serax	**Sedation:** PO: 10–15 mg tid or QID. **Severe Anxiety, Alcohol Withdrawal:** PO: 10–30 mg tid or QID. **Sedation in Elderly:** Geriatric PO: 10 mg tid (max. dose 60 mg/d).	**Capsule:** 10, 15, 30 mg **Tablet:** 15 mg	CNS AGENTS (G) Sedative-Hypnotics (SG) Intermediate-Acting Sedative Hypnotics (SG) **Cost:** Low
OXICONAZOLE Oxistat	**Tinea pedis:** Topical: Apply qd or bid for 4 weeks. **Tinea corporis, cruris:** Topical: Apply qd or bid for 2 weeks.	**Cream:** 1% **Lotion:** 1%	TOPICAL ANTI-INFECTIOUS AGENTS (G) Topical Fungicides (SG) **Cost:** Medium
Oxistat	See OXICONAZOLE		Antifungal, Topical
Oxsoralen	See METHOXSALEN		Pigment Vitiligo
OXTRIPHYLLINE Generic, Choledyl	PO: 4.7 mg/kg q8h. Pediatric PO: (9–16 yrs) and adult smokers: 4.7 mg/kg q6. Pediatric PO: (1–9 yrs) 6.2 mg/kg q6h.	**Tablet:** 100, 200 mg (equiv. to 64, 127 mg theophylline) **Tablet:** (Ext'd release) 400, 600 mg (equiv. to 254, 382 mg theophylline) **Syrup:** (pediatric) 50 mg/5 ml (equiv. to 32 mg theophylline per 5 ml) **Elixir:** 100 mg (equiv. to 64 mg theophylline per 5 ml)	CV AGENTS (G) Xanthines (SG) **Cost:** Low
Oxy10	See BENZOYL PEROXIDE		Keratolytic (Acne)

GENERIC NAME Trade Name	INDICATIONS AND DOSAGES	DOSE FORMS	GROUP (G)/SUBGROUP (SG) Relative Cost within Group
OXYBUTYNIN Generic, Ditropan	**Neurogenic Bladder Symptom Relief:** PO (Adults): 5 mg bid or tid (max. dose 5 mg QID) PO (Pediatric >5 yo): 5 mg bid (max. dose 5 mg tid)	**Tablet:** 5 mg **Syrup:** 5 mg/5 ml	ANS AGENTS (G) Parasympatholytics (SG) Quaternary Amines (SG) **Cost:** Low
OXYCODONE Generic, Roxicodone See Section III For Percodan, Percocet, Roxicet, Tylox and other mixtures	**Pain Management:** PO: Initially 5 mg q6h.	**Tablet:** 5 mg **Oral Solution:** 5 mg/5 ml, 20 mg/ml	CNS AGENTS (G) Narcotic Analgesics And Related Agents (G) Of Intermediate Potency (SG) **Cost:** Low
OXYMETAZOLINE OTC, Generic, Afrin	**Nasal Spray (Adults and children > 6 yrs):** 2–3 sprays (or 2–3 drops) of 0.05% solution in each nostril q10–12h. Pediatric Nasal Solution (2–5 y): 2–3 qtt of 0.025% solution in each nostril bid.	**Solution:** 0.025, 0.05 %.	ANS AGENTS (G) Sympathomimetics (SG) Sympathomimetics, Incomplete (SG) **Cost:** Low
OXYMETHOLONE Anadrol-50	**Anemias (pro-erythrocytic therapy):** PO: 1–2 mg/kg/d (max. dose 5 mg/kg/d); 3–6 months may be needed to evaluate efficacy.	**Tablet:** 50 mg	ENDOCRINE AGENTS (G) Androgenic/Anabolic Steroids (SG) **Cost:** Medium
OXYMORPHONE Numorphan	**Pain Management:** IV: 0.5 mg to start; increase PRN. IV, SC: 1–1.5 mg q4–6h. Rectal: 5 mg q4–6h.	**Suppositories:** 5 mg **Injection:** 1, 1.5 mg/ml	CNS AGENTS (G) Narcotic Analgesics And Related Agents (SG) Of Greatest Potency (SSG) **Cost:** High
OXYPHENBUTAZONE Generic		**Capsule.** 100 mg	ANTI-INFLAMMATORY AGENTS (G) Non-Narcotic Analgesics (SG) Other Nonnarcotic Analgesics (SSG)
OXYTETRACYCLINE Generic, Terramycin	**Infection:** PO: 250–500 mg q6h (see tetracycline). IV: 250 mg q24h or 300 mg/d in 2–3 doses. Pediatric (> 8 yrs) PO: 40–50 mg/kg/d in 4 doses. Pediatric (> 8 yrs) IM: 15–25 mg/kg/d in 2–3 doses (max. dose single dose = 250 mg).	**Capsule:** 250 mg **Injection:** 50, 125 mg/ml each with 2% lidocaine	ANTI-INFECTIOUS AGENTS Tetracyclines (SG) **Cost:** Low
OXYTOCIN Pitocin, Syntocinon	**Labor Induction:** IV: 0.001–0.002 units/min initial infusion rate; then SLOWLY increase dose at a rate of an additional 0.001–0.002 units/min q15–30min (max. dose 0.020 units/min). **Prevent Post-Partum Bleeding:** IM: 10 units after delivery of the placenta (single dose). IV: 0.01–0.04% units/ml sln PRN to control uterine atony (max. dose = 30 units in a 12h period). **Initial Milk Let-Down:** Nasal: 1 spray into one or both nostrils 2–3 min prior to nursing.	**Injection:** 10 units/ml **Nasal Spray:** 40 units/ml	CV AGENTS (G) Vasoconstrictors And Oxytocics (SG) **Cost:** High

GENERIC NAME Trade Name	INDICATIONS AND DOSAGES	DOSE FORMS	GROUP (G)/SUBGROUP (SG) Relative Cost within Group
Para-Aminosalicylic acid	See AMINOSALICYLIC ACID		Tuberculostatic
P_{1-6} E_1	**Glaucoma:** Ophthalmic: 1–2 qtt qd to QID.	**Ophthalmic Solutions:** P_1E_1 through P_6E_1 Contain pilocarpine 1, 2, 3, 4 and 6% with epinephrine bitartrate 1%	
PACLITAXEL Taxol	CANCER CHEMOTHERAPY (G) Mitotic Spindle Inhibitors (SG) Promote Tubulin Polymerization (SSG)		
Pamelor	See NORTRIPTYLINE		Tricyclic Antidepressants
PAMIDRONATE Aredia	**Hypercalcemia:** IV: 60 mg (infuse slowly over 4h minimum) up to 90 mg (given over 24h minimum); may repeat after 7 days. **Severe hypercalcemia (corr. serum calcium >13.5 mg/dL):** IV: 90 mg (infuse SLOWLY over 24 hours) may repeat after 7 days. **Paget's Disease, Osteoporosis, Multiple Myeloma:** Frequent off label use	**Injection:** 30 mg	METABOLIC AGENTS (G) Calcium Kinetics Regulators (SG) Other Calcium Regulators (SG) **Cost:** High
Pamine	See METHSCOPOLAMINE		Anticholinergic
Pamisyl	See AMINOSALICYLIC ACID		Tuberculostatic
PANCURONIUM Pavulon	**Endotracheal Intubation:** IV: 0.06–0.1 mg/kg to start; effect should be seen in 2–3 min. If additional effect required give 0.01 mg/kg.	**Injection:** 1, 2 mg/ml	GENERAL AND LOCAL ANESTHETICS (G) Neuromuscular Blocking Agents (SG) Non-Depolarizing Agents (SSG) **Cost:** Low
PanOxyl	See BENZOYL PEROXIDE		Keratolytic (Acne)
Panscol	See SALICYLIC ACID		Keratolytic
Pantopon	See ALKALOIDS OF OPIUM		Narcotic Analgetic
Panwarfin	See WARFARIN SODIUM		Anticoagulant
PAPAVERINE Generic, Pavabid, Cerespan, Genabid, Pavacot	PO: 100–300 mg q4–8h. PO (ER): 150 mg every 12 hours (max. dose: 300 q12h). IV,IM: 30–120 mg q3h as indicated (give IV over 1–2 minutes). **Impotence (off label use):** Intracavernous Injection: 2.5 to 60 mg alone or in combination with phentolamine.	**Tablet:** 30, 60, 100, 150, 200, 300 mg **Tablet:** (ER) 200 mg **Capsule:** (ER)150 mg **Injection:** 30 mg/ml	CV AGENTS (G) Vasodilators (SG) Post-Arteriolar (Antianginal and related agents) (SG) **Cost:** High
Paradione	See PARAMETHADIONE		Anticonvulsant
Parafon Forte	See CHLORZOXAZONE		Muscle Relaxant
Paral	See PARALDEHYDE		Hypnotic, Ultra Short
PARALDEHYDE Generic, Paral	**Hypnotic:** PO: 4–8 ml one time.	**Liquid:** 1 ml = 1 g	CNS AGENTS (G) Sedative-Hypnotics (SG) Ultrashort-Acting Hypnotics (SG) **Cost:** Medium

GENERIC NAME Trade Name	INDICATIONS AND DOSAGES	DOSE FORMS	GROUP (G)/SUBGROUP (SG) Relative Cost within Group
Paraplatin	See CARBOPLATIN		Cancer Chemotherapy
Parasal	See AMINOSALICYLIC ACID		Tuberculostatic
PAREGORIC Generic, Camphorated tincture of opium	**Diarrhea:** PO: 5–10 ml 1–4 times/day.	**Tincture:** 5 ml = 2 mg morphine equivalent.	CNS AGENTS (G) Narcotic Analgesics (SG) Potent But Low Total Dose (SG) **Cost:** Low
Parlodel	See BROMOCRIPTINE		Dopamine Agonist
Parnate	See TRANYLCYPROMINE		MAO Inhibitor
PAROMOMYCIN Humatin	**Intestinal Amebiasis:** PO: 25–30 mg/kg/d given in 3 doses with meal. **Hepatic Coma:** PO: 4 g/d in divided doses, treat for 5–6 days.	**Capsule:** 250 mg	ANTI-INFECTIOUS AGENTS (G) Aminoglycosides And Related (SG) **Cost:** High
PAROXETINE Paxil	**Depression:** PO: Initial dose 20 mg/d, 10 mg/d increments, at q 1wk intervals, up to max. dose of 50 mg/d. Geriatric: initial dose 10 mg/d, increase as needed (max. dose 40 mg/d).	**Tablet:** 20, 30 mg	CNS AGENTS (G) Aminergic Stimulants (SG) Specific Serotonin Uptake Inhibitors (SSRI) (SSG) **Cost:** High
Parsidol	See ETHOPROPAZINE		Anticholinergic (Parkinsonism)
PAS	See AMINOSALICYLIC ACID		Tuberculostatic
Pathocil	See DICLOXACILLIN		Lactam Antibiotic
Pavabid	See PAPAVERINE		Vasodilator
Pavacot	See PAPAVERINE		Vasodilator
Pavulon	See PANCURONIUM		Curariform
Paxil	See PAROXETINE		Specific Serotonin Uptake Inhibitors
Paxipam	See HALAZEPAM		Sedative Hypnotic
PBZ	See TRIPELENNAMINE		Antihistamine
Pedi-Dri	See UNDECYLENIC ACID		Fungicide, Topical
PEDIOTIC	**External otitis:** External auditory canal**:** 4 qtt tid to QID.	**Otic Suspension (per cc):** polymyxin B sulfate (10,000 Units), neomycin sulfate equal to 3.5 mg of neomycin base, hydrocortisone 10 mg (= 1 %)	
PEGASPARGASE Oncaspar	CANCER CHEMOTHERAPY (G) React With DNA (SG) Other Miscellaneous (SSG)		
PEG-ES	See POLYETHYLENE GLYCOL-ELECTROLYTE SOLUTIONS		Bowel Cleanser
Peganone	See ETHOTOIN		Anticonvulsant

GENERIC NAME Trade Name	INDICATIONS AND DOSAGES	DOSE FORMS	GROUP (G)/SUBGROUP (SG) Relative Cost within Group
PEMOLINE Cylert	**Attention Deficit:** Pediatric PO: (administer as single dose) 37.5 mg/d to start; increase 18.8 mg/d q1week; maintenance 56.25–75 mg/d (max. dose 112 mg/d).	**Tablet:** 18.75, 37.5, 75 mg	CNS AGENTS (G) Sympathomimetic Stimulants (SG) Other Schedule 3 Or 4 "Diet Pills" (SG) **Cost:** High
Pen-Vee K	See PENICILLIN V		Lactam Antibiotic
Penbritin	See AMPICILLIN		Lactam Antibiotic
PENBUTOLOL Levatol	**Hypertension:** PO: 20 mg qd initially and for maintenance.	**Tablet:** 20 mg	ANS AGENTS (G) Sympathoplegics (SG) Beta Adrenergic Receptor Blockers (SSG) Non-Selective (Beta 1 and Beta 2) (SSG) **Cost:** Medium
PENCICLOVIR Denavir	**Recurrent Orolabial Herpes:** Topical: cover area q2h during day for 4 days	**Cream:** 1%	DERMATOLOGIC AGENTS (G) Topical Anti-Infectious (SG) Antiviral (SSG)
Penetrex	See ENOXACIN		Quinolone Antibacterial
PENICILLAMINE Cuprimine, Depen,D-Penicillamine	**Rheumatoid Arthritis:** PO: 125–250 mg/d to start. At 1–3 month intervals, increase by 125–250 mg/d (max. dose 1–1.5 g/d). Adjust doses every 2–3 months after assessing dose effectiveness. **Wilson's Disease:** PO: 1–2 g/d in 4 divided doses (1 hr ac and at hs) (follow with 24 h urine copper determinations at baseline, shortly after starting therapy and every three months). **Cystinuria:** PO: 1–4 g/d in 4 divided doses (if history of stones, limit cystine excretion to 100 mg/day; if no history of stones then limit cystine excretion to 100–200 mg/d). Pediatric PO: 30 mg/kg/d given in 4 divided doses.	**Capsule:** 125, 250 mg **Tablet:** 250 mg	ANTI-INFLAMMATORY AGENTS (G) Gold Compounds And Antirheumatic (SG) and also ANTIDOTES AND USED IN POISONINGS (G) **Cost:** Medium
PENICILLIN G Generic, Penicillin G Sodium, Penicillin G Potassium	**250 mg equals 400,000 Units** **Mild Infections:** PO: 250–500 mg (400,000–800,000 units) QID. Pediatric PO: 25,000–80,000 units/kg/d given in 4–6 doses. **Serious Infections:** IM, IV: 6–24 million units/d. Pediatric IV: 100,000–500,000 units/kg/d in 6–12 doses. **Rheumatic Fever-Prophylaxis:** PO: 125–250 mg bid.	**Tablet:** 200,000, 250,000, 400,000, 500,000, 800,000 units. **Oral Solution:** (powder) 400,000 units per 5 ml when reconstituted **Injection:** (premixed) 1,000,000 units, 2,000,000 units, 3,000,000 units **Powder for Injection:** 1,000,000 units, 5,000,000 units, 10,000,000 units, 20,000,000 units	LACTAM ANTIBIOTICS (G) Benzyl Penicillins and First Generation Cephalosporins (SG) **Cost:** Low

GENERIC NAME Trade Name	INDICATIONS AND DOSAGES	DOSE FORMS	GROUP (G)/SUBGROUP (SG) Relative Cost within Group
Penicillin G Potassium	See PENICILLIN G		Lactam Antibiotic
PENICILLIN G PROCAINE Generic, Crysticillin, Wycillin	**General Infections:** IM: 600,000–1.2 million units/d as 1–2 doses. Pediatric IM: 25,000–50,000 units/kg/d. **Uncomplicated Gonorrhea:** IM (women): 4.8 million units (split at 2 sites); 1 g of probenecid PO 30 min prior to injection. **Syphilis:** IM: 600,000 units/d for 8 days. **Neurosyphilis:** IM: 2–4 million units/d (give with probenecid 500 mg PO QID), give for 10–14 days (some recommend 2.4 million units IM of benzathine pcn once per week for 3 weeks following initial 14 day treatment). **Congenital Syphilis:** IM: 50,000 units/kg/d for 10–14 days. **Bacterial Endocarditis (highly sensitive organisms only):** IM: 1.2 million units QID for 2–4 weeks, plus 500 mg bid streptomycin for the first 2 weeks. **Streptococcal Infections, Erysipeloid, Rat bite fever:** IM: 600,000–1.2 million units qd for minimum of 10 days. **250 mg equals 400,000 Units**	**Injection:** 300,000 units/ml, 500,000 units/ml, 600,000 units per unit dose, 1,200,000 units per unit dose, 2,400,000 units per unit dose	LACTAM ANTIBIOTICS (G) Benzyl Penicillins and First Generation Cephalosporins (SG) **Cost:** Medium
PENICILLIN V Generic, Phenoxymethyl penicillin: Pen-Voo, V-Cillin. K^+ salt: Penicillin VK, Pen-Vee K, V-Cillin-K Various others	**Mild Infections:** PO: 125–500 mg q4–6h. Pediatric PO: 20 mg/kg/d given in divided doses q6–8h. **Bacterial Endocarditis Prophylaxis (dental procedures):** PO: 500 mg Pcn V (pediatric—250 mg), q6h for 8 doses after injected penicillin 30–60 min prior to procedure.	**Tablet:** 125, 250, 500 mg **Oral Solution:** (powder) 125 mg/5 ml, 250 mg/5 ml	LACTAM ANTIBIOTICS (G) Benzyl Penicillins and First Generation Cephalosporins (SG) **Cost:** Low
Pentam300	See PENTAMIDINE		Antiparasitic Agents
PENTAMIDINE Pentam300, NebuPent	**Pneumocystis carinii (treatment):** IM, IV: 4 mg/kg once/day, treat for 14 days (infuse IV SLOWLY over 60 minutes). **Pneumocystis carinii Pneumonia (prophylaxis):** Aerosol: 300 mg q 4 weeks (give over 45 minutes).	**Powder (for injection):** 300 mg **Injection:** 300 mg/vial **Aerosol:** 300 mg/vial	ANTI-INFECTIOUS AGENTS (G) Antiparasitic Agents (SG)
Pentasa	See MESALAMINE		Prodrug for 5-ASA
PENTAZOCINE Generic, Talwin	**Pain Management:** IV: 30 mg q3–4h (max. dose 360 mg/d, not greater than 30 mg/dose). IV, SC: 30–60 mg q3–4h (max. dose 360 mg/d, not greater than 30 mg/dose). PO: 50–100 mg q3–6h (max. dose 600 mg/d). Talwin Compound: 2 caplets tid or QID. Talacen Caplets: 1 caplet q4h max. 6 per day.	**Tablet:** 50 mg **Injection:** 30 mg/ ml	CNS AGENTS (G) Narcotic Analgesics And Related Agents (SG) Mixed Agonist-Antagonist (SSG) **Cost:** High

GENERIC NAME Trade Name	INDICATIONS AND DOSAGES	DOSE FORMS	GROUP (G)/SUBGROUP (SG) Relative Cost within Group
PENTOBARBITAL Generic, Nembutal	**Hypnotic:** PO: 100 mg hs. Rectal: 120–200 mg. IV: 150–200 mg. **Daytime Sedation:** PO: 20 mg tid or QID. Pediatric PO: 2 to 6 mg/kg/d given in 2–3 doses (max. dose: 100 mg/d). **Convulsive Emergencies:** IV: 100 mg (at a rate of 50 mg/min to start; max. dose: 200–500 mg)	**Capsule:** 50, 100 mg **Suppositories:** 30, 60, 120, 200 mg **Injection:** 50 mg/ml	CNS AGENTS (G) Sedative-Hypnotics (G) Short-Acting (SG) **Cost:** Low
PENTOSTATIN POLYSULFATE Elmiron	**Interstitial Cystitis:** PO: 100 mg tid.	**Tablet:** 100 mg	
PENTOSTATIN Nipent	CANCER CHEMOTHERAPY React with DNA		
PENTOXIFYL-LINE Trental	**Intermittent Claudication:** PO: 400 mg tid with meals. If GI/CNS side effects occur decrease to 400 mg bid.	**Tablet:** (ER) 400 mg	CV AGENTS (G) Xanthines (SG) **Cost:** Medium
Pepcid	See FAMOTIDINE		H2 Antagonist
Pepto-Bismol	See BISMUTH SUBGALLATE		Antacid
Percocet	See OXYCODONE See also Section III	**Tablet:** oxycodone HCl (5 mg), acetaminophen (325 mg)	
Percodan	See OXYCODONE See also Section III	**Tablet:** oxycodone HCl (4.5 mg), oxycodone terephthalate (0.38 mg), aspirin (325 mg) **Demi:** half strength	
Perdiem	See PSYLLIUM		Bulk Laxative
PERGOLIDE Permax	**Parkinson's:** PO: 0.05 mg qd for 2 days, increase by 0.1–0.15 mg per day every third day for the next twelve days (give daily dose in 3 divided doses). After the first two weeks, daily dose may be increased by 0.25 mg every third day until therapeutic desired effect is achieved (usually around 3 mg/d).	**Tablet:** 0.05, 0.25, 1 mg	CNS AGENTS (G) Antiparkinsonian Agents (SG) Dopamine Agonist (SSG)
Pergonal	See MENOTROPINS		FSH and LH
Periactin	See CYPROHEPTADINE		Antihistamine (Appetite)
Permapen	See PENICILLIN G BENZATHINE		Lactam Antibiotic
Permax	See PERGOLIDE		Dopamine Agonist

GENERIC NAME Trade Name	INDICATIONS AND DOSAGES	DOSE FORMS	GROUP (G)/SUBGROUP (SG) Relative Cost within Group
PERMETHRIN OTC, Elimite, Nix	**Scabies:** Topical: Massage into skin from head to toe (30 g for adult). Wash after 8–12 hours. **Pediculosis capitis:** Topical: After shampoo and drying, saturate hair and scalp. Rinse after 10 minutes.	**Cream:** 5% **Liquid:** 1%	TOPICAL ANTI-INFECTIOUS AGENTS (G) (Ecto) Parasiticidal Agents (SG) **Cost:** Low
Permitil	See FLUPHENAZINE		Antipsychotic
PERPHENAZINE Generic, Trilafon	**Psychotic Disorders:** PO: 4–8 mg tid (max. dose 64 mg/d—higher doses only for hospitalized patients). IM: 5 mg q6h (max. dose 15–30 mg/d—higher doses only for hospitalized patients) in 4 to 5 divided doses. **Severely Agitated Patients:** IM: 5–10 mg initial dose; 5 mg q6h (initiate oral therapy in 1–2 d).	**Tablet:** 2, 4, 8, 16 mg **Liquid:** 16 mg/5 ml **Injection:** 5 mg/ml	CNS AGENTS (G) Antipsychotics (SG) Prominent Extrapyramidal Effects (SSG) **Cost:** Medium
Persantine	See DIPYRIDAMOLE		Antiplatelet Agent
Pertofrane	See DESIPRAMINE		TCA, Antidepressant
Pethidine	See MEPERIDINE		Narcotic Analgetic
PHENACEMIDE Phenurone	PO: starting dose 500 mg tid, dosage may be increased by 500 mg in the 2nd and 3rd week. Maintenance dosage ranges from 2 to 3 g, up to 5 g. Pediatric (5–10 yrs): Give approximately ½ the adult dose	**Tablet:** 500 mg	CNS AGENTS (G) Anticonvulsants (SG) Miscellaneous Anticonvulsants (SSG) **Cost:** Medium
PHENAPHEN	See PART V		
PHENDIMETRAZINE Generic, Plegine, Prelu-2	**Exogenous Obesity:** PO: 35 mg bid or tid (1 hour before meals). PO (Ext'd release): 105 mg qAM.	**Tablet:** 35 mg **Capsule:** 35 mg **Capsule:** (Ext'd release) 105 mg	CNS AGENTS (G) Sympathomimetic Stimulants (SG) Other Schedule 3 Or 4 "Diet Pills" (SSG) **Cost:** Low
PHENELZINE Nardil	**Endogenous Depression:** PO: 15 mg bid to start; increase rapidly to 60–90 mg/d; taper to 7.5–60 mg/d maintenance dose.	**Tablet:** 15 mg	CNS AGENTS (G) Stimulants (SG) Monoamine Oxidase Inhibitors (SSG) **Cost:** Medium
Phenergan	See PROMETHAZINE		Antipsychotic, Antihistamine
Phenergan-Demerol	See PROMETHAZINE and MEPERIDINE		Conscious Sedation
PHENINDAMINE Nolahist	**ALLERGIC (TYPE I) REACTIONS:** PO: 25 mg q4–6h (max. dose 150 mg/d). Pediatric (6–12 yrs) PO: 12.5 mg q4–6 h (max dose 75 mg/d).	**Tablet:** 25 mg	ANTI-INFLAMMATORY ETC (G) Antihistamines (H1) (SG) With Prominent Sedation (SSG) **Cost:** Medium
PHENMETRAZINE Generic, Preludin	Exogenous Obesity: PO (Ext'd release): 75 mg qAM.	**Tablet:** (Ext'd release) 75 mg	CNS AGENTS (G) Sympathomimetic Stimulants (SG) Schedule II Agents (SSG) **Cost:** High

GENERIC NAME Trade Name	INDICATIONS AND DOSAGES	DOSE FORMS	GROUP (G)/SUBGROUP (SG) Relative Cost within Group
PHENOBAR-BITAL Generic, Luminal, Solfoton	**Anticonvulsant:** PO: 60–200 mg/d (max. dose: 400 mg/d). Pediatric PO: 3–6 mg/kg/d. **Sedation:** PO, IM, IV: 30–120 mg/d in 2–3 doses. Pediatric IM: 3–5 mg/kg (max. dose 100 mg).	**Tablet:** 15, 16, 30, 60, 100 mg **Capsule:** 16 mg **Elixir:** 15 mg/5 ml, 20 mg/5 ml **Injection:** 30, 60, 65, 130 mg/ml	CNS AGENTS (G) Sedative-Hypnotics (G) Long-Acting (SG) **Cost:** Low
PHENOLPHTHA-LEIN Generic	Restrictions currently being imposed		GASTROINTESTINAL AGENTS (G) Laxatives, irritant **Cost:** Low
PHENOXYBENZA-MINE Dibenzyline	**Catecholamine Excess States** (Pheochromocytoma): PO: 10 mg bid initially; 20–40 mg bid or tid.	**Capsule:** 10 mg	ANS AGENTS (G) Sympathoplegics (SG) Alpha Adrenergic Receptor Blockers (SSG) **Cost:** High
Phenoxymethyl penicillin	See PENICILLIN V		Lactam Antibiotic
PHENSUXIMIDE Milontin	**Absence (Petit Mal) Seizures:** PO: 500–1,000 mg bid or tid (max. dose 3 g/d).	**Capsule:** 500 mg	CNS AGENTS (G) Anticonvulsants (sG) Succinimides (SSG) **Cost:** Low
PHENTERMINE Generic, Ionamin, Phentrol	**Exogenous Obesity:** PO: 8 mg tid (30 min before meals) or 15 to 37.5 mg qd.	**Tablet:** 8, 30, 37.5 mg **Capsule:** 15, 18.7, 30, 37.5 mg	Sympathomimetic Stimulants (SG) Other Schedule 3 or 4 "Diet Pills" (SSG) **Cost:** Low
PHENTOLAMINE Regitine	**Norepinephrine Extravasation:** Local infiltration: inject 5–10 mg diluted in 10 ml saline within 12 hours. **Pheochromocytoma DX (Phentolamine Blocking Test):** IV: 25 mg rapid bolus, measure BP q 30 sec for 3 min, then q 1 min for 7 min. (Positive response if systolic and diastolic BP respectively drop 35 and 25 mm Hg or more.)	**Injection:** 5 mg/ml	ANS AGENTS (G) Sympathoplegics (SG) Alpha Adrenergic Receptor Blockers (SSG) **Cost:** High
Phentrol	See PHENTERMINE		Diet Pill
Phenurone	See PHENACEMIDE		Anti-Convulsant
PHENYLBUTA-ZONE Generic, Butazolidin, Azolid	**Arthritis:** PO: initial dose 300–600 mg/d, divided into 3 or 4 doses maintenance dose 100–200 mg (do not exceed 400 mg daily). **Acute Gout:** PO: to start 400 mg followed by 100 mg q4h (use for a maximum 7 days).	**Tablet:** 100 mg **Capsule:** 100 mg	ANTI-INFLAMMATORY ETC (G) Non-Narcotic Analgesics (SG) Other Non-Narcotic Analgesics (SSG) **Cost:** High

GENERIC NAME Trade Name	INDICATIONS AND DOSAGES	DOSE FORMS	GROUP (G)/SUBGROUP (SG) Relative Cost within Group
PHENYLEPHRINE Generic, Neo-Synephrine	**Hypotension:** IV: 0.1–0.5 mg; repeat q10–15 min PRN. IV, SC: 2–5 mg (max. initial dose 5 mg; max. subsequent dose 10 mg); repeat q1–2h PRN. **Severe Hypotension/Shock:** IV: 100–180 mcg/min to raise blood pressure rapidly; then 40–60 mcg/min when blood pressure is stabilized. Not recommended. **Paroxysmal Supraventricular Tachycardia:** IV: 0.5 mg over 20–30 sec initially (max. dose: 1 mg); then 0.6–0.7 mg PRN. (Subsequent doses should not exceed preceding dose by more than 0.1–0.2 mg, and should never exceed 1 mg.)	**Injection:** 10 mg/ml **Solution, (Ophthalmic):** 2.5, 10% **Nose Drops or Nasal Spray:** 0.25, 0.5, 1.0%	ANS AGENTS (G) Sympathomimetics (SG) Predominantly Alpha Agonist Effects (SSG) Mydriatic, Non-Cycloplegic (SSG) Nasal Decongestant (SSG) **Cost:** Medium
PHENYTOIN Generic, Dilantin, DPH, Diphenylhydantoin	**Seizure Disorders; Trigeminal Neuralgia:** PO: 100 mg tid to start, increase by 100 mg/d q2–4 week; maintenance 300–400 mg/d (max. dose 600 mg/d). Pediatric PO: 5 mg/kg/d in 2–3 doses; maintenance dose 4–8 mg/kg/d (max. dose 300 mg/d). IV: 50% > established PO dosage; 1 week course only (reduce subsequent PO dose by 50% for 1 week following IM regimen). PO (Ext'd release): 300 mg qd. **Status Epilepticus:** IV: Loading dose 10–15 mg/kg to start in divided doses of 5–10 mg/kg; give SLOWLY (i.o., <50 mg/min), then 100 mg PO or IV q6–8h. Pediatric IV: Loading dose 15–20 mg/kg to start SLOWLY (at a rate not greater than 1–3 mg/kg/min, with EKG and blood pressure monitoring). Follow up with PO dosage.	**Tablet:** (chewable) 50 mg **Capsule:** 30 mg, 100 mg **Oral Suspension:** 6, 25 mg/ml **Capsule** (Ext'd release): 30, 100 mg	CNS AGENTS (G) Anticonvulsants (SG) Hydantoins And Equivalent (SSG) **Cost:** Low
PhosLo	See ORAL CALCIUM SALTS		Calcium Ion
PHYSOSTIGMINE Generic, Antilirium, Eserine	**Reverse CNS Anticholinergic Toxicity:** IM, IV: 2 mg initially. Repeat PRN for life-threatening signs. (Give IV not faster than 1 mg/min). Indication: Treatment of CNS toxicity of parasympatholytics and possibly TCA's.	**Injection:** 1 mg/ml (2 ml amps, 1 ml syringe)	ANS AGENTS (G) Cholinergic Agents (SG) Cholinesterase Inhibitors, Reversible (SSG) **Cost:** Medium

GENERIC NAME Trade Name	INDICATIONS AND DOSAGES	DOSE FORMS	GROUP (G)/SUBGROUP (SG) Relative Cost within Group
PHYTONADIONE (K1) Generic, K1-Vitamin, Vitamin K1, Methylphytyl Naphthoquinone, Mephyton, Aquamephyton	**Prothrombin Deficiency:** PO: 2.5–10 mg to initially (max. dose 50 mg); determine subsequent doses by PT measurements. Repeat dose in 12–48 hours if PT has NOT corrected. IV, SC: 2.5–10 mg to start (max. dose 50 mg); determine subsequent doses by PT measurements. Repeat in 6–8 hours if PT has NOT corrected. IV (AVOID, if possible): 2.5–10 mg initially (give SLOWLY not >1 mg/min; max. dose 50 mg); determine subsequent doses by PT measurements. **Hemorrhagic Disease of the Newborn:** Pediatric IM (Newborn): 0.5–1 mg (single dose) (give within 1h of birth and observe for PT decrease w/in 2–4h; to correct underlying cause, phytonadione given concurrently). Also consider 0.5–1 mg 2–3 wks post-birth if pregnant mother took anticoag., antibiotics, anti-TB drugs or anti seizure meds. IV (mother): 1–5 mg 12–24h prior to delivery.	**Tablet:** 5 mg **Injection:** 2, 10 mg/ml **IM Injection:** 2, 10 mg/ml	METABOLIC AGENTS: Anticoagulants And Coagulants (SG) K Vitamins (SSG) **Cost:** Low
Pilagan	See PILOCARPINE NITRATE		Cholinergic
Pilocar	See PILOCARPINE		Cholinergic
PILOCARPINE Salagen (tab) Generic, Isopto, Ocusert Pilo, Pilocar,	**Xerostomia:** PO: 5–10 mg tid (higher dose if no response to lower dose). **Increased Intraocular Pressure:** Solution: Instill 1–2 drops up to q4h. Adjust concentration (usually = 0.5–4%) and frequency based on optimal response. Gel: 0.5 inch ribbon qhs in lower conjunctival sac.	**Tablet:** 5 mg **Solution:** 0.25, 0.5, 1, 2, 3, 4, 6, 8, 10% **Gel:** 4% **Ocusert Pilo-20:** 20 mcg/h for 1 week. **Ocusert Pilo-40:** 40 mcg/h for 1 week.	ANS AND OPHTHALMIC AGENTS (G) Cholinergic Agents (SG) Choline Esters and Equivalent (SSG) Agents Used In the Treatment of Glaucoma (SSG) **Cost:** Low
PILOCARPINE NITRATE Pilagan	**Increased IOP:** Solution: Instill 1–2 drops bid-QID. **Emergency Miosis:** Solution (4%): 1–2 drops for one dose.	**Solution:** 1, 2, 4%	OPHTHALMIC AGENTS (G) Agents Used In The Treatment Of Glaucoma (SG) Parasympathomimetic (SSG) **Cost:** Medium
Pima	See POTASSIUM IODIDE		Expectorant
PIMOZIDE Orap	Initial dose 1–2 mg/d. Maintenance dose <0.2 mg/kg/d or 10 mg/d whichever is less (max. dose <0.2 mg/kg/d or 10 mg/d).	**Tablet:** 2 mg	CNS AGENTS (G) Antipsychotics (SG) Moderate Extrapyramidal Effects (SSG) **Cost:** High
Pin-Rid	See PYRANTEL		Parasiticide
Pin-X	See PYRANTEL		Parasiticide

GENERIC NAME Trade Name	INDICATIONS AND DOSAGES	DOSE FORMS	GROUP (G)/SUBGROUP (SG) Relative Cost within Group
PINDOLOL Generic, Visken	**Hypertension:** PO: 5 mg bid initially; 10–60 mg/d maintenance in 2–3 doses. Increase dose by 10 mg/d at 3–4 week intervals when needed.	**Tablet:** 5, 10 mg	ANS AGENTS (G) Sympathoplegics (G) Beta Adrenergic Blockers (SSG) Non-Selective (Beta 1 and Beta 2) Blockers (SSG) **Cost:** Medium
PIPERACILLIN Pipracil	**General Infections:** IM, IV: 3–4 g q4–6h (max. dose 24 g/d)(give IV doses over 20–30 minutes, give IM injections no more than two g per site). **Severe Infections:** IV: 12–18 g/d (200–300 mg/kg/d) given in 4–6 divided doses. **Uncomplicated Gonorrhea:** IM: 2 g (single dose) with 1000 mg PO probenecid 30 min prior to injection. **Intra-abdominal Surgery Prophylaxis:** IV: 2 g immediately prior; 2 g during surgery; then 2 g q6h for 24 hours after surgery.	**Injection:** (powder) 2, 3, 4, 40 g	LACTAM ANTIBIOTICS—PENICILLINS AND CEPHALOSPORINS Extended Gram Negative and Other Coverage (SG) No/Marginal Effectiveness In Meningitis; Some Activity vs. P. aeruginosa:(SSG) **Cost:** Low
PIPERACILLIN and **TAZOBACTAM** Zosyn	**Infection due to B-lactamase producing staphylococci:** IV: 12 g piperacillin plus 1.5 g tazobactam per day given in 4 divided doses (give IV over 30 minutes).	**Powder** (for injection): 2g piperacillin and 0.25 g tazobactam; 3g piperacillin and 0.375 g,tazobactam; 4g piperacillin and 0.5 g tazobactam	LACTAM ANTIBIOTICS—PENICILLINS AND CEPHALOSPORINS (G) Formulations Containing a Lactamase Inhibitor (SG)
Piperazine Estrone Sulfate	See ESTROPIPATE		Estrogen
PIPOBROMAN Vercyte	CANCER CHEMOTHERAPY (G) Alkylating Agents (SG) Other Alkylating Agents (SSG)		
Pipracil	See PIPERACILLIN		Lactam Antibiotic
PIRBUTEROL Maxair	**Asthma, Bronchospasm:** Adults and Children >12 yrs: 2 inhalations q4–6h. Do not exceed 12 inhalations/d	**Inhaler:** 0.2 mg/puff	RESPIRATORY AGENT (G) Beta Adrenergic Agonist for Inhalation (SG) **Cost:** Low
PIROXICAM Generic, Feldene	**Arthritic Conditions:** PO: 20 mg/d in 1–2 doses.	**Capsule:** 10, 20 mg	CNS AGENTS (G) Non-Narcotic Analgesics (G) Aspirin and Related NSAIDs (SG) **Cost:** Medium
Pitocin	See OXYTOCIN		Uterine Muscle Stimulant
Pituitrin	See POSTERIOR PITUITARY INJECTION		Used for Antidiuretic Effect
Placidyl	See ETHCHLORVYNOL		Hypnotic
Plaquenil	See HYDROXYCHLOROQUINE		Antiparasitic Agent
Platinol	See CISPLATIN		

GENERIC NAME Trade Name	INDICATIONS AND DOSAGES	DOSE FORMS	GROUP (G)/SUBGROUP (SG) Relative Cost within Group
Plegine	See PHENDIMETRAZINE		Diet Pill
Plendil	See FELODIPINE		Calcium Channel Blocker
PLICAMYCIN Mithracin	CANCER CHEMOTHERAPY (G) React With DNA (SG) Antibiotics (SSG)		
Pod-Ben-25	See PODOPHYLLUM RESIN		Lyse Warts, Papillomas
Podocon-25	See PODOPHYLLUM RESIN		Lyse Warts, Papillomas
PODOFILOX Condylox	Apply bid q12h for 3 consecutive days, then discontinue use for 4 consecutive days. This 7 day treatment cycle may be repeated up to 4 times or until wart removed.	**Topical Solution:** 0.5% podofilox	MISCELLANEOUS DERMATOLOGIC AGENTS (G)
Podofin	See PODOPHYLLUM RESIN		Lyse Warts/Papillomas
Podophyllin	See PODOPHYLLUM RESIN		Lyse Warts/Papillomas
PODOPHYLLUM RESIN Podophyllin, Pod-Ben-25, Podocon-25, Podofin	**Topical (physician application only):** Apply to wart/papilloma for 30–40 minutes, leave on for 1–4 hours, remove dried resin thoroughly with soap and water or alcohol.	**Liquid:** 25% Podophyllum Resin in tincture of benzoin.	DERMATOLOGIC AGENTS (G) Miscellaneous (SG) Lyse Warts/Papillomas (SG)
Polaramine	See DEXCHLORPHENIRAMINE		Antihistamine
POLY-PRED	**Ophthalmic:** 1 or 2 gtt q3–4h (may need to give q 30 min. initially in severe infections).		**Ophthalmic Suspension (per cc):** neomycin sulfate (equal to 3.5 mg of neomycin base), polymyxin B sulfate (10,000 Units), prednisolone acetate (0.5%)
Polycillin	See AMPICILLIN		Lactam Antibiotic
POLYETHYLENE GLYCOL-ELECTROLYTE SOLUTION PEG-ES, GoLYTELY, NuLYTELY, Colyte	**Bowel Cleansing:** PO: 240cc q 10 min until 4.0 L taken (fast 3–4 hours prior to taking soln). Nasogastric Tube: 1.2–1.8 L/hr, give 4.0 L total.	**Oral Solution:** *GoLYTELY* powder for 4L soln (= 236 g PEG 3350; 22.7 g NaSulfate, 6.7 g $NaHCO_3$; 5.9 g NaCl; 3 g KCl). *NuLYTELY* powder for 4 L soln (= 420 g PEG 3350; 5.7 g $NaHCO_3$; 11.2 g NaCl; 1.48 g KCl). *Colyte:* powder (1 gal size = 227.1 g PEG 3350; 21.5 g NaSulfate, 6.4 g $NaHCO_3$; 5.5 g NaCl; 2.8 g KCl) & (4L size = 240 g PEG 3350; 22.7 g NaSulfate, 6.7 g $NaHCO_3$; 5.4 gm NaCl; 3 g KCl).	GASTROINTESTINAL AGENTS (G) Laxatives And Bowel Cleansers (G) Isosmotic Oral Solution (SG) **Cost:** High
Polymox	See AMOXICILLIN		Lactam Antibiotic
Polymyxin	See POLYMYXIN B		Polymyxin Antibiotic

GENERIC NAME Trade Name	INDICATIONS AND DOSAGES	DOSE FORMS	GROUP (G)/SUBGROUP (SG) Relative Cost within Group
POLYMYXIN B Polymyxin	Solution: Instill 1–3 drops (10,000–25,000 units/ml) q1h. Decrease frequency as response develops. Ointment: Apply small amount q3–4h.	**Powder for solution:** 500,000 units polymyxin B sulfate.	OPHTHALMIC (G) Antibacterial (SG) **Cost:** Low
POLYSPORIN	**Infection:** Ophthalmic: 0.25–.05 inch ribbon q 3–4 h. Topical: Apply 1–3 times /d.		**Ophthalmic Ointment** (per g): polymyxin B sulfate (10,000 Units), bacitracin zinc (500 Units). **Topical Powder and Ointment** (per g): polymyxin B sulfate (10,000 Units), bacitracin zinc (500 units).
POLYTHIAZIDE Renese	**Hypertension:** PO: 2–4 mg/d. **Edema:** PO: 1–4 mg/d.	**Tablet:** 1, 2, 4 mg	RENAL AGENTS (G) Sodium Diuretics (SG) Thiazide Diuretics (SSG) **Cost:** Medium
POLYTRIM	See TRIMETHOPRIM X		Antibacterial (Urinary)
Pondimin	See FENFLURAMINE		Diet Pill
Ponstel	See MEFENAMIC ACID		Non-Narcotic Analgetic
Pontocaine	See TETRACAINE		Local Anesthetic
POSTERIOR PITUITARY INJECTION Pituitrin	**Post op Ileus:** PO: 10 units SC or IM	**Injection:** 20 units/1 ml vial	ENDOCRINE AGENTS (G) Posterior Pituitary Hormones (Antidiuretic) (SG)
POTASSIUM CHLORIDE Generic, K-Dur, Klor-Con, Micro-K, Slow-K, K-lor, Cena-K, Klorvess	**Potassium Deficiency:** PO: 40–150 mEq/d. Prevention of hypokalemia (adjunct to potassium-wasting diuretics): PO: 16–30 mEq/d. **Severe Potassium Deficits (K+ < 2.0 mEq/l):** IV: Up to 40 mEq/h (max. concentration [K+] = 80 mEq/l), max. dose 400 mEq/d (use lower doses and monitor closely for potassium intoxication). **Moderate Potassium Deficits (K+ > 2.5 mEq/l):** IV: Up to 10 mEq/h (max. concentration [K+] = 40 mEq/l); max. dose 200 mEq/d.	**Tablet:** (Ext'd release) 6.7, 8, 10 mEq **Tablet:** (Ext'd release) 750, 1500 mg **Tablet:** (effervescent) 20, 25, 50 mEq **Capsule:** (Ext'd release) 600, 750 mg **Powder:** 15, 20, 25 mEq/packet **Liquid:** 20, 30, 40, 45 mEq/15 ml	METABOLIC AGENTS (G) Specific Ions (SG) **Cost:** Medium
POTASSIUM IODIDE Generic, Pima, SSKI	**Expectorant:** PO: to start 300–1000 mg pc, bid or tid, optimal dose is 1–1.5 g tid. Pediatric PO: 50% of adult dose of potassium iodide. **Sporotrichosis (cutaneous):** PO (SSKI): 0.3 g tid pc initially, increase as tolerated or to 1.5 mg tid.	**Solution:** 1 g potassium iodide per ml. **Tablet:** (controlled action) 135 mg potassium iodide and 25 mg niacinamide hydroiodide. **Syrup:** 325 mg potassium iodide per 5 ml.	RESPIRATORY AGENTS (G) Expectorants and Mucolytic Agents (SG) **Cost:** Low

GENERIC NAME Trade Name	INDICATIONS AND DOSAGES	DOSE FORMS	GROUP (G)/SUBGROUP (SG) Relative Cost within Group
POTASSIUM PHOSPHATE Generic	**Phosphate Supplementation During TPN:** IV: 10–15 mM of phosphorous/Liter TPN solution.	**Injection:** 3 mM phosphate + 4.4 mEq potassium/ml (5, 10, 15, 30, 50 ml)	METABOLIC AGENTS (G) Specific Ions (SG)
PRALIDOXIME Generic, Protopam	**Organophosphate intoxication:** After or with large doses of atropine. 1–2 g IV over 15–30 minutes. Repeat hourly. IV (autoinjector) or SC if necessary.	**Autoinjector:** 600 mg in 2 ml **Emergency kit:** 1 g vials and diluent.	ANTIDOTES AND USED IN POISONINGS (G)
Pramine	See IMIPRAMINE		Antidepressant (TCA)
PRAMOXINE OTC, Tronothane, Proxine, Tronolane, others	**Topical:** 0.5–1%	**Liquid:** 1% **Cream:** 0.5%, 1% **Gel:** 1%	GENERAL AND LOCAL ANESTHETICS (G) Local Anesthetics (SG) Topical (Mucosal) Only (SSG) **Cost:** Low
Pravachol	See PRAVASTATIN		Lipid Lowering Drug
PRAVASTATIN Pravachol	PO: 10–20 mg q hs initially, maintenance dose 10 to 40 mg/d in single or divided doses. PO (elderly): 10 mg q hs.	**Tablet:** 10, 20, 40 mg	METABOLIC AGENTS (G) LIPID LOWERING DRUGS (SG) HMG-CoA Reductase Inhibitors (SSG) **Cost:** Medium
PRAZEPAM Centrax	**Sedation:** PO: 20–60 mg/d in two or more divided doses. Geriatric PO: 10–15 mg/d in two or more divided doses to start, increase SLOWLY PRN (max. dose 40 mg/d).	**Tablet:** 5, 10 mg **Capsule:** 5, 10, 20 mg	CNS AGENTS (G) Sedative-Hypnotics (SG) Intermediate-Acting (SSG) **Cost:** Medium
PRAZIQUANTEL Biltricide	**Schistosomiasis Infections:** PO: 20 mg/kg/d given in 3 doses, each dose 4–6 hours apart (do not chew tablets). **Clonorchiasis:** PO: 3 doses of 25 mg/kg each as a one day treatment (do not chew tablets).	**Tablet:** 600 mg	ANTIPARASITIC AGENTS (G) **Cost:** Very High
PRAZOSIN Generic, Minipress	**Hypertension:** PO: 1 mg bid or tid initially; 6–15 mg/d maintenance in 2–3 doses (max. dose 40 mg/d). **Prostatism:** 1 mg bid or tid.	**Capsule:** 1, 2, 5 mg	ANS AGENTS (G) Sympathoplegics (SG) Alpha Adrenergic Receptor Blockers (SSG) **Cost:** Low
PRAZOSIN-DIURETIC COMBINATION Minizide	**Hypertension:** PO:	**Capsules:** Combination in fixed proportion of prazosin/polythiazide: 1/0.5, 2/0.5,5:/0.5 mg.	ALPHA ADRENERGIC BLOCKER (SG) AND SODIUM DIURETIC (SG)
Pred-G	**Ophthalmic (suspension):** 1 qtt bid to QID; for initial 2 to 4 d, may give up to 1 qtt every hour. **Ophthalmic (ointment):** Apply a small amount (½ in.) to the conjunctival sac 1–3 times/d.		**Ophthalmic Suspension:** gentamicin sulfate (0.3%), prednisolone acetate (1.0%) **Ophthalmic Ointment:** gentamicin sulfate (0.3%), prednisolone acetate (0.6%)

GENERIC NAME Trade Name	INDICATIONS AND DOSAGES	DOSE FORMS	GROUP (G)/SUBGROUP (SG) Relative Cost within Group
PREDNISOLONE Generic, Prelone, Meticorten, others	PO (Prednisolone): 5–60 mg/d. Intraarticular (acetate): 4–100 mg/injection. Intraarticular (tebutate): 4–30 mg/injection. Intraarticular (phosphate): 2–20 mg/injection. IV/IM (phosphate): 4–60 mg/d. IV (acetate): 4–60 mg/d.	**Tablet:** 5 mg **Syrup:** 15 mg/5 ml **Acetate (suspension):** 25, 50 mg/ml **Tebutate (suspension):** 20 mg/ml **Phosphate (injectable soln):** 20 mg/ml **Phosphate (oral soln):** 5 mg/ml	ENDOCRINE AGENTS (G) Anti-Inflammatory Steroids (SG) **Cost:** Low
PREDNISONE Generic, Orasone, Deltasone	PO: 5–60 mg/d.	**Tablet:** 1, 2.5, 5, 10, 20, 50 mg **Oral Solution:** 5 mg/5 ml, 5 mg/ml **Syrup:** 5 mg/ml	ENDOCRINE AGENTS (G) Anti-Inflammatory Steroids (SG) **Cost:** Low
Pregnyl	See HUMAN CHORIONIC GONADOTROPIN (FSH)		
Prelone	See PREDNISOLONE		Corticosteroid
Prelu-2	See PHENDIMETRAZINE		Diet Pill
Preludin	See PHENDIMETRAZINE		Diet Pill
Premarin	See CONJUGATED ESTROGENS		Estrogens
Prepidil	See DINOPROSTONE		Uterine Stimulating Prostaglandin
Presamine	See IMIPRAMINE		TCA, Antidepressant
Pretz-D	See EPHEDRINE		Sympathomimetic
Prevacid	See LANSOPRAZOLE		Inhibit Gastric Acid Secretion
PRILOCAINE Citanest	Infiltration: 4%. Peripheral Nerve Block: 4%.	**Injection:** 4% **Injection:** 4% with 1:200,000 epinephrine	GENERAL AND LOCAL ANESTHETICS (G) Local Anesthetics (G) Injectable Only (SG) **Cost:** Low
Prilosec	See OMEPRAZOLE		Inhibitor Of Gastric Acid Secretion
Primaclone	See PRIMIDONE		Anticonvulsant
Primacor	See MILRINONE		Vasodilator and Inotropic as Xanthines
PRIMAQUINE PHOSPHATE	Doses are expressed as primaquine base; 26.5 mg phosphate = 15 mg base (0.53 mg phosphate = 0.3 mg base). **Acute Vivax Malaria:** PO: 15 mg/d for 14 days (given concurrently with chloroquine). Pediatric PO: 0.3 mg(base)/kg/d for 14 days (max. single dose 15 mg(base) per dose). **Malaria Prophylaxis:** PO (chloroquine with primaquine combination): 1 tablet q7d, start at least 1 day prior to entering endemic area, continue for 8 weeks after leaving endemic area.	**Tablet:** 15 mg **Combination Form: Chloroquine with Primaquine Tablet:** chloroquine 300 mg base, primaquine 45 mg base	ANTI-INFECTIOUS AGENTS (G) Antiparasitic Agents (G) **Cost:** Low

GENERIC NAME Trade Name	INDICATIONS AND DOSAGES	DOSE FORMS	GROUP (G)/SUBGROUP (SG) Relative Cost within Group
Primaxin	See IMIPENEM WITH CILASTATIN		Penicillin with Lactamase Inhibitor
PRIMIDONE Generic, Mysoline, Desoxyphenobarbital	**Seizure Disorders:** PO (patients not previously dosed): 100–125 mg qd for 3 days; then 100–125 mg bid for 3 days; then 100–125 mg tid for 3 days; maintenance 250 mg tid-QID (max. dose 2000 mg/d). Pediatric PO (<8 y.o.) (patients not previously dosed): 50 mg qhs for 3 days; then 50 mg bid for 3 days; then 100 mg bid for 3 days; maintenance 125–250 mg tid (or 10–25 mg/kg/d in divided doses).	**Tablet:** 50, 250 mg **Suspension:** 250 mg/5 ml	CNS AGENTS (G) Anticonvulsants (SG) Sedative-Hypnotics (SSG) **Cost:** Low
Principen	See AMPICILLIN		Lactam Antibiotic
Prinivil	See LISINOPRIL		ACE Inhibitor
PRINZIDE	**Hypertension:** PO: 1–2 tablets qd and adjust within the limits imposed.	**Tablet:** Lisinopril with hydrochlorothiazide in proportions of 10/12.5, 20/12.5, 20/25 mg	ACE INHIBITOR (SG) AND THIAZIDE DIURETIC (SG)
Priscoline	See TOLAZOLINE		Alpha Adrenergic Blocker
Privine	See NAPHAZOLINE		Sympathomimetic, Nasal
Pro-Banthine	See PROPANTHELINE		Parasympatholytics
Probalan	See PROBENECID		Uricosuric
Proampacin	See AMPICILLIN		Lactam Antibiotic
PROBENECID Generic, Benemid, Probalan	**Gout Associated Hyperuricemia:** PO: 0.25 g bid for 7 days, then 0.5 g bid (maintain good hydration, alkalinize urine w/ K-citrate (7.5 g/d) or NaBicarb (3–7.5 g/day). After 6 mo. w/o an attack attempt to decrease dosage by 0.5 m/d each 6 mo. Watch urate serum levels; if these start to rise, decrease dose no further. **Adjunct to Pcn/Cephalosporin Tx:** PO: 2 g/d given in 2 or more divided doses. **Uncomplicated Gonorrhea:** PO: 1 g probenecid (given 30 min prior to IM penicillin G Procaine 4.8 million units (split at 2 sites)). **Neurosyphilis:** PO: 500 mg probenecid QID; give for 10–14 days (along w/ 2–4 million units/day of aqueous procaine penicillin G).	**Tablet:** 500 mg	METABOLIC AGENTS (G) Used In The Treatment Of Gout (SG) Slow Renal Excretion Of Penicillin (SG) **Cost:** Low
PROBUCOL Lorelco	**Hyperlipidemia:** PO: 500 mg with AM and PM meals.	Removed from U.S. market	METABOLIC AGENTS (G) Other Lipid Lowering Agents (SSG)

GENERIC NAME Trade Name	INDICATIONS AND DOSAGES	DOSE FORMS	GROUP (G)/SUBGROUP (SG) Relative Cost within Group
PROCAINAMIDE Generic, Procan, Pronestyl, Sub-Quin	**Arrhythmias:** PO: Tablet: One tablet q3h of size closest approximating 2.5 mg/lb **Ventricular Tachycardia:** IV: 100 mg q5min (rate not >25–50 mg/min) until a total of 500 mg given, arrhythmia suppressed, BP decreases >15 mmHg, QRS widens >50%, or PR interval increases. May repeat dose after 10 minutes or more have passed (max. dose 1000 mg). IV: (alternate dosing method) 500–600 mg given over 30 minutes at a rate of 20 mg/min (max. single dose 1000 mg). IV Maintenance doses: 2–6 mg/min (IV maint. dose range 200–1000 mg/d; adjust according to clinical situation and levels; therapeutic levels = 3–10 mcg/ml for procainamide plasma level; and therapeutic NAPA plasma levels = 10–30 mcg/ml). IV: 50 mg/kg/d divided in 4–8 doses given q3–6h (convert to PO ASAP, if more than 3 injections are needed use blood levels and clinical response to adjust further doses).	**Tablet:** 250, 375, 500 mg **Capsule:** 250, 375, 500 mg **Tablet:** (Ext'd release) 250, 500, 750, 1000 mg **Injection:** 100 mg/ml, 500 mg/ml	CV AGENTS (G) Antiarrhythmic Agents (G) Group I (SG) **Cost:** Medium
PROCAINE Generic, Novocain	**Infiltration:** 0.25–0.5%. **Peripheral Nerve Block:** 0.5–2%.	**Injection:** 1, 2, 10%	LOCAL ANESTHETICS (G) Injectable Only (SG) **Cost:** Low
Procan	See PROCAINAMIDE		Antiarrhythmic
PROCARBAZINE Matulane	CANCER CHEMOTHERAPY (G) React With DNA (SG) Other Miscellaneous (SSG)		
Procardia	See NIFEDIPINE		Calcium Channel Blocker
PROCHLOR-PERAZINE Compazine	**Nausea and Vomiting:** PO: 5–10 mg tid-QID PO (Ext'd release): 15 mg qAM or 10 mg bid. Rectal: 25 mg bid IM: 5–10 mg q3–4h (max. dose 40 mg/d) IV: 2.5–10 mg SLOWLY (rate not faster than 5 mg/minute, max. single dose = 10 mg; max. daily dose 40 mg/d) Pediatric PO, Rectal (20–29 lbs): 2.5 mg qd-bid (max. dose 7.5 mg/d). Pediatric PO, Rectal (30–39 lbs): 2.5 mg bid-tid (max. dose 10 mg/d). Pediatric PO, Rectal (40–85 lbs): 2.5 mg tid; or 5 mg bid (max. dose 15 mg/d). IM: 0.06 mg/pound one dose only. **Psychotic Disorders:** PO: 5–10 mg tid or QID to start; maintenance 50–150 mg/d. IV: 10–20 mg q2–4h PRN, maintenance dose 10–20mg q4–6h; when possible convert to PO maintenance. Pediatric PO, Rectal (6–12 years): 2.5 mg bid or tid to start; maintenance 20–25 mg/d (max. dose 25 mg/d) **Anxiety:** PO: 5 mg tid or QID. PO (Ext'd release): 10 mg q12–24h.	**Tablet:** 5, 10, 25 mg **Capsule:** (Ext'd release) 10, 15, 30 mg **Syrup:** 5 mg/5 ml **Suppositories:** 2.5, 5, 25 mg **Injection:** 5 mg/ml	CNS AGENTS (G) Antipsychotics (SG) Prominent Extrapyramidal Effects (SSG) **Cost:** Low

GENERIC NAME Trade Name	INDICATIONS AND DOSAGES	DOSE FORMS	GROUP (G)/SUBGROUP (SG) Relative Cost within Group
Procrit	See EPOETIN ALPHA		Hematopoietic Hormone
PROCYCLIDINE Kemadrin	**Parkinsonism:** PO: 2.5 mg tid to start; maintenance 4–5 mg tid or QID. **Drug-Induced Extrapyramidal Disorders:** PO: 2.5 mg tid to start; increase 2.5 mg/d qd; maintenance 10–20 mg/d in divided doses.	**Tablet:** 5 mg	CNS AGENTS (G) Antiparkinsonian Agents (G) Anticholinergics (SG) **Cost:** Medium
Profasi	See HUMAN CHORIONIC GONADOTROPIN (FSH)		
Profenal	See SUPROFEN		NSAID, Ocular
Profilate	See ANTIHEMOPHILIC FACTOR VIII (Non-recombinant)		Hemostatic
Progest-M	See PROGESTERONE		Progestin
PROGESTERONE Oil: Generics, Bay Progest, Femotrone in Oil, Gesterol 50, Powder: Generics, Progest-M	**Amenorrhea:** IM: 5–10 mg/d for 6–8 days (expect withdrawal bleeding 4–7 days after last injection). **Abnormal Uterine Bleeding:** IM: 5–10 mg/d for 6 doses. (Expect bleeding termination in 6 days.)	**Injection:** 50 mg/ml **Powder:** 1, 2, 4, 5, 8, 10, 16, 25, 50, 100, 1000 g	ENDOCRINE AGENTS (G) Progestins (SG) **Cost:** Low
Proglycem	See DIAZOXIDE		Hypotensive Agent
Prograf	See TACROLIMUS		Immunomodulator (Transplants)
Prohim	See YOHIMBINE		Alpha Adrenergic Blocker
Prokine	See SARGRAMOSTIM GLYCOSYLATED GM-CSF		Myeloid Stimulation
Proleukin	See ALDESLEUKIN		Immunomodulator (Cancer Chemotherapy)
Prolixin	See FLUPHENAZINE		Antipsychotic
Proloid	See THYROGLOBULIN		Thyroid Replacement
Proloprim	See TRIMETHOPRIM		Antibacterial
PROMETHAZINE Generic, Phenergan	**Motion Sickness:** PO, rectal: 25 mg bid (take 30–60 minutes before departure, then in 8–12 h). Pediatric PO, rectal: 12.5 to 25 mg bid PRN. **Nausea/Vomiting:** PO, IM, IV or rectal dosage: 12.5–25 mg every 4–6 hours PRN (IV rate not to exceed 25 mg/min). Pediatric rectal (>2 yrs.): 0.25–0.5 mg/kg q4–6h, PRN. **Allergy/Pruritus:** PO, rectal: 12.5 mg PO or PR tid and 25 mg hs. **Pediatric PO, rectal:** (>2 yrs): 6.25–12.5 mg tid. **Sedation:** PO, IM, IV or rectal dosage: 25–50 mg hs (IV rate not to exceed 25 mg/min; PO should not exceed 25 mg/ml concentration). Pediatric PO, rectal (>2 yrs): 0.5 mg/pound hs. **Preoperative Sedation:** See under conscious sedation.	**Tablet:** 12.5, 25, 50 mg **Syrup:** 6.25, 25 mg per 5 ml **Injection:** 25, 50 mg per ml **Suppositories:** 12.5, 25, 50 mg	CNS AGENTS (G) Antipsychotics (SG) Moderate Extrapyramidal Effects (SSG) **Cost:** Low

GENERIC NAME Trade Name	INDICATIONS AND DOSAGES	DOSE FORMS	GROUP (G)/SUBGROUP (SG) Relative Cost within Group
Promethazine-Meperidine	See CONSCIOUS SEDATION		Narcotic-Antipsychotic Combination
Pronestyl	See PROCAINAMIDE		Antiarrhythmic
PROPAFENONE Rythmol	**Ventricular Arrhythmias:** Start with 150 mg every q8h; increase at 3–4 day (or longer) intervals to 225 q8h (max. dose 300 mg q8).	**Tablet:** 150, 225, 300 mg	Antiarrhythmic Agents (SG) Group I Antiarrhythmic Agents (SSG) **Cost:** Very High
PROPANTHELINE Generic, Pro-Banthine	**Peptic Ulcer, Hypermotility:** PO: 15 mg tid, take 30 min ac, and 30 mg at hs. Geriatric PO: 7.5 mg tid.	**Tablet:** 7.5, 15 mg	ANS AGENTS (G) Parasympatholytics (SG) Quaternary Amines (SSG) **Cost:** Low
PROPARACAINE Generic, AK-Taine, Alcaine, Ophthaine, Ophthetic	**Deep Anesthesia:** Solution: 1 drop q5–10 minutes (max. dose: 7 consecutive doses). **Suture Removal:** Solution: 1 or 2 drops 2 or 3 minutes before removal. **Foreign Body Removal:** Solution: 1 to 2 drops prior to procedure. **Tonometry:** Solution: 1 to 2 drops just prior to measurement.	**Ophthalmic Solution:** 0.5%	LOCAL ANESTHETICS (G) Topical Only (SG)
Propine	See DIPIVEFRIN		Sympathomimetic
Proplex T	See COAGULANT FACTOR IX		Hemostatic
PROPOXYPHENE Generic, Darvon, Darvon-N, Profene, Dolene	**Pain:** PO (HCl): 65 mg q4h (max. dose 390 mg/d). PO (Darvon-N = napsylate salt): 100 mg q4h (max. dose 600 mg/d). **Capsule** (HCL). 32, 65 mg	**Tablet** (napsylate): 100 mg **Suspension** (napsylate): 10 mg/ml (**Note:** The HCL (65 mg) and the napsylate (100 mg) contain the same amount of propoxyphene base.)	Narcotic Analgesics And Related Agents (SG) Purely Stimulant Effects (SSG) **Cost:** Low
PROPOXYPHENE HCl WITH ACET-AMINOPHEN OR ASPIRIN Generic, E-Lor, Genagesic, Wygesic		**Tablet:** 65 mg of the base with 650 mg of acetaminophen **Capsules:** with 390 mg aspirin and 32 mg caffeine	
PROPOXYPHENE NAPSYLATE AND ACETAMIN-OPHEN TABS Generic, Darvo-cet N-50, 100, Propacet 100		**Tablet:** 32 or 65 mg of the base and 325 or 650 mg of acetaminophen	

GENERIC NAME Trade Name	INDICATIONS AND DOSAGES	DOSE FORMS	GROUP (G)/SUBGROUP (SG) Relative Cost within Group
PROPRANOLOL Generic, Inderal, Betachron	**Hypertension:** PO: 40 mg bid initially; 80–240 mg/d maintenance in 2–3 doses (max dose: 640 mg/d). PO (Ext'd release): 80 mg qd initially; 120–160 mg qd maintenance (max dose: 640 mg/d). **Angina:** PO: 80–320 mg/d in 2–4 divided doses. PO (Ext'd release): 80 mg qd initially; 160 mg qd maintenance (max dose: 320 mg/d). **Arrhythmias:** PO: 10–30 mg tid-QID given ac and hs. **Migraine (Prophylaxis):** PO: 40 mg bid initially; 160–240 mg/d maintenance in 2–4 doses. PO (Ext'd release): 80 mg qd. **IHSS:** PO: 20–40 mg tid or QID given ac and hs. PO (Ext'd release): 80–160 mg qd. **Post-MI:** PO: 180–240 mg/d in 2–4 doses (max. dose: 320 mg/d). **Emergency beta blockade:** IV: 0.5–3 mg SLOWLY (rate < 1 mg/min); may repeat (once) in 2 min; wait at least 4h until next dose. **Pediatric HTN:** Pediatric PO: 1 mg/kg/d initially; 1–4 mg/kg/d maintenance in 2–3 doses. **Essential tremor:** PO: 40 mg bid initially, maintenance 120–240 mg/d in 2–4 divided doses (max. dose: 320 mg/d).	**Tablet:** 10, 20, 40, 60, 80, 90 mg **Capsule:** (Ext'd release) 60, 80, 120, 160 mg **Oral Solution:** 4 mg/ml, 8 mg/ml **Oral Solution:** (concentrate) 80 mg/ml **Injection:** 1 mg/ml	Sympathoplegics (SG) Beta Adrenergic Receptor Blockers (SSG) Non-Selective blockers (SSG) **Cost:** Low
Propulsid	See CISAPRIDE		Increase esophageal muscle tone
PROPYL-HEXEDRINE (INHALER) OTC, Generic, Benzedrex	**Intranasal (adults and children >5 yrs):** 1–2 inhalations in each nostril (while blocking the other nostril) not more than every 2 hours (do not use more than 3 days).	**Inhaler:** 250 mg propylhexedrine	RESPIRATORY AGENTS (G) Sympathomimetic Nasal (Topical) Decongestants (SG) **Cost:** Low
PROPYLTHIO-URACIL Generic, PTU	**Hyperthyroidism:** PO: 300–400 mg/d to start (rarely 600–900 mg/d); maintenance 100–150 mg/d. Pediatric PO (6–10 years): 50–150 mg/d to start. Pediatric PO (>10 years): 150–300 mg/d to start.	**Tablet:** 50 mg	ENDOCRINE AGENTS (G) Thyroid and Antithyroid Agents (SG) Anti-Thyroid Agents and Related (SSG) **Cost:** Low
Proscar	See FINASTERIDE		Testosterone Antagonist
ProSom	See ESTAZOLAM		Short-Acting Hypnotics
Prostacyclin	SEE EPOPROSTENOL		Pulmonary Vasodilator
Prostaglandin E1	See ALPROSTADIL		Vasodilator PG
Prostaglandin E2	See DINOPROSTONE		Uterine Stimulating PG

GENERIC NAME Trade Name	INDICATIONS AND DOSAGES	DOSE FORMS	GROUP (G)/SUBGROUP (SG) Relative Cost within Group
Prostaglandin, 15 methyl PGF2a	See CARBOPROST		Uterine Stimulating PG
Prostaglandin, isopropyl-PGF2a	See LATANOPROST		IOP Lowering Agent
Prostaphlin	See OXACILLIN		Lactam Antibiotic
Prostigmin	See NEOSTIGMINE		Cholinesterase Inhibitor
Prostin-15 mg Prostaglandin	See CARBOPROST		Uterine Stimulating
ProstinE2 Prostaglandin	See DINOPROSTONE		Uterine Stimulating
PROTAMINE SULFATE Generic	**Heparin Overdose Or To Terminate Action During Surgery:** IV: 1 mg protamine sulfate (basic) neutralizes approx. 90 USP units heparin (acidic). (Give slowly at a rate <50 mg/10 min). (max. single dose: 50 mg.)	**Injection:** 10 mg/ml	METABOLIC AGENTS (G) Anticoagulants And Coagulants (SG) Heparin and Related Agents (SSG) **Cost:** Very High
Protamine Zinc Insulin	See INSULINS		
PROTIRELIN Thypinone, Relefact TRH	**Adjunct To Hypothyroidism Diagnosis:** IV: 500 mcg as a single dose, obtain TSH immediately prior to and 30 minutes after infusion.	**Injection:** 500 mcg/ml	ENDOCRINE AGENTS (G) Thyroid And Antithyroid Agents (SG) Thyroid Stimulating Hormone (SSG)
Protopam	See PRALIDOXIME		Antidote to ChE Inhibitor
Protostat	See METRONIDAZOLE		Antibacterial, Parasiticide
PROTRIPTYLINE Vivactil	**Endogenous Depression:** PO: 15–40 mg/d to start in 3–4 doses; maintenance 15–60 mg/d. **Geriatric/adolescent PO:** 5 mg tid to start; maintenance up to 20 mg/d.	**Tablet:** 5, 10 mg	CNS AGENTS (G) Tricyclic Antidepressants (SG) **Cost:** Medium
Protropin	See SOMATREM		Growth Hormone, Recombinant
Proventil	See ALBUTEROL		Sympathomimetic, Beta 2 Selective
Provera	See MEDROXYPROGESTERONE		Progestins
Provocholine	See METHACHOLINE		Cholinergic
Proxine	See PRAMOXINE		Antidote to ChE Inhibition
Prozac	See FLUOXETINE		Stimulant
PSEUDOEPHED-RINE OTC, Generic, Sudafed	Adults: 60 mg q4–6h (max. dose 240 mg in 24 hours). Pediatric (6–12 yrs): 30 mg q4–6h (max. dose 120 mg in 24 hours). Pediatric (2–5 yrs): 15 mg q4–6h (max. dose 60 mg in 24 hours).	**Tablet:** 30 (OTC), 60, 240 mg **Tablet:** (Ext'd release) 120 mg **Capsule:** 60 mg **Capsule:** (Ext'd release) 120 mg **Liquid:** 3, 6 mg/ml **Drops:** 7.5 mg/0.8 ml	ANS AGENTS (G) Sympathomimetics (SG) Sympathomimetics, Mixed Alpha and Beta Agonist Effects (SSG) **Cost:** Low

GENERIC NAME Trade Name	INDICATIONS AND DOSAGES	DOSE FORMS	GROUP (G)/SUBGROUP (SG) Relative Cost within Group
PSYLLIUM Generic, OTC, Serutan, Metamucil	PO: 1 heaping tsp in 240 ml water, 1–3 times daily with meals.	Countless preparations and mixtures of psyllium, most containing 3.4 gm of psyllium/ tsp. See label of each preparation.	GASTROINTESTINAL AGENTS (G) Laxatives And Bowel Cleansers (SG) Bulk (SSG) **Cost:** Medium
Pteroylglutamic Acid	See FOLIC ACID		Vitamin
PTU	See PROPYLTHIOURACIL		Antithyroid
Pulmicort	See BUDESONIDE		Corticosteroid
Pulmozyme	See DORNASE ALFA		Mucolytic
Purge	See CASTOR OIL		Irritant Laxative
Purinethol	See MERCAPTOPURINE		Cancer Chemotherapy
Pyopen	See CARBENICILLIN		Lactam Antibiotic
PYRANTEL Pin-Rid, Antiminth, Pin-X, Reese's Pinworm	**Ascariasis, Enterobiasis:** PO: 11 mg/kg as a single dose (max. total dose 1 g). (May give with food.)	**Liquid:** 50, 144 mg pyrantel per ml **Capsule** (soft gel): 180 mg **Oral Suspension:** 50 mg/ml	ANTI-INFECTIOUS AGENTS (G) Antiparasitic Agents (SG) **Cost:** High
PYRAZINAMIDE	**Tuberculosis (given in combination):** Adults PO (single dose/day): 15–30 mg/kg/d (max. dose 2000 mg/d).	**Tablet:** 500 mg	ANTI-INFECTIOUS AGENTS (G) Antituberculous Agents (SG) Antituberculous Second Line Agents (SSG) **Cost:** High
PYRIDOSTIG-MINE Mestinon, Re-gonol	**Myasthenia Gravis:** PO: 600 mg/day doses spaced to provide maximum relief. (range 60–1500 mg/d). PO (Sustained release): 180–540 mg qd or bid	**Tablet:** 60 mg **Tablet:** (Ext'd release) 180 mg **Syrup:** 12 mg/ ml **Injection:** 5 mg/ ml	ANS AGENTS (G) Cholinergic Agents (SG) Cholinesterase Inhibitors, Reversible (SG) **Cost:** High
PYRILAMINE Generic, Nisaval, Mepyramine	PO: 25–50 mg tid or QID.	**Tablet:** 25 mg	ANTI-INFLAMMATORY (G) Antihistamines (H1 Antagonists) (SG) With Prominent Sedation (SSG) **Cost:** Low

GENERIC NAME Trade Name	INDICATIONS AND DOSAGES	DOSE FORMS	GROUP (G)/SUBGROUP (SG) Relative Cost within Group
PYRIMETH-AMINE Daraprim	**Malaria (prophylaxis):** PO (adults and children >10 yrs): 25 mg/week. **Malaria Treatment (susceptible strains only, adjunct to other treatment):** PO: (adults and children >10 yrs): 50 mg/d for 2 days if used alone; 25 mg/d if used in combination. **Toxoplasmosis:** PO: 50–75 mg/d initially (give with 1–4 g sulfapyrimidine); treat for 1–3 weeks then reduce dose to initial level and treat for 4–5 weeks more.	**Tablet:** 25 mg	ANTI-INFECTIOUS AGENTS (G) Antiparasitic Agents (SG) **Cost:** Medium
QUAD	See FLOXURIDINE		
QUAZEPAM Doral	PO: 15 mg qhs to start, maintenance 7.5–15 mg qhs.	**Tablet:** 7.5, 15 mg	CNS AGENTS (G) Sedative-Hypnotics (SG) Intermediate-Acting (SSG) **Cost:** Medium
Quelicin	See SUCCINYLCHOLINE		Curariform
Questran	See CHOLESTYRAMINE		Bile Acid Binding Resins
QUINACRINE Atabrine	**Giardiasis:** PO: 100 mg q8h for 5–7 days. Pediatric PO: 7 mg/kg/d in 3 doses for 5 days with meals (max. dose 300 mg/d). **Beef, Pork or Fish Tapeworm:** PO: 200 mg, for 4 doses given q10 minutes, give each dose with 600 mg Na+ bicarbonate. **Pediatric PO (11–14 yrs):** 150 mg, for 3–4 doses given q10 minutes, give each dose with 300 mg Na+ bicarbonate. **Pediatric PO (5–10 yrs):** 100 mg, for 3–4 doses given q10 minutes, give each dose with 300 mg Na+ bicarbonate	**Tablet:** 100 mg	ANTI-INFECTIOUS AGENTS (G) Antiparasitic Agents (SG) **Cost:** Medium
Quinidex	See QUINIDINE		Antiarrhythmic Agent
Quinaglute	See QUINIDINE		Antiarrhythmic Agent
QUINAPRIL Accupril	**Hypertension:** PO: 10 mg qd to start; 20–80 mg/d maintenance in 1 or 2 divided doses. (5 mg qd to start in patients on diuretics). **Congestive Heart Failure:** PO: 5 mg bid to start; 10–20 mg bid maintenance (if serum sodium <130 mEq/L, initial dose is 2.5 mg/d).	**Tablet:** 5, 10, 20, 40 mg	CV AGENTS (G) Vasodilators (SG) ACE Inhibitors (SSG) **Cost:** Medium
QUINESTROL Estrovis	**Post-Menopausal Estrogen Replacement, Menopausal Symptoms, Atrophic Vaginitis & Related Conditions, Hypogonadism (female):** PO: 100 mcg/d for 7 days, on day 14 of treatment initiate 100 mcg/wk doses (max. maintenance dose: 200 mcg/wk).	**Tablet:** 100 mcg	ENDOCRINE AGENTS (G) Estrogens (SG) **Cost:** High

GENERIC NAME Trade Name	INDICATIONS AND DOSAGES	DOSE FORMS	GROUP (G)/SUBGROUP (SG) Relative Cost within Group
QUINETHAZONE Hydromox	**Hypertension:** PO: 50–100 mg qd., may require 50 mg bid (max. dose 150–200 mg/d).	**Tablet:** 50 mg	RENAL AGENT (G) Sodium Diuretics (SG) Thiazide Diuretics (SSG) **Cost:** High
QUINIDINE Generic, Quinaglute, Cardioquin, Duraquin, Dura-Tabs, Cin-Quin, Quinora, Quinidex Extentabs	**(Note:** 200 mg of sulfate = 267 mg gluconate = 267 mg polygalacturonate—all doses expressed as sulfate unless otherwise indicated.) **Premature Atrial/Ventricular Contractions:** PO: 200–300 mg q6–8h. PO (Ext'd release): 300–600 mg q8–12h. **Atrial Fibrillation Conversion (digitalized pts.):** PO: 200 mg q2–3h, give for 5 to 8 doses; increase daily until sinus rhythm restored (max. dose: 3 to 4 grams/day). **Paroxysmal Supraventricular Tachycardia:** PO (sulfate): 400–600 mg q2–3h until episode is terminated. **Parenteral Dosing:** IM (gluconate): Loading dose 600 mg, then 200–400 mg q2h or PRN. IV (gluconate): Administer dilute sln SLOWLY (i.e., not to exceed 16 mg/min) until desired effect achieved while continuously monitoring BP, EKG and clinical signs.	**Tablet:** 200, 300 mg **Tablet:** (Ext'd release) 300, 324 mg **Injection:** 50 mg/ml	CV AGENTS (G) Antiarrhythmic Agents (SG) Group I (SSG) **Cost:** Low
QUININE Generic	**Chloroquine-Resistant Malaria:** PO: 650 mg q8h for 5–7 days. **Nocturnal Leg Cramps:** PO: 260–300 mg hs.	**Capsule:** 64.8, 65, 200, 260, 300, 325 mg **Tablet:** 162.5, 260 mg	ANTI-INFECTIOUS AGENTS (G) Antiparasitic Agents (SG) **Cost:** Low
Quinora	See QUINIDINE		Antiarrhythmic
RAMIPRIL Altace	**Hypertension:** PO: 2.5 mg qd to start, 2.5–20 mg/d maintenance in 1 or 2 divided doses (in patient on diuretics 1.25 mg qd to start).	**Capsule:** 1.25, 2.5, 5, 10 mg	CV AGENTS (G) Vasodilators (SG) ACE Inhibitors (SSG) **Cost:** Medium
RANITIDINE Zantac	**Duodenal or Gastric Ulcer:** PO: 100–150 mg bid (or 300 mg qhs); after acute stage, may maintain at 150 mg qhs. IV, IV: 50 mg q6–8h (Infuse IV sln SLOWLY over 15–20 min). **Hypersecretory Conditions:** PO: 150 mg bid.	**Tablet:** 150, 300 mg **Injection:** 0.5 mg/ml, 25 mg/ml	GASTROINTESTINAL AGENTS (G) Inhibitors Of Acid Secretion (SG) H2 Antagonists (SSG)
Recombinate	See ANTIHEMOPHILIC FACTOR VIII RECOMBINANT		Hemostatic
Redux	See DEXFENFLURAMINE		Diet Pill, Atypical
Regestol	See DOCUSATE		Stool Softener
Regitine	See PHENTOLAMINE		Alpha Adrenemic Blocker
Reglan	See METOCLOPRAMIDE		Antiemetic

GENERIC NAME Trade Name	INDICATIONS AND DOSAGES	DOSE FORMS	GROUP (G)/SUBGROUP (SG) Relative Cost within Group
Regonol	See PYRIDOSTIGMINE		Cholinesterase Inhibitor
Regular Insulin	See INSULIN INJECTION		
RegulaxSS	See DOCUSATE		Stool Softener
Reioamine	See DIMENHYDRINATE		Antihistamine
Rela	See CARISOPRODOL		Muscle Relaxant
Relafen	See NABUMETONE		Non-Narcotic Analgesics
Relefact TRH	See PROTIRELIN		Thyroid Stimulating Agent
REMIFENTANIL Ultiva	**Adjunct to general anesthesia:**	IV: powder 1, 2, 5 mg	CNS AGENTS (G) Narcotic Analgesics (SG)
Renese	See POLYTHIAZIDE		Sodium Diuretic
Renoquid	See SULFACYTINE		Antibacterial, Urinary
Rescriptor	See DELAVIRDINE		ANTIVIRAL, HIV
Resectisol	See MANNITOL		Osmotic Agent
RESERPINE Generic, Serpasil, Sandril	**Hypertension:** PO: 0.5 mg/d initially for 1–2 weeks; reduce to 0.1–0.25 mg/d maintenance.	**Tablet:** 0.1, 0.25, 1.0 mg	ANS AGENTS (G) Sympathoplegics (SG) Centrally-Acting Adrenergic Inhibitors (SSG) **Cost:** Low
Respbid	See THEOPHYLLINE		Xanthine Bronchodilator
Restoril	See TEMAZEPAM		Ultrashort-Acting Hypnotic
Retin A	See TRETINOIN		Acne And Psoriasis
Retrovir	See ZIDOVUDINE		Reverse Transcriptase Inhibitor
Rev Eyes	See DAPIPRAZOLE		Alpha Adrenergic Antagonist
Reversol	See EDROPHONIUM		Cholinesterase
ReVia	See NALTREXONE		Narcotic Antagonist
Rexolate	See SODIUM SALICYLATE		Non-Narcotic Analgetic
Resulin	See TROGLITAZONE		Oral Antidiabetic
RHo (D) IMMUNE GLOBULIN Generic, RhoGAM, Gamulin Rh, HypRho-D, Rhesonativ	**Postpartum Prophylaxis:** IM: One vial (approx. 300 mcg) within 72 hours of delivery (more may be needed depending on volume of fetomaternal hemorrhage). **Antepartum Prophylaxis:** IM: One vial (approx. 300 mcg) at 26 to 28 weeks gestation and one vial within 72 hours after delivery.	**Injection vial:** approx. 300 mcg	ANTI-INFLAMMATORY ETC AGENTS (G) Immunomodulators (SG) Rh Neutralizing Antibody
RhoGAM	See RHo(D)IMMUNE GLOBULIN		Rh Antibody
RIBAVIRIN Virazole	**Respiratory Infections (due to Respiratory Syncytial Virus):** Aerosol Inhalation: Treat with aerosol generator for 12–18 hours/day (minimum 3 days, maximum 7 days) as a component of a full treatment program; use 20 mg/ml concentration as starting solution—ave. aerosol concentration over ½ day = 190 mcg/liter of air.	**Powder:** (for reconstitution for aerosol): 6g powder/100 ml vial	ANTI-INFECTIOUS AGENTS (G) Antiviral Agents (SG) **Cost:** Very High
Ridaura	See AURANOFIN		Antirheumatic goldcompound
Rifadin	See RIFAMPIN		Antituberculous

GENERIC NAME Trade Name	INDICATIONS AND DOSAGES	DOSE FORMS	GROUP (G)/SUBGROUP (SG) Relative Cost within Group
RIFAMATE	**Tuberculosis:** PO: 2 capsules/d, 1 hour before or 2 h after a meal.		**Capsule:** rifampin (300 mg), isoniazid (150 mg)
RIFAMPIN Rifadin, Rimactane	**Tuberculosis (Initial Therapy, Given In Combination):** Adults (single dose/day): 600 mg/d. Adults (two doses/week): 10 mg/kg twice per week (max. dose 600 mg/ week). Pediatric (single dose/day): 10–20 mg/kg/d (max. dose 600 mg/d). **Meningitis Carriers (Prophylaxis or Asymptomatic):** PO: 600 mg qd for 4 days. Pediatric PO (1–12 yrs): 10–20 mg/ kg/d for 4 days (max. dose: 600 mg/ d).	**Capsule:** 150, 300 mg **Injection:** (powder) 600 mg	Antituberculous Agents (SG) Agents of First Choice (SSG) **Cost:** Low
Rimactane	See RIFAMPIN	Antituberculous	
RIMANTADINE Flumadine	**Influenza A Prophylaxis or Treatment:** PO: 100 mg bid.	**Tablet:** 100 mg **Syrup:** 50 mg/5 ml	ANTIVIRAL AGENT (SG) AND Sympathomimetic Stimulant (SG)
Riopan	See MAGALDRATE		Antacid
Risperdal	See RISPERIDONE		Atypical Antipsychotic
RISPERIDONE Risperdal	**Antipsychotic:** PO: Initial dose 1 mg bid, with increments of 1 mg bid on second and third day to target dose of 3 mg bid. dose range 4–16 mg/day.	**Tablet:** 1, 2, 3, 4 mg **Oral solution:** 1 mg/ml	ANTIPSYCHOTICS (G) Atypical Antipsychotics (SG) **Cost:** High
Ritalin	See METHYLPHENIDATE		Sympathomimetic Stimulant
RITODRINE Generic,Yutopar	**Inhibit Uterine Contractions:** PO: 10 mg q 2h for 24 hours, then 10–20 mg q 4–6 h (max dose 120 mg/d). IV: 0.1 mg/min initially; maintenance usually 0.15–0.35 mg/min.	**Tablet:** 10 mg **Injection:** 10 mg/ml, 15 mg/ ml	CNS AGENTS (G) Sympathomimetics (SG) Beta 2 Selective (SSG) **Cost:** Low
RITONAVIR	**HIV Infection:** 600 mg bid with reverse transcriptase Inhibitor.		ANTI-INFECTIOUS AGENTS (G) Antiviral Agents (SG) Protease Inhibitor (SSG)
Robaxin	See METHOCARBAMOL		Muscle Relaxants
Robinul	See GLYCOPYRROLATE		Anticholinergic
Robitussin	See PART III		
Rocaltrol	See CALCITRIOL		D Vitamin
Rocephin	See CEFTRIAXONE		Lactam Antibiotic
ROCURONIUM Zemuron	**Rapid sequence intubation:** IV: 0.6–1.2 mg/kg **Tracheal intubation:** IV: initial dose 0.6 mg/kg, maintenance doses 0.1, 0.15 and 0.2 mg/kg administered at 25% recovery of control (see package insert for further dosing details).	**Injection:** 10 mg/ml	GENERAL ANESTHETICS (G) Neuromuscular Blocking Agents (SG) Non-Depolarizing Agents (SSG) **Cost:** High
Rogaine	See MINOXIDIL		Alpha Adrenergic Blocker
Romazicon	See FLUMAZENIL		Antagonize sedation of benzodiazepines

GENERIC NAME Trade Name	INDICATIONS AND DOSAGES	DOSE FORMS	GROUP (G)/SUBGROUP (SG) Relative Cost within Group
Roquine	See CHLOROQUINE		Antimalarial Antirheumatic
Rowasa	See MESALAMINE		Prodrug for 5-Aminosalicylic Acid
Roxicodone	See OXYCODONE		Narcotic Analgesic
RU486	See MIFEPRISTONE		Progestin Antagonist
Rubesol 1000	See CYANOCOBALAMIN		Vitamin (B_{12})
Rythmol	See PROPAFENONE		Antiarrhythmic Agent
S-P-T Porcine	See THYROID DESICCATED (USP)		Thyroid Hormone
Salacid	See SALICYLIC ACID		Non-Narcotic Analgesic
Salbutamol	See ALBUTEROL		Beta Adrenergic Agonist
Salflex	See SALSALATE		Non-Narcotic Analgesic
Salicyl-salicylate	See SALSALATE	Non-Narcotic Analgesic	
SALICYLIC ACID Generic, Salacid, Panscol	Topical: Apply once in evening to affected area and place under occlusion; remove the next morning (hydrate skin prior to application for 5 minutes).	**Ointment:** 3%, 25%, 60% **Cream:** 10%, 60% **Lotion:** 3% **Solution:** 13.6%, 17%, 26% **Liquid:** 12.6%, 16.7%, 17%, 20% **Gel:** 6%, 12%, 17%, 20% **Kit:** 17%	DERMATOLOGIC AGENTS (G) Keratolytic (SG) **Cost:** High
SALMETEROL Serevent	**Asthma/Bronchospasm:** Inhalation (adults and children >12 yrs): 2 puffs (42 mcg) bid (give approx. 12 hours apart). **Prevention of Exercise-Induced Bronchospasm:** Inhalation: 2 puffs at least 30–60 minutes before exercise.	**Aerosol:** 25 mcg salmeterol base from actuator per puff.	RESPIRATORY AGENTS (G) Sympathomimetics (Beta-Agonists) (SG) For Deep Inhalation (SSG)
Salmon-Calcitonin	See CALCITONIN		Inhibit Osteoclastic Activity
SALSALATE Generic, Disalcid, Salflex, Salicyl-salicylate	**Pain:** PO: 1000 tid or 1500 bid (max dose 3000 mg/d in 2–4 doses).	**Capsule:** 500 mg **Tablet:** 500, 750 mg	ANTI-INFLAMMATORY ETC AGENTS (G) Non-Narcotic Analgesics (SG) Other Salicylates (SSG) **Cost:** Low
Saluron	See HYDROFLUMETHIAZIDE		Sodium Diuretic
Sandimmune	See CYCLOSPORINE		Immunosuppressant
Sandostatin	See OCTREOTIDE		Inhibits Release Of Many Internal Secretions
Sandril	See RESERPINE		Hypotensive
Sanorex	See MAZINDOL		Diet Pill
Sansert	See METHYSERGIDE		Vasoconstrictor

GENERIC NAME Trade Name	INDICATIONS AND DOSAGES	DOSE FORMS	GROUP (G)/SUBGROUP (SG) Relative Cost within Group
SAQUINAVIR Invirase	**HIV Infection:** 600 mg tid together with a reverse transcriptase inhibitor	**Capsule:** 200 mg.	ANTI-INFECTIOUS AGENTS (G) Antiviral Agents (G) HIV Protease Inhibitor (SG) **Cost:** Very Great
SARGRAMOSTIM GLYCOSYLATED GM-CSF, Leukine, Prokine	**Myeloid Reconstitution (post bone marrow transplantation):** IV: 250 mcg/square meter/day for 21 days, give as 2 h infusion starting 2–4 h after bone marrow infusion.	**Powder for reconstitution/ injection:** 250, 500 mcg	ANTI-INFLAMMATORY ETC AGENTS (G) Hemopoietic Colony—Stimulating Factors (SG) **Cost:** Very Great
Scabene	See LINDANE		Ectoparasiticide
SCOPOLAMINE Generic, Hyoscine	**Preanesthetic:** IM, SC, IV: 0.32–0.65 mg one dose **Refraction:** In Conjunctival Sac (Adults): Instill 1–2 drops 1 hour before refraction. **Uveitis:** In Conjunctival Sac (Adults): Instill 1–2 drops up to q6h. **Motion sickness, Prevention:** PO: 0.6–1 mg at onset of motion.	**Ophthalmic Solution:** 0.25% **Transdermal patch:** Not currently available. **Injection:** 0.3, 0.4, 0.86, 1.0 mg/ml **Tablets:**	ANS AGENTS (G) Parasympatholytics (SG) Tertiary Amines (SSG) **Cost:** Low
SECOBARBITAL Generic, Seconal	**Hypnotic:** PO: 100 mg hs IM: 100–200 mg hs IV: 50–250 mg. **Pre-Procedural Sedation:** PO: 200–300 mg 1–2 hours before procedure. **Pediatric PO:** 2–6 mg/kg 1–2 hours before procedure (max. dose 100 mg). **Pediatric IM:** 3–5 mg/kg (max. dose 100 mg) **Capsule:** 100 mg	**Injection:** 50 mg/ml	CNS AGENTS (G) Sedative-Hypnotics (G) Short-Acting Hypnotics (SG) **Cost:** Low
Seconal	See SECOBARBITAL		Hypnotic
Sectral	See ACEBUTOLOL		Beta Adrenergic Blocker
Seldane	See TERFENADINE		Antihistamine
SELEGILINE Eldepryl, L-Deprenyl	**Parkinsonism:** PO: 10 mg/d in divided doses of 5 mg each taken at breakfast and lunch.	**Capsules:** 5 mg	CNS AGENTS (G) Antiparkinsonian Agents (SG) Inhibitor of MAO, Type B (SSG) **Cost:** High
SELENIUM SULFIDE Generic, OTC, Selsun	**Seborrheic dermatitis:** Shampoo: massage 5–10 ml into scalp, rinse off after 2–3 minutes in place; use 2 applications/week for 2 weeks then taper down to q2–4weeks to maintain control. **Tinea versicolor:** Topical: apply for 10 minutes daily for 1 week.	**Shampoo:** 1%, 2.5% **Lotion:** 1%, 2.5%	DERMATOLOGIC AGENTS (G) **Cost:** Low
Selsun	See SELENIUM SULFIDE		Controls Seborrhea
Sensorcaine	See BUPIVACAINE		Local Anesthetic
Septra	TRIMETHOPRIM and SULFAMETHOXAZOLE		Antibacterial

GENERIC NAME Trade Name	INDICATIONS AND DOSAGES	DOSE FORMS	GROUP (G)/SUBGROUP (SG) Relative Cost within Group
SEPTRA IV INFUSION	**Severe Urinary Tract Infections and Shigellosis:** IV: 8–10 mg/kg/d (based on trimethoprim) in 2–4 equally divided doses q 6, 8 or 12 h; give for up to 14 days for UTI and 5 days for shigellosis. **P. carinii Pneumonia:** IV: 15–20 mg/kg/d (based on trimethoprim) in 3–4 equally divided doses q 6–8 h by IV infusion for up to 14 days.		**Injection** (per 5 cc): sulfamethoxazole (400 mg), trimethoprim (80 mg)
Ser-Ap-Es	**Hypertension:** PO: 1–2 tablet tid.		**Tablet:** reserpine (0.1 mg), hydralazine HCl (25 mg), hydrochloro- thiazide (15 mg)
Serax	See OXAZEPAM		Intermediate-Acting Sedative
Serentil	See MESORIDAZINE		Antipsychotic
Serevent	See SALMETEROL		Beta Adrenergic Agonist
Seromycin	See CYCLOSERINE		Tuberculostatic
Serophene	See CLOMIPHENE		Stimulate Ovulation
Serpasil	See RESERPINE		Hypotensive
SERTRALINE Zoloft	PO: Initial 50 mg qd, maintenance 50–200 mg/d	**Tablet:** 50, 100 mg	CNS AGENTS (G) Sympathomimetic Stimulants (SG) Other Unscheduled (SSG) **Cost:** High
Serzone	See NEFAZODONE		Equivalent to TCA Antidepressants
Simron	See FERROUS GLUCONATE		Ferrous Ion
SIMVASTATIN Zocor	PO: 5–10 mg q PM initially (use lower dose if LDL <190 mg), maintenance dose 5 to 40 mg/d in single or divided doses. Adjust therapy q 4 weeks. PO (elderly): starting 5 mg/d, maximum LDL reductions may be achieved with 20 mg/d	**Tablet:** 5, 10, 20, 40 mg	METABOLIC AGENTS (G) Hypocholesterolemic agents (SG) HMG-CoA Reductase Inhibitors (SSG)
Sinemet	See LEVODOPA-CARBIDOPA MIXTURE		Dopamine Precursor
Sinequan	See DOXEPIN		Tricyclic Antidepressants
Skelaxin	See METAXALONE		Muscle Relaxant
Slo-Bid	See THEOPHYLLINE		Xanthine
Slow-K	See POTASSIUM CHLORIDE		Supplementary K Ion
Soda	See SODIUM BICARBONATE		Antacid
SODIUM BICARBONATE OTC, Soda, Baking Soda,	**Gastric Hyperacidity:** PO:1 level tsp in 1/3 glass water or 1 tab q 6–24 h. (Range = 0.3–2 g 1 to 4 times a day.)	**Tablet:** 350, 520, 650	GASTROINTESTINAL AGENTS (G) Antacids (SG) Acid Neutralizing (SSG) **Cost:** Low
SODIUM NITRITE Generic	**Cyanide intoxication:** 300 mg (10 ml of 3% soln) over 2–4 min.	Available in cyanide emergency packs	ANTIDOTES AND USED IN POISONINGS (G)

GENERIC NAME Trade Name	INDICATIONS AND DOSAGES	DOSE FORMS	GROUP (G)/SUBGROUP (SG) Relative Cost within Group
SODIUM PHOSPHATE Generic, OTC, Fleet Phospho-Soda	PO: 20–30 ml (mix with glass water). Pediatric PO: 5–15 ml.	**Solution:** (18 g sodium phosphate; 48 g sodium biphosphate per 100 ml; 96.4 mg sodium/20 ml)	GASTROINTESTINAL AGENTS (G) Laxatives And Bowel Cleansers (SG) Bulk and Saline Laxatives (SSG) **Cost:** High
SODIUM SALICYLATE Generic	**Analgesia:** PO: 325 to 650 mg q4h	**Tablet:** (Enteric) 325, 650 mg	ANTI-INFLAMMATORY ETC (G) Non-Narcotic Analgesics (SG) Aspirin and Related NSAIDs (SSG) **Cost:** Low
SODIUM THIOSULFATE Generic	**Cyanide Intoxication:** 12.5 g IV over 10 min period after induction of methemoglobinemia.	1 or 2.5 g in 10 ml	ANTIDOTES AND USED IN POISONINGS (SG)
Sofarin	See WARFARIN SODIUM		Anticoagulant
Solaquin	See HYDROQUINONE		Skin Lightener
Solfoton	See PHENOBARBITAL		Sedative
Solganal	See AUROTHIOGLUCOSE		Antirheumatic Gold Compound
Solu-Cortef	See HYDROCORTISONE		Corticosteroid
Solu-Medrol	See METHYLPREDNISOLONE		Corticosteroid
Soma	See CARISOPRODOL		Muscle Relaxant
SOMATOTROPIN (GH) Humatrope, Nutropin Human GH (recombinant)	**GH Inadequacy Induced Growth Failure:** SC, IM (Humatrope): Up to 0.06 mg/kg (0.16 IU/kg) 3 times/week. SC (Nutropin): 0.3 mg/kg/week given daily in equally divided doses. **Chronic renal insufficiency (CRI):** SC (Nutropin): 0.35 mg/kg/week given daily in equally divided doses.	**Injection:** (powder) 5 mg (aprox. 13 IU) per vial, 10 mg (aprox. 26 IU) per vial	ENDOCRINE AGENTS (G) Anterior Pituitary Hormones (SG) **Cost:** High
SOMATREM Protropin	Human GH plus one Amino Acid (recombinant) **GH Inadequacy Induced Growth Failure:** SC, IM: Up to 0.1 mg/kg (0.26 IU/kg) 3 times per week.	**Injection:** (powder) 5 mg (aprox. 13 IU) per vial, 10 mg (aprox. 26 IU) per vial	ENDOCRINE AGENTS (G) Anterior Pituitary Hormones (SG) **Cost:** High
Soprodol	See CARISOPRODOL		Muscle Relaxant
Sorate	See ISOSORBIDE DINITRATE		Vasodilator
Sorbide-TD	See ISOSORBIDE DINITRATE		Vasodilator
Sorbitrate	See ISOSORBIDE DINITRATE		Vasodilator
SOTALOL Betapace	**Ventricular Arrhythmias:** PO: 80 mg bid initially; 160–320 mg/d maintenance in 2–3 doses (max dose: 640 mg/d).	**Tablet:** 80, 160, 240 mg	ANS AGENTS (G) Sympathoplegics (SG) Non-Selective (Beta 1 and 2) Blockers (SSG) **Cost:** High
SPARFLOXACIN Zagam	**Infections:** PO: 400 mg on first day then 200 mg/d	**Tablet:** 200 mg	ANTI-INFECTIOUS AGENTS (G) Quinolone Antibacterial (SG)
Sparine	See PROMAZINE		Antipsychotic
Spectazole	See ECONAZOLE		Antifungal, Topical

GENERIC NAME Trade Name	INDICATIONS AND DOSAGES	DOSE FORMS	GROUP (G)/SUBGROUP (SG) Relative Cost within Group
SPECTINO-MYCIN Trobicin	**Gonorrhea:** IM: 2 g (5 ml) follow with oral course of doxycycline (give 4 g in geographic areas where resistant gonorrhea is prevalent). Pediatric IM (>45kg): should receive adult dosages. Pediatric IM (<45kg): 40 mg/kg IM once.	**Injection:** (powder) 400 mg spectinomycin per ml when reconstituted	ANTI-INFECTIOUS (G) Miscellaneous Antibacterials (SG) **Cost:** High
Spectrobid	See BACAMPICILLIN		Lactam Antibiotic
SPIRONOLAC-TONE Generic, Aldac-tone	**Diagnosis of Primary Hyperaldosteronism:** PO: (long test) 400 mg/d (administer 3–4 wk; test positive if hypokalemia and BP correct to normal). PO: (short test) 400 mg/d (administer for 4d; if serum K increases with tx, then decreases after tx ended, test is presumptively positive). **Edema:** PO: 50–100 mg/d, in 1 or 2 divided doses. **Hypokalemia:** PO: 25–100 mg/d. **Hypertension:** PO: 50–100 mg/d.	**Tablet:** 25, 50, 100 mg	RENAL AGENTS (G) Sodium Diuretics (G) Potassium-Sparing Diuretics (SG)
SPIRONOLAC-TONE/HCTZ COMBINATION Generic Aldactazide-25	**Diuresis:** PO: 1–4 tabs/d Single or divided doses. **Hypertension:** PO in combination with other hypotensives.	**Tablet:** Combination of spironolactone 25 mg and hydrochlorothia-zide 25 mg. Combination of 50/50 available as Aldactazide-50	RENAL AGENTS (G) Aldosterone Antagonist(SSG) (K Retaining Diuretic) **Cost:** Medium
Sporanox	See ITRACONAZOLE		Antifungal, Topical
Sprinkle	See THEOPHYLLINE		Xanthine Bronchodilator
SSKI	See POTASSIUM IODIDE		Expectorant
Stadol	See BUTORPHANOL		Narcotic Agonist-Antagonist
STANOZOLOL Winstrol	**Hereditary Angioedema:** PO: 2 mg tid, initially, then taper over 1–3 months to 2 mg/d or 2 mg qod. Off label use as for other anabolics.	**Tablet:** 2 mg	ENDOCRINE AGENTS (G) Androgenic/Anabolic Steroids (SG) **Cost:** High
STAVUDINE Zerit, d4T	**HIV Infection:** PO (>59 kg): 40 mg q12h. PO (<60 kg): 30 mg q12h.	**Capsule:** 15, 20, 30, 40 mg	ANTI-INFECTIOUS AGENTS (G) Antiviral Agents (SG) Reverse Transcriptase Inhibitor (SSG)
Stelazine	See TRIFLUOPERAZINE		Antipsychotic
Sterapred	See PREDNISOLONE		Corticosteroid
Stoxil	See IDOXURIDINE		Antiviral
Streptase	See STREPTOKINASE		Thrombolytic

GENERIC NAME Trade Name	INDICATIONS AND DOSAGES	DOSE FORMS	GROUP (G)/SUBGROUP (SG) Relative Cost within Group
STREPTOKINASE Kabikinase, Streptase	**Acute Myocardial Infarction:** IV: 1.5 million units over 60 min. **Deep Vein Thrombosis, Pulmonary Emboli:** IV: 250,000 units over 30 minutes; then 100,000 units/h for 24–72 hours (72 h for DVT, 72–24 h for art. thrombus or embolism, and 24 h for pulmonary embolism. Follow with heparin IV infusion.	**Injection:** (powder) 250,000, 600,000, 750,000, 1,500,000 IU/vial	METABOLIC AGENTS (G) Anticoagulants And Coagulants (SG) Thrombolytic Agents (SG) **Cost:** Low compared with other 'lytics
STREPTOMYCIN Generic, Streptomycin Sulfate	**Infections (when less toxic alternates not available):** IM: 0.5–2 g/d in 2–4 doses (max. dose 2 g/d; desirable peak serum levels 15–25 mcg/ml). Pediatric IM: 20–40 mg/kg/d in 2–4 doses (avoid excessive doses in children). **Tuberculosis (adjunct therapy for resistant TB):** IM: 15 mg/kg/d (max. single dose 1.0 g); or 25–30 mg/kg twice per week (max. single dose 1.5 g); or 25–30 mg/kg three times per week (max. single dose 1.5 g); (max. single dose over total therapy should be less than 120 g). **Tularemia:** IM: 1–2 g/d in 2–4 doses for 7–14 days or until patient afebrile for 5–7 days. **Plague:** IM: 2 g/d in 2 divided doses (treatment for 10 days minimum recommended). **Bacterial Endocarditis (penicillin-sensitive alpha and non-hemolytic streptococci):** IM: 1 g bid for 1 week, then 0.5 g bid for 2nd week (given as adjunct to penicillin). Geriatric (>60 yrs) IM: 0.5 g q12h for 2 weeks (given as adjunct to penicillin).	**Injection:** 400 mg/ml	ANTI-INFECTIOUS AGENTS (G) Aminoglycoside Antibiotics (SG) **Cost:** Low
STREPTOZOCIN Zanosar	CANCER CHEMOTHERAPY (G) Alkylating Agents (SG) Nitrosoureas (SSG)		
Sub-Quin	See PROCAINAMIDE		Antiarrhythmic
Sublimaze	See FENTANYL		Narcotic Analgetic
SUCCINYLCHOLINE Generic, Anectine, Quelicin, Sucostrin, Suxinyl	**Intubation, Electroconvulsant Therapy:** IV: 0.3–1.1 mg/kg (over 10–30 sec); effect should be seen within 1 min. **Prolonged Muscular Relaxation:** IV: 0.3–1.1 mg/kg (over 10–30 sec) to start, then 0.04–0.07 mg/kg PRN.	**Injection:** 20, 50, 100 mg/ml **Injection:** (powder) 100 mg **Infusion:** (powder) 500 mg, 1 g	GENERAL ANESTHETICS AND ADJUNCTS (G) Neuromuscular Blocking Agents (SG) Depolarizing Agent (SSG)
Sucostrin	See SUCCINYLCHOLINE		Curariform
SUCRALFATE Carafate	**Duodenal Ulcer:** PO: 1 g QID 1 hour before meals and hs; continue 4–8 weeks. **Maintenance Therapy:** PO: 1 g bid.	**Tablet:** 1 g **Suspension:** 1 g per 10 ml	GASTROINTESTINAL AGENTS (G) Antacids (SG) Surface and Mixed Activity (SG) **Cost:** Medium

GENERIC NAME Trade Name	INDICATIONS AND DOSAGES	DOSE FORMS	GROUP (G)/SUBGROUP (SG) Relative Cost within Group
Sucrets	See DYCLONINE		Local Anesthetic
Sudafed	See PSEUDOEPHEDRINE		Sympathomimetic
Sufenta	See SUFENTANIL		Narcotic Analgesic
SUFENTANIL Sufenta	**Analgesic, Adjunct to Anesthesia:** IV: 1–2 mcg/kg initial dose. Maintenance 10–25 mcg given as needed to maintain analgesia.	**Injection:** 50 mcg/ml	Narcotic Analgesics (SG) Of Intermediate Potency (SSG) **Cost:** High
Sulamyd	See SULFACETAMIDE		Antibacterial
Sular	See NISOLDIPINE		Calcium Channel Blocker
SULCONAZOLE Exelderm	**Tinea pedis, corporis, cruris, versicolor:** Topical: Apply to affected areas qd-bid for 3 weeks.	**Cream:** 1% **Lotion:** 1%	DERMATOLOGIC AGENTS (G) Topical Fungicides (SG) **Cost:** Medium
SULFACETA-MIDE Generic, Sulamyd	**Ointment:** Apply 1.25–2.5 cm q6h. **Solution:** Instill 1–2 drops q1–3h.	**Ointment:** 10%. **Solution:** 10, 15, 30%	OPHTHALMIC AGENTS (G) Antibacterial (SG) **Cost:** Low
SULFACYTINE Renoquid	**Urinary tract infections:** PO: 500 mg initial dose then 250 QID (give for 10 days).	**Tablet:** 250 mg	ANTI-INFECTIOUS AGENTS (G) Sulfonamides (SG)
SULFADIAZINE Generic	**Sulfadiazine Responsive Infections:** PO: 2–4 g loading dose then 4–8 g/d given in 4–6 divided doses. **Prevention Of Recurrent Rheumatic Fever:** PO (weight >30 kg): 1 g/d Pediatric PO (weight <30 kg): 0.5 g/d (do not use to treat initial episode of streptococcal infections).	**Tablet:** 500 mg	ANTI-INFECTIOUS AGENTS (G) Sulfonamides (SG) **Cost:** Low
SULFADOXINE and **PYRIMETH-AMINE** Fansidar	**Acute Malaria Attack (may be given alone or as adjunct given with quinine):** PO: 2–3 tablets as a single dose. Pediatric PO (9–14 yrs): 2 tablets single dose. Pediatric PO (4–8 yrs): 1 tablet single dose. **Malaria Prophylaxis (take 1–2 days prior to departure and continue for 4–6 weeks after return from malarious area):** PO: 1 tablet/week; or 2 tablets q second week. Pediatric PO (9–14 yrs): 3/4 tablet/week; or 1 and tablets q second week. Pediatric PO (4–8 yrs): tablet/week; or 1 tablets q o week.	**Tablet:** 500 mg sulfadoxine and 25 mg pyrimethamine	ANTIPARASITIC AGENTS (G) **Cost:** Medium
SULFAMETHOX-AZOLE Generic, Gantanol, Urobak	**Infections:** PO: 2 g to start, then 1 g bid (max. dose 1 g tid). Pediatric PO: 50–60 mg/kg to start, then 25–30 mg/kg bid (max. dose 75 mg/kg/d).	**Tablet:** 500 mg **Oral Suspension:** 500 mg/5 ml	ANTI-INFECTIOUS AGENTS (G) Sulfonamides (SG) **Cost:** Low

GENERIC NAME Trade Name	INDICATIONS AND DOSAGES	DOSE FORMS	GROUP (G)/SUBGROUP (SG) Relative Cost within Group
SULFASALAZINE Azulfidine	**Ulcerative Colitis:** PO (initial regimen): 3–4 g/d in evenly divided doses, (above 4 g/d toxicity increases). PO (maintenance): 500 mg QID.	**Tablet:** 500 mg **Enteric Tablet:** 500 mg **Oral Suspension:** 250 mg/5 ml	ANTI-INFLAMMATORY AGENTS (G) Prodrug for 5-ASA (SG) **Cost:** Low
SULFINPYRA-ZONE Anturane	PO: 200–400 mg/d in 2 divided doses (max. dose 800 mg/d).	**Tablet:** 100 mg **Capsule:** 200 mg	METABOLIC AGENTS (G) Anticoagulants And Coagulants (SG) Antiplatelet Agents (SSG) **Cost:** High
SULFISOXAZOLE Generic, Gantrisin	**Ophthalmic Infections:** Topical: **Ointment:** Apply small amount 1–3 times/d & hs. Solution: Instill 2–3 drops up to 3 times/d (more can be used). **Urinary Tract Infections:** PO: Adult 1 g QID. Pediatric: Over two months of age, 120 mg/kg/d in 4–6 doses. **Solution:** 4%	**Ointment:** 4%	ANTI-INFECTIOUS AGENTS (G) Sulfonamides (SG) **Cost:** Low
SULINDAC Generic, Clinoril	**Pain:** PO: 150–200 mg bid (max. dose 400 mg/d). **Acute Gout:** PO: 200 mg bid for 7 days (may go 14 days).	**Tablet:** 150, 200 mg	ANTI-INFLAMMATORY ETC AGENTS Non-Narcotic Analgesics (SG) Aspirin and Related NSAIDs (SSG) **Cost:** Medium
SUMATRIPTAN Imitrex	**Migraine Headaches:** SC: Up to 6 mg; if effective, may repeat dose after 1 hour (max dose in 24 hours: two 6 mg injections separated by at least one hour). PO: 25–100 mg initial dose at headache onset; repeat q 2h PRN up to a maximum of 300 mg/d.	**Tablet:** 25, 50 mg **Injection:** 12 mg/ml	CV AGENTS (G) Vasoconstrictors And Oxytocics (G) Cost: Very High
Sumycin	See TETRACYCLINE		Antibiotic
Suprax	See CEFIXIME		Lactam Antibiotic
SUPROFEN Profenal	**Solution:** 2 drops q4h while awake (on the day prior to surgery), then 2 drops at 3, 2, and 1 hour pre-operatively.	**Solution:** 1%	OPHTHALMIC AGENTS (G) Anti-Inflammatory, Non-Steroidal (SG)
Surelac	See LACTASE		Enzyme
Surmontil	See TRIMIPRAMINE		Tricyclic Antidepressant
Survanta	See BERACTANT		Lung Surfactant
Susprin	See IBUPROFEN		Non-Narcotic Analgetic
Sustaire	See THEOPHYLLINE		Xanthine Bronchodilator
Suxinyl	See SUCCINYLCHOLINE		Curariform
Symmetrel	See AMANTADINE		Antiviral Agent, Stimulant
Synalgos-DC	See DIHYDROCODEINE		Narcotic Analgetic
Synarel	See NAFARELIN		Antagonizes LH-RF
Synthroid	See LEVOTHYROXINE		Thyroid Replacement
Syntocinon	See OXYTOCIN		Oxytocic
Syprine	See TRIENTINE		Copper Chelator
Syraprim	See TRIMETHOPRIM		Antibacterial

GENERIC NAME Trade Name	INDICATIONS AND DOSAGES	DOSE FORMS	GROUP (G)/SUBGROUP (SG) Relative Cost within Group
SYRUP OF IPECAC OTC, Generic	**Induce Vomiting:** PO: 15–30 ml. Repeat in 20 minutes if no emesis, or move to lavage. PO: Children (1–12 yrs): 5–10 ml of syrup.	1.5% available OTC to keep in home. 2% kept Rx only at manufacturer's option.	ANTIDOTES AND USED IN POISONINGS (G)
Tace	See CHLOROTRIANISENE		Estrogen
TACRINE Lognex	**Alzheimer's Disease:** PO: Initial 40 mg/d (10 mg QID). May increase to 20 mg QID after six weeks of treatment at 40 mg/d if no significant increase in LFT's. After this, at 6 week intervals may increase to 120 mg/d then 160 mg/d (max. dose 160 mg/d).	**Capsule:** 10, 20, 30, 40 mg	CNS AGENTS (G) Cholinergic Agents (SG) Cholinesterase Inhibitor, Central (SSG) **Cost:** Very High
TACROLIMUS Prograf, FK 506	**Inhibit Graft Rejection:** PO: 0.05–0.1 mg/kg/d given as continuous IV infusion (wait at least 6h after transplant to start infusion) then convert to oral doses as soon as possible. IV: 0.15–0.3 mg/kg/d given in 2 divided doses q12h (give first dose 8–12 h after discontinue IV; wait at least 6h after transplant to give first dose).	**Capsules:** 1,5 mg **Injection:** 5 mg/ml	ANTI-INFLAMMATORY ETC AGENTS (G) Immunomodulators (SG)
Tagamet	See CIMETIDINE		H2 Antagonist
Talacen	PO: 1 tablet q 4 h, PRN pain.		**Tablet:** pentazocine (equal to 25 mg pentazocine base), acetaminophen (650 mg)
Talwin Compound	**Pain:** PO: 1–2 caplets tid or QID, PRN		**Caplet:** pentazocine 12.5 mg, aspirin (325 mg)
Talwin NX	**Pain:** PO: 1 tablet q3–4h.		**Tablet:** pentazocine 50 mg, naloxone 0.5 mg
Talwin	See PENTAZOCINE		Mixed Agonist-Antagonist
TAMOXIFEN Nolvadex, Tamoxifen	**Breast Cancer:** PO: 10–20 mg bid (morning and evening).	**Tablet:** 10 mg	ENDOCRINE AGENTS (G) Antiestrogen (SG) **Cost:** Low
Tao	See TRIACETYLOLEANDOMYCIN		Macrolide Antibiotic
Tapazole	See METHIMAZOLE		Antithyroid
Taractan	See CHLORPROTHIXENE		Antipsychotic
Tavist	See CLEMASTINE		Antihistamine
Taxol	See PACLITAXEL		Cancer Chemotherapy
Tazidime	See CEFTAZIDIME		Lactam Antibiotic
Tazicef	See CEFTAZIDIME		Lactam Antibiotic
Teebacin	See AMINOSALICYLIC ACID		Non-Narcotic Analgetic
Teebaconin	See ISONIAZID		Tuberculostatic
Tegison	See ETRETINATE		Osteoclast Inhibitor
Tegopen	See CLOXACILLIN		Lactamase Resistant Penicillin
Tegretol	See CARBAMAZEPINE		Anticonvulsant
Temaril	See TRIMEPRAZINE		Antipsychotic, Antipruritic

GENERIC NAME Trade Name	INDICATIONS AND DOSAGES	DOSE FORMS	GROUP (G)/SUBGROUP (SG) Relative Cost within Group
TEMAZEPAM Generic, Restoril	**Hypnotic:** PO: 15–30 mg at hs.	**Capsule:** 7.5, 15, 30 mg	CNS AGENTS (G) Sedative-Hypnotics (SG) Ultrashort-Acting Hypnotic (SSG) **Cost:** Low
Temovate	See CLOBETASOL		Anti-Inflammatory Steroids, Topical
Tenex	See GUANFACINE		Centrally-Acting Adrenergic Inhibitors
TENIPOSIDE VM 26,Vumon	CANCER CHEMOTHERAPY (G) Mitotic Spindle Inhibitors (SG) Other Mitotic Spindle Inhibitors (SSG)		
TENORETIC 50,100	**Hypertension:** Adjust dose within the limits imposed by fixed combination.	**Tablet:** Atenolol 50 or 100 mg, chlorthalidone 25 mg	BETA ADRENERGIC BLOCKER AND DIURETIC COMBINATION (G)
Tenormin	See ATENOLOL		Cardioselective Beta 1 Blocker
Tensilon	See EDROPHONIUM		Cholinesterase Inhibitor
Tenuate	See DIETHYLPROPION		Anorexic
Terazol	See TERCONAZOLE		Topical Fungicide
TERAZOSIN Hydrin	**Hypertension:** PO: Initial dose 1 mg hs, maintenance dose range 1–5 mg/d (max. dose 20 mg/d); higher doses may benefit from twice daily dosing to minimize side effects. **Benign Prostatic Hyperplasia:** PO: Initial dose 1 mg hs, maintenance dose range 1–10 mg/d (max. dose 20 mg/d).	**Tablet:** 1, 2, 5, 10 mg	ANS AGENTS (G) Sympathoplegics (G) Alpha Adrenergic Receptor Blockers (SG) **Cost:** Medium
TERBINAFINE Lamisil	**Interdigital tinea pedis, Tinea cruris:** Topical: Apply bid to affected area, treat for 7–28 days. **Onychomycosis:** PO: 250 mg q d for 6 weeks (finger) or 12 weeks (toes) and evaluate after new growth.	**Cream:** 1% **Tablets: 250 mg**	DERMATOLOGIC AGENTS (G) Topical Anti-Infectious Agents (SG) Topical, Systemic Fungicides (SSG) **Cost:** Low
TERBUTALINE Brethine, Bricanyl	**Asthma, Bronchospasm:** PO: 2.5–5 mg tid (max. dose 15 mg/d in adults). Pediatric (12–15 yrs) PO: 2.5 mg tid (max. dose 7.5 mg/d). SC: 0.25 mg, repeat in 15–30 min once only (max. dose 0.5 mg/4 h).	**Tablet:** 2.5, 5 mg **Injection:** 1 mg/ml	ANS AGENTS (G) Sympathomimetics (SG) Beta 2 Selective (SSG) **Cost:** Low
TERCONAZOLE Terazol	**Vaginosis:** Suppository: Administer one suppository qd hs for 3 consecutive days. Cream: 0.4%: administer one applicatorful qd for 7 consecutive days. Cream 0.8%: administer one applicatorful qd for 3 consecutive days.	**Vaginal Cream:** 0.4%, 0.8% **Vaginal Suppositories:** 80 mg	ANTI-INFECTIOUS AGENTS (G) Topical Fungicides (SG) **Cost:** Medium

GENERIC NAME Trade Name	INDICATIONS AND DOSAGES	DOSE FORMS	GROUP (G)/SUBGROUP (SG) Relative Cost within Group
TERFENADINE Seldane	**Allergic (Type I) Reactions:** PO: 60 mg q12h. Pediatric (6–12 yrs) PO: 30–60 mg bid. Pediatric (3–6 yrs) PO: 15 mg bid.	**Tablet:** 60 mg	ANTI-INFLAMMATORY ETC AGENTS (G) Antihistamines (H1) Mild Sedation (SG) **Cost:** Very High
Terramycin	See OXYTETRACYCLINE		Antibiotic
Teslac	See TESTOLACTONE		Antiestrogen
Tessalon	See BENZONATATE		Antitussive
Testandro	See TESTOSTERONESUSPENSION		Androgen
TESTOLACTONE Teslac	**Breast Cancer Palliation** (postmenopausal women)**:** PO: 250 mg QID for 7 months.	**Tablet:** 50 mg	ENDOCRINE AGENTS (G) Antiestrogen (SG)
TESTOSTERONE TRANSDERMAL Androderm	**Androgen Replacement Therapy:** Two patches applied to skin at bedtime.	**Patch:** 2.5 mg	ENDOCRINE AGENTS (G) Androgenic/Anabolic Steroids (SG) **Cost:** High
TESTOSTERONE CYPIONATE Generic, Depo-Testosterone, Duratest-100	**Androgen Replacement Therapy:** IM: 50–400 mg q 2–4 weeks.	**Injection:** 100, 200 mg/ml	ENDOCRINE AGENTS (G) Androgenic/Anabolic Steroids (SG) **Cost:** Low
TESTOSTERONE ENANTHATE Generic, Delatestryl, Durathate, Everone 200, Andro L.A. 200	**Androgen Replacement Therapy:** IM: 50–400 mg q 2–4 weeks.	**Injection:** 100, 200 mg/ml	ENDOCRINE AGENTS (G) Androgenic/Anabolic Steroids (SG) **Cost:** Low
TESTOSTERONE PROPIONATE Generic	**Androgen Replacement Therapy:** IM. 25–50 mg qd.	**Injection:** 100 mg/ml	ENDOCRINE AGENTS (G) Androgenic/Anabolic Steroids (SG) **Cost:** Low
TESTOSTERONE SUSPENSION Generic, Testandro	**Androgen Replacement Therapy:** IM: 25–50 mg 2–3 times weekly.	**Injection:** 25, 50, 100 mg/ml	ENDOCRINE AGENTS (G) Androgenic/Anabolic Steroids (SG) **Cost:** Low
Testred	See METHYLTESTOSTERONE		Androgen
TETRACAINE Generic, Pontocaine	**Solution:** 1 or 2 drops (duration 15–20 min). Not for prolonged use.	**Ointment:** 0.5% **Solution:** 0.5%	OPHTHALMIC PREPARATIONS (G) Local Anesthetics (G) **Cost:** Low

GENERIC NAME Trade Name	INDICATIONS AND DOSAGES	DOSE FORMS	GROUP (G)/SUBGROUP (SG) Relative Cost within Group
TETRACYCLINE Generic, Achromycin, Panmycin, Sumycin, others	**Infections:** PO: from 250 mg q6h to 500 mg q6–12h depending on severity. IM 250 mg q24h or 300 mg/d in 1–2 divided doses. IV 250–500 mg q12h. Pediatric: >8 yrs. PO: 25–50 mg/kg/d in 4 divided doses. **Brucellosis:** PO: 500 mg q6h for 3 weeks, add 1 g IM streptomycin bid for 1st week. **Syphilis (Penicillin allergic patients-primary, secondary or latency <1 year):** PO 500 mg q6h for 15d. **Uncomplicated Gonorrhea:** PO: 500 mg q6h for 7d following parenteral treatment with lactam antibiotics. **Adjunct for Pelvic Inflammatory Disease:** PO: 500 mg q6h for 10–14d following parenteral treatment with lactam antibiotics. **Non-Gonococcal Urethritis, Chlamydia, Prophylaxis after Rape or Other Unprotected Contact:** PO: 500 mg q6h for 7d **Acne:** PO: 250 mg 1–4 times/d depending upon severity and response. **Lymphogranuloma Venereum:** PO: 500 mg q6h for 14d. Apply 1 to 4 times daily to infected area. Cover with sterile bandage as appropriate.	**Capsule:** 100, 250, 500 mg **Tablet:** 250, 500 mg **IM Powder:** 100, 250 mg **IV Powder:** 250, 500 mg **Oral Suspension:** 125 mg/5 ml **Ointment:** 3%, 1% **Suspension:** 1%	ANTI-INFECTIOUS CHEMOTHERAPY (G) Tetracycline Antibiotics (SG) **Cost:** Low OPHTHALMIC PREPARATIONS (G) Antibacterial (SG) **Cost:** High
Tetrahydro-cannabinol	See DRONABINOL		Sedative
TETRAHYDRO-ZOLINE Tyzine	Adults and children (>6 yrs): 2–4 qtt of 0.1 % solution in each nostril q 3–4h PRN; or 3–4 sprays in each nostril q4h PRN. Pediatric Nasal Solution (2–6 y.o.): 2–3 qtt of 0.05% solution in each nostril q 4–6h PRN.	**Solution:** 0.1, 0.05%	ANS AGENTS (G) Sympathomimetics (SG) Sympathomimetics, Incomplete (SSG) **Cost:** Medium
Thalitone	See CHLORTHALIDONE		Sodium Diuretic
THC	See DRONABINOL		Sedative
Theo-Dur	See THEOPHYLLINE		Bronchodilator

GENERIC NAME Trade Name	INDICATIONS AND DOSAGES	DOSE FORMS	GROUP (G)/SUBGROUP (SG) Relative Cost within Group
THEOPHYLLINE Generic, Theo-Dur, Slo-Bid, Bronkodyl, Aquaphyllin, Slo-Phyllin, Sprinkle, Elixophyllin, Respbid, Sustaire, Accurbron	**Bronchospasm (rapid effect):** PO: 5 mg/kg initial dose, then maintenance as follows: 3 mg/kg q8h (non smokers); 2 mg/kg q8h (>60 yrs., cor pulmonale); 1–2 mg/kg q12h (CHF) (max. dose [use in conjunction with serum theophylline levels] 13 mg/kg/d). Pediatric PO (1–9 yrs): 5 mg/kg loading dose, then 4 mg/kg 6h maintenance (max. dose [use in conjunction with serum theophylline levels] 24 mg/kg/d). Pediatric PO (9–12 yrs): 5 mg/kg loading dose, then 3 mg/kg 6h maintenance (max. dose [use in conjunction with serum theophylline levels] 20 mg/kg/d). Pediatric PO (12–16 yrs): 5 mg/kg loading dose, then 3 mg/kg 6h maintenance (max. dose [use in conjunction with serum theophylline levels] 18 mg/kg/d) **Bronchospasm (chronic maintenance therapy):** PO: initial dose 400 mg/d OR 16 mg/kg/d [whichever is less] given in divided doses q 6 to 8 h to start; then increase dose q 3 days by 25% as tolerated and as needed (max maintenance dose 900 mg/d OR 13 mg/kg/d [whichever is less]); therapeutic serum theophylline concentration = 10–20 mcg/ml. PO (Ext'd release): 200 mg q12h to start, after 3 days increase to 300 mg q12h (max dose [use only in conjunction with serum theophylline levels] 13 mg/kg/d OR 400–450 mg q 12 h [whichever is less]); therapeutic serum theophylline concentration = 10–20 mcg/ml. PO (24h Release: Theo-24): 200 mg q12h to start, after each 3 days may increase daily dose by 100 mg PRN (max dose [use in conjunction with serum theophylline levels] 13 mg/kg/d OR 900 mg/d [whichever is less]); therapeutic serum theophylline concentration = 10–20 mcg/ml.	**Tablet:** 100, 125, 200, 250, 300 mg **Tablet:** (Ext'd release) 100, 200, 250, 300, 400, 450, 500 mg **Capsule:** 100, 200 mg **Capsule:** (Ext'd release) 50, 60, 65, 75, 100, 125, 130, 200, 250, 260, 300 mg **Syrup:** 80 mg/15 ml, 150 mg/15 ml **Elixir:** 80 mg/15 ml **Solution:** 80 mg/15 ml **Oral Solution:** 150 mg/15 ml	CV AGENTS (G) Xanthines (SG) **Cost:** Low
TheraCys	See BCG		Immunomodulator

GENERIC NAME Trade Name	INDICATIONS AND DOSAGES	DOSE FORMS	GROUP (G)/SUBGROUP (SG) Relative Cost within Group
THIABENDAZOLE Mintezol	**Intestinal Strongyloides stercoralis, Cutaneous Larva Migrans, Necator americanus (hookworm):** PO (>70 kg): 1.5 g bid for 2 days (repeat once if cutaneous larva migrans lesions still present after 2 days of therapy). PO (13.6–70 kg): 22 mg/kg bid for 2 days (repeat once if cutaneous larva migrans lesions still present after 2 days of therapy). **Trichinosis:** PO (>70 kg): 1.5 g bid for 2–4 days. PO (13.6–70 kg): 22 mg/kg bid for 2–4 days. **Visceral Larva Migrans:** PO (>70 kg): 1.5 g bid for 7 days. PO (13.6–70 kg): 22 mg/kg bid for 7 days.	**Tablet:** (chewable) 500 mg **Oral Suspension:** 500 mg/5 ml	ANTI-INFECTIOUS AGENTS (G) Antiparasitic Agents (SG) **Cost:** High
THIETHYLPERA-ZINE Torecan, Nor-zine	**Nausea, Vomiting:** PO, rectal: 10–30 mg/d in divided doses. IV: 2 ml (10 mg) 1–3 times/day.	**Tablet:** 10 mg **Suppository:** 10 mg **IM Injection:** 5 mg/ml	GASTROINTESTINAL AGENTS (G) Antiemetics (Minor) (SG) **Cost:** High
THIOGUANINE 6-TG	CANCER CHEMOTHERAPY (G) Antimetabolites (SG) Purine Analogues (SSG)		
THIORIDAZINE Generic, Mellaril	**Psychotic Disorders:** PO, IM: 150–300 mg/d to start in 2–4 doses (max. dose 800 mg/d). Pediatric PO (2–12 yrs): 0.5–3 mg/kg/d.	**Tablet:** 10, 15, 25, 50, 100, 150, 200 mg **Concentrate:** 30, 100 mg/ml **Suspension:** 5, 20 mg/ml	CNS AGENTS (G) Antipsychotics (SG) Moderate Extrapyramidal Effects (SSG) **Cost:** Medium
THIOTEPA	CANCER CHEMOTHERAPY (G) Alkylating Agents (SG) Nitrogen Mustards (SSG)		
THIOTHIXENE Generic, Navane	**Psychotic Disorders:** PO: 2 mg tid to start; maintenance 15–30 mg/d (max. dose 60 mg/d). IV: 4 mg bid-QID to start; maintenance 15–30 mg/d.	**Capsule:** 1, 2, 5, 10, 20 mg **Injection:** (IM) 2 mg/ml **Solution:** 5 mg/ml **Concentrate:** 5 mg/ml	CNS AGENTS (G) Antipsychotics (SG) Prominent Extrapyramidal Effects (SSG) **Cost:** Low
Thiuretic	See HYDROCHLOROTHIAZIDE		Sodium Diuretic
Thorazine	See CHLORPROMAZINE		Antipsychotic
Thypinone	See PROTIRELIN		Thyroid Stimulant
ThyrarBovine	See THYROID DESICCATED (USP)		Thyroid Replacement
THYROGLOBULIN Proloid	**Hypothyroidism (without myxedema):** PO: 30 mg/d to start, increase by 30 mg q2–3 weeks PRN. Maintenance 60–180 mg/d. **Hypothyroidism with Chronic Myxedema:** PO: 15 mg/d (decrease dosage if angina occurs).	**Tablet:** 30, 60, 90, 120, 180 mg	ENDOCRINE AGENT (G) Thyroid Replacements (SG) **Cost:** Medium

GENERIC NAME Trade Name	INDICATIONS AND DOSAGES	DOSE FORMS	GROUP (G)/SUBGROUP (SG) Relative Cost within Group
THYROID DESICCATED (USP) Generic, Armour Thyroid, Thyrar Bovine, S-P-T Porcine, Thyroid USP, Thyroid Strong	**Hypothyroidism (Without Myxedema):** PO: 15 mg/d to start, increase by 30 mg q2–3 weeks PRN. Maintenance 60–180 mg/d **Hypothyroidism With Chronic Myxedema:** PO: 15 mg/d (decrease dosage if angina occurs).	**Tablet:** 15, 30, 60, 90, 120, 180, 240, 300 mg **Capsule:** 60, 120, 180, 300 mg **Tablet:** (thyroid strong) 30, 60, 120, 180 mg (50% more potent than thyroid USP tabs)	ENDOCRINE AGENT (G) Thyroid Replacements (SG) **Cost:** Low
Thyroid Stimulating Hormone	See THYROTROPIN		
Thyroid Strong	See THYROID DESICCATED		Thyroid Replacement
Thyroid USP	See THYROID DESICCATED		Thyroid Replacement
Thyrolar	See LIOTRIX		Thyroid Replacement
THYROTROPIN Thytropar, TSH, Thyroid Stimulating Hormone	IM, SC: 10 IU for 1 to 3 days, give radioiodine study 24h after last dose.	**Injection:** (powder) 10 IU of thyrotropic activity/vial	ENDOCRINE AGENT (G) Thyroid Stimulating Hormone (G)
Thytropar	See THYROTROPIN		Thyroid Stimulating Hormone
Tiazac	See DILTIAZEM		Calcium Channel Blocker
Ticar	See TICARCILLIN		Lactam Antibiotic
TICARCILLIN Ticar	**Urinary Tract Infections (uncomplicated):** IM, IV: 1000 mg q6h. **Severe Infections:** IV: 200–300 mg/kg/d in 4–8 doses. Pediatric IV: 200–300 mg/kg/d in 4–6 doses.	**Injection:** (powder) 1, 3, 6, 20, 30 g	LACTAM ANTIBIOTICS (G) Extended Gram Negative Coverage (SG) No/Marginal Effectiveness In Meningitis or vs. P. aeruginosa (SSG) **Cost:** Medium
TICARCILLIN and **CLAVULANIC ACID** Timentin	**Systemic and Urinary Tract Infections:** IV: (>60 kg): 3.1 g (of ticar.) q4–6h, administer over 30 minutes. IV: (<60 kg): 200–300 mg/kg/d (of ticar.) given in divided doses every 4 to 6 hours. **Infections (gynecologic):** IV (moderate severity): 200 mg/kg/d in divided doses q 6 h by IV infusion. IV (severe): 300 mg/kg/d in divided doses q 4 h by IV infusion.	**Injection:** (powder) (contains 4.75 mEq sodium/g) 3g ticarcillin (as disodium) and 0.1 g clavulanic acid in 3.1 g vials **Solution:** 3g ticarcillin (as disodium) and 0.1 g clavulanic acid in 100 ml frozen vials	PENICILLIN AND A LACTAMASE INHIBITOR **Cost:** Medium
Tice Bacillus Calmette-Guerin	See BCG		Immunomodulator
Ticlid	See TICLOPIDINE		Antiplatelet Agent

GENERIC NAME Trade Name	INDICATIONS AND DOSAGES	DOSE FORMS	GROUP (G)/SUBGROUP (SG) Relative Cost within Group
TICLOPIDINE Ticlid	PO: 250 mg bid (with food).	**Tablet:** 250 mg	METABOLIC AGENTS (G) Anticoagulants And Coagulants (SG) Antiplatelet Agents (SSG)
Ticon	See TRIMETHOBENZAMIDE		Antinauseant
Tigan	See TRIMETHOBENZAMIDE		Antiemetic
Tilade	See NEDOCROMIL		Mast Cell Stabilizer
TILUDRONATE Skelid	**Paget's Disease:** PO: 400 mg/d for 90 days	**Tablet:** 200 mg	METABOLIC AGENTS (G) Calcium Kinetics Regulators (SG) Inhibit Osteoclastic Activity (SSG) **Cost:** Very expensive
Timentin	See TICARCILLIN and CLAVULANIC ACID		Penicillin Plus Lactamase Inhibitor
TIMOLIDE	**Hypertension:** PO: 1–2 tablets/d	**Tablet:** timolol (10 mg), hydrochlorothiazide (25 mg)	BETA BLOCKER AND DIURETIC COMBINATION (G)
TIMOLOL Blocadren, Timoptic	**Hypertension:** PO: 10 mg bid initially; 20–60 mg/d maintenance in 1–2 doses. **Post-MI:** PO: 10 mg bid. **Migraine:** Initial dose 10 mg bid, maintenance dose range 10–30 mg qd (give larger doses in divided doses). **Glaucoma:**	**Tablet:** 5, 10, 20 mg; **Ophthalmic Solution:** 0.25%, 0.5%	ANS Agents (G) Sympathoplegics (SG) Beta Adrenergic Blockers (SG) OPHTHALMIC PREPARATION (G) **Cost:** High
Timoptic	See TIMOLOL		Beta-Adrenergic Receptor Blockers
Tinactin	See TOLNAFTATE		Antifungal
Tindal	See ACETOPHENAZINE		Antipsychotic
TIOCONAZOLE OTC, Vagistat	**Vaginal Candidiasis:** Intravaginal: 1 applicatorful intravaginally at bedtime.	**Ointment:** 6.5% in single dose applicator.	ANTI-INFECTIOUS AGENTS (G) Topical Fungicides (SG) **Cost:** Medium
TIZANIDINE Zanaflex	**Relieve Spasticity:** PO: Initially 4 mg hs increasing to maximum of 36 mg/d in 3 doses	**Tablet:** 4 mg	CNS AGENTS (G) Muscle Relaxants (SG) **Cost:** Very expensive
TOBRAMYCIN Tobrex	**Serious Infections:** IM, IV: Initial dose 2 mg/kg q 8h and maintenance 1.7 mg/kg q 8h for 7–10 d. Pediatric: IV, IM: 6–7.5 mg/kg/d in 3–4 divided doses. Monitor levels. **Ointment:** Apply 1 cm 2–3 times/d. **Solution:** Instill 1–2 drops q4h (q30–60 min for severe infections). **Injection:** 10, 40 mg/kg	**Ointment:** 0.3% **Solution:** 0.3%	ANTI-INFECTIOUS AGENT (G) Aminoglycoside Antibiotic (SG) and Ophthalmologic Anti-Infective Prep (SG **Cost:** High
Tobrex	See TOBRAMYCIN		Antibacterial
TOCAINIDE Generic, Tonocard	**Ventricular Arrhythmias:** PO: 400 mg to start, maintenance 400–600 mg tid (max. dose 2400 mg/day).	**Tablet:** 400, 600 mg	CV AGENT (G) Antiarrhythmic Agents (SG) Group I Antiarrhythmic (SSG) **Cost:** High
Tofranil	See IMIPRAMINE		Antidepressant (TCA)

GENERIC NAME Trade Name	INDICATIONS AND DOSAGES	DOSE FORMS	GROUP (G)/SUBGROUP (SG) Relative Cost within Group
TOLAZAMIDE Generic, Tolinase	**Diabetes:** PO: Initial dose: 100 mg/d if fasting blood sugar <200 mg%; 250 mg/d if fasting blood sugar >200 mg% (max. dose 1000 mg/d). Give dose q12h if >500 mg/d.	**Tablet:** 100, 250, 500 mg	ENDOCRINE AGENTS (G) Oral Antidiabetic Agents (SG) Sulfonylurea (SSG) **Cost:** Low
TOLAZOLINE Priscoline	IV: 1–2 mg/kg over 10 min, then 1–2 mg/kg/h.	**Injection:** 25 mg/ml.	ANS AGENTS (G) Sympathoplegics (SG) Alpha Adrenergic Blockers (SSG) **Cost:** Very High
TOLBUTAMIDE Generic, Orinase, Oramide	**Diabetes:** PO: 0.25–2 g/d in 1–2 doses (max. dose 3 g/d).	**Tablet:** 250, 500 mg	ENDOCRINE AGENTS (G) Oral Antidiabetic Agents (SG) Sulfonylurea (SSG) **Cost:** Low
Tolinase	See TOLAZAMIDE		Oral Antidiabetic
TOLMETIN Generic, Tolectin	**Pain:** PO: 400 mg tid to start; maintenance 600–1800 mg/d in 3–4 doses. Pediatric PO: 20 mg/kg in 3 or 4 divided doses to start; maintenance 15–30 mg/kg/d.	**Tablet:** 200, 600 mg **Capsule:** 400 mg	ANTI-INFLAMMATORY AGENTS (G) Non-Narcotic Analgesics (G) Aspirin and Related (SG) **Cost:** Low
TOLNAFTATE Generic, OTC, Aftate, Tinactin, Tolnate	Topical: Apply bid for 2–3 weeks (may extend up to 4–6 weeks). (Use powders only as adjunctive therapy.)	**Cream:** 1% **Solution:** 1% **Gel:** 1% **Powder:** 1% **Spray Powder:** 1% **Spray Liquid:** 1%	DERMATOLOGIC AGENTS (G) Topical Fungicides (SG) **Cost:** Low if generic
Tonocard	See TOCAINIDE		Antiarrhythmic
Topicort	See DESOXIMETASONE		Anti-Inflammatory Steroid, Topical
TOPIRAMATE Topamax	**Partial Seizures (Adjunctive Use Only): PO:** Initially 50 mg/day increased to 200–400 mg/day.	**Tablets:** 25, 100, 200 mg	CNS Agents (G) Anticonvulsants (SG) Miscellaneous Anticonvulsants (SSG)
Topamax	See TOPIRAMATE		Anticonvulsant
Topotecan			Cancer Chemotherapy
Toprol	See METOPROLOL		Beta Adrenergic Blocker
Toradol	See KETOROLAC		Non-Narcotic Analgetic
Torecan	See THIETHYLPERAZINE		Phenothiazine Antinauseant
Tornalate	See BITOLTEROL		Beta Adrenergic Blocker
TORSEMIDE Demadex	**Congestive heart failure:** PO, IV: 10–20 mg qd. **Chronic Renal Failure:** PO, IV: 20 mg qd. **Hypertension:** PO: 5 mg qd; after 4–6 weeks increase to10 mg qd as needed.	**Tablet:** 5, 10, 20, 100 mg **Injection:** 10 mg/ml	RENAL AGENTS (G) Sodium Diuretics (G) Potent ("Loop") Diuretics (SG) **Cost:** High
Tracrium	See ATRACURIUM		Curariform
Tral	See HEXOCYCLIUM		Parasympatholytic (Anticholinergic)

GENERIC NAME Trade Name	INDICATIONS AND DOSAGES	DOSE FORMS	GROUP (G)/SUBGROUP (SG) Relative Cost within Group
TRAMADOL Ultram	Pain: 100 mg q6h as needed.	**Tablet:** 50 mg	CNS AGENTS (G) Narcotic Analgesics (SG) Of Lowest Potency (SSG) **Cost:** High
Trandate	See LABETALOL		Alpha *and* Beta Adrenergic Blocker
TRANDOLAPRIL Mavik	**Hypertension:** PO: Initially 1 or 2 mg once daily, then 2–4 mg qd.	**Tablet:** PO: 1, 2, 4 mg	CV AGENTS (G) Vasodilator (SG) ACE Inhibitor (SSG)
TRANEXAMIC ACID Cyklokapron	**Dental Procedures In Hemophiliacs:** IV: 10 mg/kg given immediately prior to procedure; after surgery, give 25 mg/kg PO tid or QID for 2 to 8 days. PO: (Alternate Regimen): give 25 mg/kg orally, tid or QID beginning 1 day prior to surgery. **Patients Unable To Take PO Medication:** IV: 10 mg/kg tid or QID.	**Tablet:** 500 mg **Injection:** 100 mg/ml	METABOLIC AGENTS (G) Anticoagulants And Coagulants (SG) Other Hemostatic Agents (SSG)
Trans-Retinoic Acid	See TRETINOIN		Keratolytic
Transderm-Nitro	See NITROGLYCERIN		Vasodilator
Trantoin	See NITROFURANTOIN		Antibacterial
Tranxene	See CLORAZEPATE		Sedative Hypnotic
TRANYLCYPROMINE Parnate	**Endogenous Depression:** PO: 10 mg bid to start; maintenance 10–30 mg/d (max. dose 60 mg/d).	**Tablet:** 10 mg	CNS AGENTS (G) Stimulant (SG) Monoamine Oxidase Inhibitors (SSG) **Cost:** Medium
Trasylol	See APROTININ		Hemostatic
TRAZODONE Generic, Desyrel	**Endogenous Depression:** PO: 150 mg/d to start in 2–4 doses; maintenance 150–400 mg/d (max. dose 600 mg/d).	**Tablet:** 50,100, 150, 300 mg	CNS AGENTS (G) Tricyclic Antidepressants (SG) **Cost:** Low
Trecator SC	See ETHIONAMIDE		Tuberculostatic
Tremin	See TRIHEXYPHENIDYL		Parasympatholytic
Trental	See PENTOXIFYLLINE		Xanthine Equivalent
TRETINOIN Retin A, Renova trans-Retinoic Acid	Apply 2–5 times/wk (Cover entire area).	**Cream:** 0.025%, 0.05%, 0.1% **Gel:** 0.025%, 0.01% **Liquid:** 0.05% **Capsules:** PO: 10 mg (As Vesanoid for Promyelocytic Leukemia)	DERMATOLOGIC AGENTS (G) Kerato-lytic-plastic Agents (SG) Acne and Psoriasis (SSG) **Cost:** Very High
Trexan	See NALTREXONE		Narcotic Antagonist
Tri-Sulfa	See TRIPLE SULFA		Antibacterial

GENERIC NAME Trade Name	INDICATIONS AND DOSAGES	DOSE FORMS	GROUP (G)/SUBGROUP (SG) Relative Cost within Group
TRIACETIN Fungoid, Ont-Clear Nail	**Fungal Infections Including Onychomycosis:** Topical (cream, solution): Apply tid for up to 4 weeks. If no improvement, review the diagnosis. Topical (Tincture): brush on to affected areas tid. Topical (Spray): spray onto affected nails for 1–2 seconds.	Available as liquid solution, in a nonaqueous vehicle and in a vanishing cream base.	DERMATOLOGIC AGENTS (G) Topical Fungicides (SG) **Cost:** Medium
TRIACETYLOLE-ANDOMYCIN Tao	**Streptococcal Infection:** PO: 250–500 mg QID for 10 days.	**Capsule:** 250 mg	ANTI-INFECTIOUS AGENTS (G) Macrolide Antibiotics (SG) **Cost:** High
TRIAMCINOLONE Generic, Aristocort, Kenacort, Trilone, Trilog	PO: 8–48 mg/d. Intraarticular (diacetate): 5–40 mg/injection. IV (diacetate): 40 mg/week (average). IV (acetonide): 2.5–60 mg/d. Intraarticular (hexacetonide): 2–20 mg/injection. Intraarticular (acetonide): 2.5–40 mg/injection.	**Tablet:** 1, 2, 4, 8 mg **Syrup:** 4 mg/5 ml **Diacetate (suspension):** 40 mg/ml **Hexacetonide (suspension):** 5, 20 mg/ml **Acetonide (suspension):** 3, 10, 40 mg/ml	ANTI-INFLAMMATORY AGENTS ETC (G) Anti-inflammatory Steroids (SG) **Cost:** Low
TRIAMCINOLONE ACETONIDE Generic, Aristocort, Kenalog	Apply to affected area 2 times a day.	**Ointment:** 0.5% **Cream:** 0.5% **Medium Potency:** **Ointment:** 0.025%, 0.1% **Cream:** 0.1% **Lotion:** 0.1% **Low Potency:** **Lotion:** 0.025% **Cream:** 0.025% **Aerosol:** (2 sec. spray)	DERMATOLOGIC AGENTS (G) Antiinflammatory Steroids (SG) **Cost:** Low
TRIAMTERENE Dyrenium, In Dyazide	**Edema:** PO: 100 mg bid to start; 100–300 mg qd or qod maintenance (max. dose 300 mg/d).	**Capsule:** 50, 100 mg	RENAL AGENTS (G) Potassium-Sparing Diuretics (SG) **Cost:** Medium
Triavil	See AMITRIPTYLINE		Antidepressant (TCA)
TRIAVIL 2–25 4–25 4–50	**Schizophrenia:** PO: 1 tablet bid and adjust		**Tablet:** Perphenazine combined with amitriptyline 2/25 mg, 4/25 mg and 4/50 mg
TRIAZOLAM Generic, Halcion	**Hypnotic:** PO: 0.125–0.5 mg hs. Geriatric PO: 0.125 mg hs initially; max. dose: 0.25 mg hs.	**Tablet:** 0.125, 0.25 mg	CNS AGENTS (G) Sedative-Hypnotics (SG) Ultrashort-Acting Hypnotics (SSG) **Cost:** Medium
Triban	See TRIMETHOBENZAMIDE		Antiemetic
TRICHLORMETHI-AZIDE Generic, Naqua, Diurese	**Hypertension, Edema:** PO: 2–4 mg qd	**Tablet:** 2, 4 mg	RENAL AGENTS (G) Thiazide Diuretics (sSG) **Cost:** Low

GENERIC NAME Trade Name	INDICATIONS AND DOSAGES	DOSE FORMS	GROUP (G)/SUBGROUP (SG) Relative Cost within Group
Tridesilon	See DESONIDE		Corticosteroid, Topical
Tridil	See NITROGLYCERIN		Vasodilator
TRIENTINE Syprine	**Wilson's Disease:** PO: 750–1250 mg/d in 2–4 doses (Max 2 g/d).	**Capsule:** 250 mg	ANTIDOTES AND USED IN POISONINGS (G)
TRIFLUOPERAZINE Generic, Stelazine	**Psychotic Disorders:** PO: initial 2–5 mg bid; maintenance 15–20 mg/d (max. dose 40 mg/d) IM: initial 1–2 mg q4–6h; maintenance <6 mg/d (max. 10 mg/d) in 4 or 6 divided doses.	**Tablet:** 1, 2, 5, 10 mg **Liquid:** 10 mg/ml **Injection:** 2 mg/ml	CNS AGENTS (G) Antipsychotics (SG) Prominent Extrapyramidal Effects (SSG) **Cost:** Low
TRIFLURIDINE Viroptic	**HSV 1&2 (IDU & VIRA-A resistant):** Solution: 1 drop q2h while awake (max. dose: 9 doses/d); rx until full reepitheliazation occurs, and other rx for additional 7 days with 1 drop q4h (max. dose: 5 doses/d).	**Solution:** 1.0%	OPHTHALMOLOGIC AGENTS (G) Anti-Viral Agents (SG) **Cost:** High
TRIHEXYPHENIDYL Generic, Artane	**Parkinsonism:** PO: 1–2 mg/d to start; increase 2 mg/d q3–5d; maintenance 6–10 mg/d in 3–4 doses. **Drug-Induced Extrapyramidal Disorders:** PO: 1 mg to start, then 5–15 mg/d.	**Tablet:** 2, 5 mg **Capsule:** (Ext'd release) 5 mg **Liquid:** 2 mg/5 ml	CNS AGENTS (G) Antiparkinson Agents (SG) Anticholinergics (SG) **Cost:** Medium
Triiodothyronine	See LIOTHYRONINE (T3)		Thyroid Hormone
Trilafon	See PERPHENAZINE		Tricyclic Antidepressant
Trilog	See TRIAMCINOLONE		Anti-inflammatory Steroid
Trilone	See TRIAMCINOLONE		Anti-inflammatory Steroid
Trimanual	See TRIMETHOPRIM		Antibacterial, Antimalarial
TRIMEPRAZINE Temaril	PO: 2.5 QID. PO: (Ext'd release) 5 mg bid.	**Tablet:** 2.5 mg **Spansules:** 5 mg **Syrup:** 2.5 mg/5 ml	CNS AGENTS (G) Antihistamines (H1) (G) With Prominent Sedation (SG) **Cost:** High
TRIMETHAPHAN Arfonad	**Production of Hypotension:** IV: start drip at a rate of 3 to 4 ml/min (3 to 4 mg/min) then individualize. Indications: Rapid control of hypertensive crises, hypotensive anesthesia.	**Injection:** 50 mg/ml	ANS AGENTS (G) Sympathoplegics (SG) Ganglionic Blockers (SSG) **Cost:** Very High
TRIMETHOBENZAMIDE Generic, Tigan	**Nausea, Vomiting:** PO: 250 mg q6–8h. Rectal: 200 mg q6–8h. IV: 200 mg q6–8h. Pediatric PO (30–90 lbs.): 100–200 mg q6–8h.	**Capsule:** 100, 250 mg **Suppositories:** 200 mg **Pediatric Suppositories:** 100 mg **Injection:** 100 mg/ml	GASTROINTESTINAL AGENTS (G) Antiemetics (Minor) (SG) **Cost:** High
TRIMETHOPRIM Generic, Trimpex, Proloprim, Metremia, Syraprim, Trimanual	**Urinary Tract Infections:** PO: 100 mg bid for 10 days; or 200 mg qd for 10 days. **Ophthalmic Infections:** solution: 1 drop q 3 h (max 6 doses/d) for 7–10 days	**Tablet:** 100, 200 mg **Solution:** 1 mg/ml	ANTI-INFECTIOUS AGENTS (G) Agents Related to Sulfonamides (SG) **Cost:** Medium

GENERIC NAME Trade Name	INDICATIONS AND DOSAGES	DOSE FORMS	GROUP (G)/SUBGROUP (SG) Relative Cost within Group
TRIMETHOPRIM and SULFAMETHOXAZOLE Bactrim, Septra, TMP/SMX, Co-trim, Sulfatrim, Bethaprim	**Bacterial Infections:** PO: one "DS" tab bid	**Tablet:** 80 mg TMP, 400 mg SMX (one unit). "DS" or double strength contain two units. Half strength also available. **Oral Suspension:** 40 mg TMP, 200 mg SMX/5 ml **Injection:** IV: 40 mg TMP, 200 mg SMX/5 ml or 160 TMP/800 SMX in 10 ml for dilution	ANTI-INFECTIOUS AGENTS (G) Agents Related to Sulfonamides (SG) Sulfonamide-Trimethoprim Mixture (SSG)
TRIMETREXATE Neutrexin	**P. carinii Pneumonia:** Injection: Must be given with leucovorin. Folate antagonist.	See labeling for dosage detail	ANTI-INFECTIOUS AGENTS (G) Parasiticides (SG)
TRIMIPRAMINE Generic, Surmontil	**Endogenous Depression:** PO: 75 mg/d to start in 2–4 doses; maintenance 50–150 mg/d (max. dose 200 mg/d). Geriatric/adolescent PO: 50 mg/d to start in 2–4 doses; maintenance 100 mg/d.	**Capsule:** 25, 50, 100 mg	CNS AGENTS (G) Tricyclic Antidepressants (SG) **Cost:** Medium
Trimox	See AMOXICILLIN		Lactam Antibiotic
Trimpex	See TRIMETHOPRIM		Antibacterial
Triostat	See LIOTHYRONINE (T3)		Thyroid Hormone
TRIOXSALEN Generic, Trisoralen	**Vitiligo:** PO (Adults and children >12 yrs): 10 mg daily, take dose 2 to 4 hours before UV exposure.	**Tablet:** 5 mg	MISCELLANEOUS DERMATOLOGIC AGENTS (G)
TRIPELENNAMINE Generic, PBZ	PO: 25–50 mg q4–6h (max. dose 600 mg/d). PO: (Sustained release) adults 100 mg qam and qpm (max. dose 100 mg q8h).	**Tablet:** 25, 50 mg **Tablet:** (ER) 100 mg **Elixir:** 25 mg/5 ml of base per 5 ml)	ANTI-INFLAMMATORY ETC AGENTS (G) Antihistamines (H1) (SG) Prominent Sedation (SSG) **COST:** Low
TRIPLE SULFAS	An obsolete but still official preparation available in vaginal dose forms. Not to be confused with Multiple Sulfas or Trisulfapyrimidines		
TRIPROLIDINE OTC, Generic, Actidil, Actifed	PO (>12 yrs): 2.5 mg q4–6h (do not exceed 4 doses per day). Pediatric (6–12 yrs) PO: 1.25 mg q4–6h (do not exceed 4 doses per day).	**Tablet:** 2.5 mg **Syrup:** 1.25 mg/5 ml	ANTI-INFLAMMATORY ETC AGENTS (G) Antihistamines (H1) (SG) Prominent Sedation (SSG) **Cost:** Medium
Trisoralen	See TRIOXSALEN		Repigment Vitiligo
TRISULFAPYRIMIDINES Generic, Tri-Sulfa	**Infections:** PO: 2–4 g initially then 2–4 g/d given in 3–6 divided doses.	**Tablet:** 167 mg each of sulfadiazine, sulfamerazine and sulfamethazine	ANTI-INFECTIOUS AGENTS (G) Sulfonamides (SG) **Cost:** Low

GENERIC NAME Trade Name	INDICATIONS AND DOSAGES	DOSE FORMS	GROUP (G)/SUBGROUP (SG) Relative Cost within Group
Trobicin	See SPECTINOMYCIN		Antibiotic Used for Gonorrhea
TROGLITAZONE Resulin	**Type II Insulin resistant diabetes:** PO: Initially 200 mg/d, then to 400–600 mg/d prn	Consult most recent labeling before using	ENDOCRINE AGENTS (G) Oral Antidiabetic Agents (SG) Cost; High
Tronothane	See PRAMOXINE		Local Anesthetic, Topical
TROPICAMIDE Generic, Mydriacyl	**Mydriasis:** Solution (0.5–1%): Instill 1–2 drops 15–20 minutes before procedure, repeat in 30 min PRN. **Cycloplegia:** Solution (1%): Instill 1–2 drops.	**Solution:** 0.5, 1%	OPHTHALMIC PREPARATIONS (G) Cycloplegic Mydriatics (SG) **Cost:** Low
TSH	See THYROTROPIN		Thyroid Stimulating Hormone
TUBOCURARINE Generic, Delacurarine	**Surgery:** IV: 40–60 units to start, then 20–30 units in 3–5 min PRN. Alternate dosage: 1.1 units/kg.	**Injection:** 3 mg/ml	GENERAL ANESTHETICS AND ADJUNCTS (G) Neuromuscular Blocking Agents (SG) Non-Depolarizing (Competitive) Agents (SSG) **Cost:** Medium
TUINAL 100,200 Mg	**Hypnosis:** PO: 1 capsule hs.		**Capsule:** amobarbital 50 or 100 mg combined with secobarbital 50 or 100 mg.
Tums	See CALCIUM CARBONATE		Antacid
Tylenol	See ACETAMINOPHEN		Non-Narcotic Analgetic
Tylox	See OXYCODONE		Oxycodone-APAP Mixture
Type A Botulinum Toxin	See Under Botulinum Toxin		
Tyzine	See TETRAHYDROZOLINE		Nasal and Ocular Decongestant
Ultane	See SEVOFLURANE		General Anesthetic
Ultiva	See REMIFENTANIL		Narcotic Analgesic
Ultracef	See CEFADROXIL		Lactam Antibiotic
Ultralente U	See EXTENDED INSULIN ZINC SUSPENSION		
Ultram	See TRAMADOL		Narcotic Analgetic, Unscheduled
UNASYN	**Infection:** IM, IV: 1.5–3.0 g q6h. (Note: give IM by deep injection; give IV by injection or infusion (over at least 10–15 min).	**Injection** (powder): 1 g ampicillin 0.5 g sulbactam sodium) **Injection:** (powder): 3.0 g (2 g ampicillin sodium, 1 g sulbactam sodium)	ANTI-INFECTIOUS AGENTS (G) Lactam Antibiotics (SG) Formulations Containing a Lactamase Inhibitor (SSG)
UNDECYLENIC ACID Generic, OTC, Desenex, Cruex, Pedi-Dri	Topical: ointment, liquid or cream apply bid (powders are adjunctive treatment only).	Available as powder, ointment, cream, liquid, foam and soap	DERMATOLOGIC AGENTS (G) Topical Fungicides (SG) **Cost:** Low
Unifiber	See METHYLCELLULOSE		Bulk Laxative
Unipen	See NAFCILLIN		Lactamase Resistant Penicillin

GENERIC NAME Trade Name	INDICATIONS AND DOSAGES	DOSE FORMS	GROUP (G)/SUBGROUP (SG) Relative Cost within Group
UREA Ureaphil	**Increased ICP, IOP:** IV: administer as a 30% solution SLOWLY, rate not to exceed 4 ml/minute (max. dose 120g/d). Adults: 1 to 1.5 g/kg.	**Injection:** 40 g/150 ml	RENAL AGENTS (G) Osmotic Diuretics (SG) **Cost:** High
Ureaphil	See UREA		(Hyper)Osmotic Agent
Urecholine	See BETHANECHOL		Cholinergic
Urex	See METHENAMINE		Urinary Antibacterial
Urobak	See SULFAMETHOXAZOLE		Antibacterial
UROFOLLI-TROPIN (FSH) Metrodin	**Induce Ovulation:** IM: 75 IU/d urofollitropin initially, give for 7–12 days; follow w/5,000–10,000 U of HCG, one day after the last urofollitropin dose (observe qod for signs of excess ovarian stimulation and/or enlargement—do NOT give HCG if ovaries unusually enlarged on last day of therapy). May repeat sequence twice with larger (double) urofollitropin dose if ovulation w/o pregnancy occurred.	**Injection:** (powder) 0.83 mg (75 IU FSH activity) per amp	ENDOCRINE AGENTS (G) Anterior Pituitary Hormones (SG)
UROKINASE Abbokinase	IV: 2000 units/lb, initial dose; then 2000 units/lb/hr.	**Injection** (powder): 5000 and 250,000 IU/vial.	Metabolic Agents (G) Anticoagulants And Coagulants (SG) Thrombolytic Agents (SSG) **Cost:** High
Uroqid	See METHENAMINE		Urinary "Antiseptic"
URSODIOL Actigall	**Dissolution of radiolucent gallstones:** PO: 8–10 mg/kg/day given in 2–3 divided doses.	**Capsule:** 300 mg	MISCELLANEOUS GI AGENTS (G) Gallstone Dissolving Agents (SG)
Uticort	See BETAMETHASONE BENZOATE		Anti-inflammatory Steroid
V-Cillin	See PENICILLIN V		Lactam Antibiotic
Vagistat	See TIOCONAZOLE		Vaginal Candidiasis
VALACYCLOVIR Valtrex	**Herpes Zoster (in immunocompromised adults):** PO: 1 g tid for 7 days.	**Caplets:** 500 mg	ANTI-INFECTIOUS AGENTS (G) Antiviral Agents,Systemic (SG)
Valergen	See ESTRADIOL VALERATE		Estrogen
Valisone	See BETAMETHASONE VALERATE		Anti-inflammatory Steroid
Valium	See DIAZEPAM		Sedative-Hypnotic
VALPROIC ACID Generic, Depakene, Divalproex, Depakote	**Seizure Disorders:** PO: 15 mg/kg/d to start, each week add 5–10 mg/kg/d; maintenance 30–60 mg/kg/d in 1–3 doses (if > 250 mg/d, give in divided doses).	**Manic Phase, Manic Depressive State:** **Tablet:** (Ext'd release) 125, 250, 500 mg **Capsule:** 250 mg **Capsule:** (sprinkle) 125 mg **Syrup:** 50 mg/ml	CNS AGENTS (G) Anticonvulsants (SG) **Cost:** High

GENERIC NAME Trade Name	INDICATIONS AND DOSAGES	DOSE FORMS	GROUP (G)/SUBGROUP (SG) Relative Cost within Group
Valtrex	See VALACYCLOVIR		Antiviral
Vanceril	See BECLOMETHASONE		Anti-inflammatory Steroids
Vancocin	See VANCOMYCIN		Antibiotic Resistant to Staph Lactamase
VANCOMYCIN Generic, Vancocin, Lyphocin	**Bacterial Infections:** PO, IV: 500 mg q6h or 1 g q12h. Pediatric PO, IV: 40 mg/kg/d in 3–4 divided doses (max dose 2 g/d). **Endocarditis Prophylaxis (Dental):** IV: 1 g SLOWLY (over 60 min) 1 hour prior to procedure. Pediatric IV: 20 mg/kg SLOWLY (over 60 min) 1 hour prior to procedure. **Endocarditis Prophylaxis (GI/GU procedures in penicillin allergic patient):** IV: 1 g SLOWLY (over 60 min) + 1 mg/kg gentamicin IV or IM (max. dose 80 mg) 1 hour prior to procedure; may repeat once after initial dose. Pediatric IV: 20 mg/kg SLOWLY (over 60 min) + 2 mg/kg gentamicin IV or IM 1 hour prior to procedure; may repeat once after initial dose.	**Injection:** (powder) 0.5, 1, 5, 10 g **Oral Solution:** (powder) 1, 10 g **Pulvules:** 125, 250 mg	ANTI-INFECTIOUS AGENTS (G) Lactam Antibiotics (SG) Penicillins Resistant to Staphylococcal Lactamase(SSG) **Cost:** High
Vantin	See CEFPODOXIME		Lactam Antibiotic
Vascor	See BEPRIDIL		Calcium Channel Blocker
VASERETIC 10–25	**Hypertension:** PO: 1–2 tablet qd.	**Tablet:** enalapril (10 mg) and hydrochlorothiazide (25 mg)	ACE INHIBITOR (G) AND SODIUM DIURETIC (G)
VASOCIDIN	**Ophthalmic Solution:** 2 qtt q 4 h. Increase the interval between doses as condition improves. **Ophthalmic Ointment:** Apply 0.25–0.5 inch ribbon tid or QID during the day and 1–2 times at night.		**Ophthalmic Solution:** sulfacetamide sodium (10%), prednisolone acetate (0.25%) **Ophthalmic Ointment:** sulfacetamide sodium (10%), prednisolone acetate (0.5%)
Vasodilan	See ISOXSUPRINE	Beta Adrenergic Agonist	
VASOPRESSIN (8-Arginine Vasopressin) Pitressin (synthetic)	**Diabetes Insipidus:** IM, SC: 5–10 units q8–12h PRN.	**Injection:** 20 pressor units/ml	ENDOCRINE AGENT (G) Antidiuretic Hormone (SG)
Vasoprin	See ISOXSUPRINE		Beta Adrenergic Agonist
Vasotec	See ENALAPRIL		ACE Inhibitor
Vasoxyl	See METHOXAMINE		Alpha Adrenergic Agonist
VECURONIUM Norcuron	**Surgery:** IV: 0.08–0.1 mg/kg to start, 0.01–0.015 mg/kg maintenance PRN (usually at 15–30 min).	**Injection:** (powder) 10 mg	GENERAL ANESTHETICS AND ADJUNCTS (G) Neuromuscular Blocking Agents (SG) Non-Depolarizing Agents (SSG) **Cost:** High
Velban	See VINBLASTINE		Cancer Chemotherapy

GENERIC NAME Trade Name	INDICATIONS AND DOSAGES	DOSE FORMS	GROUP (G)/SUBGROUP (SG) Relative Cost within Group
Velosef	See CEPHRADINE		Lactam Antibiotic
Velosulin Human	See INSULIN INJECTION		Regular Insulin
Veltane	See BROMPHENIRAMINE		Antihistamine
VENLAFAXINE Effexor	PO: 75 mg/d in 2–3 divided doses; increase PRN by 75 mg q4d (max. dose 375 mg/day).	**Tablet:** 25, 37.5, 50, 75, 100 mg	CNS AGENTS (G) Sympathomimetic Stimulants (SG) Other Unscheduled (SSG) **Cost:** High
Ventolin	See ALBUTEROL		Sympathomimetic, Beta 2 Selective
VePesid	See ETOPOSIDE		Cancer Chemotherapy
Veracillin	See DICLOXACILLIN		Lactamase Resistant Penicillin
VERAPAMIL Generic, Calan, Isoptin, Verelan	**Angina:** **Hypertension:** **Supraventricular Tachycardia:** **Atrial Fibrillation (digitalized patients):** See discussion, Part 1	**Tablet:** 40, 80, 120 mg **Tablet:** (Ext'd release) 120, 180, 240 mg **Capsule:** (Ext'd release) 120, 180, 240 mg **Injection:** 5 mg/ 2 ml	CV AGENTS (G) Vasodilators (G) Calcium Channel Blockers (SG) **Cost:** Low
Vercyte	See PIPOBROMAN		
Verelan	See VERAPAMIL		Calcium Channel Blocker
Vermox	See MEBENDAZOLE		Parasiticide
Versed	See MIDAZOLAM		Sedative-Hypnotic
Vesanoid	See TRETINOIN		CANCER CHEMOTHERAPY
Vesicholine	See BETHANECHOL		Cholinergic
Vibramycin	See DOXYCYCLINE		Tetracycline Antibiotic
Vicks Inhaler (Nasal)	See L-DESOXYEPHEDRINE (Inhaler)		Sympathomimetic
Vicodin	See HYDROCODONE		Narcotic
VIDARABINE Vira-A	**Herpes Simplex (conjunctival and corneal infections):** Ointment: ½ inch ribbon q3h (max. dose: 5 doses/day). (Discontinue if no improvement in 7 days or if not reepithelialized in 21 days. Continue bid rx for 7 days after full resolution.)	**Ointment:** 3%	OPHTHALMIC AGENTS (G) Anti-Viral Agents (SG) **Cost:** High
Videx	See DIDANOSINE		Antiviral
VINBLASTINE Generic Velban	CANCER CHEMOTHERAPY (G) Mitotic Spindle Inhibitors (SG) Promote Tubulin Depolymerization (SSG)		
VINCRISTINE Generic Oncovin	CANCER CHEMOTHERAPY (G) Mitotic Spindle Inhibitors (SG) Promote Tubulin Depolymerization (SSG)		

GENERIC NAME Trade Name	INDICATIONS AND DOSAGES	DOSE FORMS	GROUP (G)/SUBGROUP (SG) Relative Cost within Group
VINORELBINE Navelbine	CANCER CHEMOTHERAPY (G) Mitotic Spindle Inhibitors (SG) Promote Tubulin Depolymerization (SSG)		
Vira-A	See VIDARABINE		Antiviral
Virazole	See RIBAVIRIN		Antiviral
Virilon	See METHYLTESTOSTERONE		Androgen/Anabolic
Viroptic	See TRIFLURIDINE		Antiviral
Visken	See PINDOLOL		Non-Selective, Beta 1 and 2 Blocker
Vistaril	See HYDROXYZINE		Antihistamine, Antipsychotic
Vitamin A Acid	See TRETINOIN		Keratolytic
Vitamin D3	See CALCITRIOL		Active form of D Vitamin
Vitamin K1	See PHYTONADIONE(K1)		Coagulant
Vitamin B12	See CYANOCOBALAMIN		
Vivactil	See PROTRIPTYLINE		Tricyclic Antidepressant
Voltaren	See DICLOFENAC		Non-Narcotic Analgesics
Voxsuprine	See ISOXSUPRINE		Beta Adrenergic Agonist
Vumon	See TENIPOSIDE		
WARFARIN SODIUM Generic, Coumadin, Panwarfin, Sofarin	**Anticoagulation:** PO: 10 mg/d for 2 to 4 days initially, maintenance dose usually 2–10 mg/d (adjust dosage to PT or INR determinations).	**Tablet:** 1, 2, 2.5, 5, 7.5, 10 mg	METABOLIC AGENTS (G) Anticoagulants And Coagulants (SG) Inhibitors of Prothrombin Synthesis (SSG) **Cost:** Low
Wellbutrin	See BUPROPION		Sympathomimetic Stimulant
Wigraine	See ERGOTAMINE		Vasoconstrictor
WinRho SD	See RHo(D) IMMUNE GLOBULIN (HUMAN)		Rh Antibody
Winstrol	See STANOZOLOL		Androgen/Anabolic
Wycillin	See PENICILLIN G PROCAINE		Lactam Antibiotic
Wymox	See AMOXICILLIN		Lactam Antibiotic
Wytensin	See GUANABENZ		Centrally Acting Sympathoplegic
Xalatan	See Latanoprost		IOP Lowering Prostagland
Xanax	See ALPRAZOLAM		Sedative Hypnotics
Xerac B.P.	See BENZOYL PEROXIDE		Keratolytic
Xylocaine	See LIDOCAINE		Local Anesthetic
XYLOMETAZOLINE OTC, Otrivin	**Nasal Decongestion:** Adults (>6 yrs): 2–3 drops or sprays (0.1%) in each nostril q8–10h. Pediatric (2 to 6 yrs): 2–3 drops (0.05%) in each nostril q8–10h.	**Solution:** 0.05%, 0.1%	ANS AGENTS (G) Sympathomimetics, Incomplete (SG) **Cost:** Medium
Yocon	See YOHIMBINE		Vasodilator
Yodoxin	See IODOQUINOL		Parasiticide

GENERIC NAME Trade Name	INDICATIONS AND DOSAGES	DOSE FORMS	GROUP (G)/SUBGROUP (SG) Relative Cost within Group
YOHIMBINE Generic, Yohimex, Prohim, Yovital, Actibine, Yocon	**Erectile Impotence (unlabeled use):** PO: ½ to 1 tablet tid.	**Tablet:** 5.4 mg	ANS AGENTS (G) Sympathoplegics (SG) Alpha Adrenergic Receptor Blockers (SSG) **Cost:** Medium
Yohimex	See YOHIMBINE		Vasodilator
Yovital	See YOHIMBINE		Vasodilator
Yutopar	See RITODRINE		Beta Adrenergic Agonist
ZAFIRLUKAST Accolate	**Chronic Asthma:** PO: 20 mg bid 1 hr before or 2 hrs after meals	**Tablet:** 20 mg	ANTI-INFLAMMATORY, ETC (G) Leukotriene Antagonist (SG) **Cost:** Expensive
ZALCITABINE Hivid, ddC	**HIV Infection:** PO: 0.75 mg q8h (given in combination with 200 mg zidovudine q8h).	**Tablet:** 0.375, 0.75 mg	ANTI-INFECTIOUS AGENTS (G) Antiviral Agents (G) **Cost:** Medium
Zanosar	See STREPTOZOCIN		
Zantac	See RANITIDINE		H2 Antagonist
Zarontin	See ETHOSUXIMIDE		Anticonvulsant (Petit Mal)
Zaroxolyn	See METOLAZONE		Sodium Diuretic
Zebeta	See BISOPROLOL		Beta Adrenergic Blocker
Zefazone	See CEFMETAZOLE		Lactam Antibiotic
Zemuron	See ROCURONIUM		Curariform
Zerit	See STAVUDINE		Antiviral
ZESTORETIC	**Hypertension:** Adjust dose within limits imposed by the fixed proportions	**Tablet:** Contain lisinopril and hydrochlorothiazide in proportions of 10 mg/12.5 mg, 20 mg/12.5 mg,20 mg/25 mg	ACE INHIBITOR (G) AND SODIUM DIURETIC (G)
Zestril	See LISINOPRIL		
ZIAC	**Hypertension:** Adjust dose within the limits imposed by the fixed proportions	**Tablet:** Contain bisoprolol and hydrochlorothiazide in proportions of 2.5 mg/6.25 mg, 5.0 mg/ 6.25, 10.0 mg/6.25	BETA BLOCKER (G) AND SODIUM DIURETIC (G)
ZIDOVUDINE AZT, Retrovir, Azidothymidine	**Symptomatic HIV Infection:** PO: 200 mg q4h to start, after 1 month may reduce dose to 100 mg q4h. **Asymptomatic HIV Infection:** PO: 100 mg q4 h (while awake; 500 mg/d) **HIV Parenteral Treatment:** IV: 1–2 mg/kg (infused over 1 hour) q4h.	**Capsule:** 100 mg **Injection:** 10 mg/ml **Syrup:** 50 mg/ ml	ANTIINFLAMMATORY AGENTS (G) Antiviral Agents (G) **Cost:** Medium (PO), High (IV)

GENERIC NAME Trade Name	INDICATIONS AND DOSAGES	DOSE FORMS	GROUP (G)/SUBGROUP (SG) Relative Cost within Group
ZILEUTON Zyflo	**Chronic Asthma:** PO: 600 mg QID	**Tablet:** 600 mg	RESPIRATORY AGENTS (G) Antiallergic Agents, Non-Steroidal (SG) Lipoxygenase Inhibitor (SSG) **Cost:** Moderate
Zinacef	See CEFUROXIME		Lactam Antibiotic
Zinecard	See DEXRAZOXANE		Cardioprotective
Zithromax	See AZITHROMYCIN		Macrolide Antibiotic
Zocor	See SIMVASTATIN		HMG-CoA Reductase Inhibitors
Zofran	See ONDANSETRON		Antiemetic
Zoladex	See GOSERELIN		Blocks Release of LH-RF
Zolicef	See CEFAZOLIN		Lactam Antibiotic
Zoloft	See SERTRALINE		Sympathomimetic Stimulant
ZOLPIDEM Ambien	**Sedation:** PO: 10 mg hs (Max. dose: 10 mg; note: in elderly or debilitated, initial dose = 5 mg)	**Tablet:** 5, 10 mg	CNS AGENTS (G) Sedative-Hypnotics (SG) Ultrashort-Acting Hypnotics (SSG) **Cost:** High
Zolyse	See CHYMOTRYPSIN		Lyse Zonular Fibers
Zosyn	See PIPERACILLIN and TAZOBACTAM		Penicillin plus inhibitor of lactamase
Zovirax	See ACYCLOVIR		Antiviral Agent
Zypan	See BUPROPION		Sympathomimetic Stimulant
Zyflo	See ZILEUTON		Lipoxygenase Inhibitor (Asthma)
Zyloprim	See ALLOPURINOL		Inhibit Uric Acid Synthesis
Zyprexa	See OLANZAPINE		Atypical Antipsychotic

PART III

COMBINATIONS OF PRESCRIPTION DRUGS

This section is concerned with identifying medications in which one tablet or capsule or spoonful or other dosage unit combines two or more agents with a fixed proportion between the components. Part II has identified and provided trade names for many combinations, including those discussed below as examples of combinations that should not be used.

JUSTIFIABLE COMBINATIONS

There are many situations in which multiple drugs must be given to reach the therapeutic goal. In tuberculosis, AIDS, *Helicobacter* infections and septicemias, for examples, the use of multiple agents is obligatory. In hypertension, congestive heart failure or manifest coronary artery disease, combinations of drugs are invariable. In these combined therapies, the drugs are ordered separately, and the dosage and time of administration of the several drugs can be varied independently.

In some situations, it may be pharmacologically rational and convenient to patient and prescriber to combine the required drugs. Examples would include formulations of a penicillin with a lactamase inhibitor (Augmentin), combinations of trimethoprim and sulfamethoxazole (generic, Septra, Bactrim) and the oral contraceptives.

IRRATIONAL OR MARKET MOTIVATED COMBINATIONS

Examples of combinations that do not allow for the individualization of dosage would include: The combinations (in treating hypertension) of a vasodilator and a diuretic (Aldoclor, Capozide, Corzide, Ziac) and others. The use (in anesthesia) of Innovar, combining a very short acting narcotic and a very long acting neuroleptic or antipsychotic. Combining an antipsychotic and a tricyclic antidepressant under the mistaken assumption that one would lessen side effects of the other (Etrafon, Triavil).

However, the objection of the professional is also the increased cost. As with all products, the brand or proprietary name can be trademarked or copyrighted and used by only one purveyor indefinitely. Thus, even after a patent has expired, a product can be protected from price competition if a successful promotional effort can maintain the name recognition and "product loyalty." However, prescription drugs are still regulated commodities and rarely vary in quality or quantity from their labeled content, that is, generic prescribing is now an established idea.

CODEINE AND OTHER NARCOTICS IN SCHEDULE 2 OR 3 MIXTURES

Codeine, hydrocodone and dihydrocodeine prescribed as such are in Schedule 2 and subject to regulations (triplicate forms) that some physicians find onerous. If codeine is prescribed in limited doses in combination with other active ingredients, the preparations fall within Schedule 3 (See Appendix B). Indeed, if the amounts of narcotic are small enough, as in cough syrups, they are "exempt" from federal if not state regulations.

The usual **codeine** tabs contain 15, 30 or 60 mg (#2, #3 or #4) combined with 300 mg of aspirin or 325 of acetaminophen (APAP). Elixirs and suspensions (12 mg/5 ml) are available. There are countless generic providers, but many trade names continue in used. Tylenol (APAP) and Empirin (ASA) with codeine are still heavily promoted and familiar, but, fortunately, the pharmacist will now substitute a generic. Fioricet, Phenaphen and Fiorinal cause problems, because they also contain a barbiturate of which the prescriber is often unaware.

Hydrocodone is equivalent to codeine 60 mg if it is given in the usual 5 mg dose. That dose in combination with 500 mg of APAP or 500 mg of ASA is available as a generic or as Anexsia 5/500, Lorcet 5/500, Vicodin, Lortab ASA and at least eighteen other names. Preparations containing 7.5 mg are generic, Lortab 7.5/500, Lorcet Plus, and Vicodin ES (for *E*xtra *S*trength). A 10/650 combination is also available. In the higher doses hydrocodone is held to be more habituating than codeine.

Dihydrocodeine (16 mg combined with ASA as a generic or as Synalgos-DC or DHC Plus) is less potent and used a an antitussive rather than an analgetic.

Oxycodone is a narcotic of medium potency included in Part II. In the distant past, it was regulated like codeine and the combinations used then for convenience in prescribing still persist even though all are now Schedule II. Available as generics, Percocet (APAP), Roxicet, Tylox, Percodan (ASA) and others.

USED FOR UPPER RESPIRATORY COMPLAINTS

The combinations summarized in this section are not technically intriguing, and they are available (except for the narcotic cough medicines noted below) OTC as well as by prescription. Moreover, there are many purveyors marketing every possible combination, dosage and dosage forms of the several standard components and the resulting collection of data and names is too large to provide you in any affordable format. Some mixtures are heavily advertised and relatively expensive. However, next to each such product on the shelf in the pharmacy are "house brands" at a lower price.

COLD REMEDIES

Compared to nasal drops, sprays and inhalers, these mixtures in most situations are simply expensive sources of aspirin, acetaminophen or ibuprofen. The antihistamines and sympathomimetics may dry secretions, but have no effect on the duration of the URI and often cause lassitude or tremulousness depending on the dose, preparation and individual. Examples are taken from a compilation of over 700 names

Decongestant-Analgesic

(Dristan, Coldrine, Ornex, Dimetapp Sinus, Sinutab).

Decongestant-Antihistamine

(Actifed, Isoclor, Isoclor Liquid, Contac, Ornade Spansules, Codimal LA, Actifed, Relief, Dimetapp Extentabs, Tavist-D).

Antihistamine-Analgesic

Coricidin, Percogesic

Decongestant-Antihistamine-Analgesic

Actifed Plus, Alka-Seltzer Plus, Coricidin D, Congestant D, Dimetapp Cold and Flu, Gendecon.

Decongestant-Antihistamine-Anti-Cholinergic

Rhinolar, Extendryl Jr, Atrohist

ANTITUSSIVES

Non-Narcotic Mixtures

All contain dextromethorphan plus one to three of a decongestant, antihistamine and analgesic.

Drixoral, Dristan, Triaminic Sore Throat Formula, Cardec DM drops, Ornex Dimetane DX, Carbinoxamine Compound Syrup or Drops, Comtrex, Tylenol Cold and Flu Powder, Triaminic DM, Promethazine-DM (liquid, syrup), Robitussin Pedi Cough and Cold, Vicks Pedi, Formula 44D, Cheracol Plus, Dimetapp DM, Promethazine DM.

Schedule 5 Narcotic ("exempt") Combinations

Require prescriptions in most jurisdictions. Contain codeine 10mg/dose unit plus an antihistamine.
Promethazine (Phenergan) with codeine, tab and liquid, bromodiphenhydramine w/Codeine.
Codeine plus an antihistamine and a decongestant Novahistine DH, Dimetane DC.
Note that plain codeine is available in many dose forms.

Mixtures Containing Schedule 3 Narcotics

These preparations contain full doses of codeine (COD) or hydrocodone (HCD) with a decongestant (D), antihistamine (A) or the nominal expectorant guaifenesin (G).
Codamine Ped Syrup HCD 2.5 mg, D
Codamine, Detussin HCD 5.0 mg, D

Nucofed, COD 20 mg, D
Tussionex Pennkinetic HCD 10 mg, A Endagen-HD, Chlorgest, Codimal HCD 1.7 mg, A
Nucotuss Expectorant Syrup COD 20 mg, D, G
1.7 mg Triaminic Expectorant DH HCD 1.7 mg, D, A, G
ETC

EXPECTORANT COMBINATIONS

If guaifenesin is added to any of the above mixtures of an antihistamine, a decongestant and/or dextromethorphan, it becomes in the judgment of its purveyor an expectorant. For example, Cheracol D cough liquid, Benylin expectorant, Novahistine DMX, ETC.

The decongestant in all of the above is most often pseudoephedrine or phenylpropanolamine. The antihistamine is most often chlorpheniramine but also promethazine, doxylamine, diphenhydramine, triprolidine or carbinoxamine. Guaifenesin is a soothing, mucilaginous substance of questioned efficacy. Effect of DM on cough is comparable to a small dose of codeine.

APPENDIX A
ABBREVIATIONS

ac	before meals	mg	milligrams
ACE	Angiotensin converting enzyme	MI	myocardial infarct
AChE	acetylcholine esterase	microg	microgram
APL	acute promeylocytic leukemia	ml	milliliters
bid	two times per day	mM	millimolar
caps	capsules	N/A	not available
CHF	congestive heart failure	ng	nanogram
CMV	cytomegalovirus	NIDDM	non-insulin dependent diabetes
d	day(s)	pc	after meals
d/c	discontinue	PG	prostaglandin
dl, dL	deciliter (= 100 ml)	PO	oral administration
DVT	deep vein thrombosis	PR	rectal administration
ER	emergency room	PRN	as needed
g	grams	pt	patients
h, hr	hour(s)	q	every
HCT	hematocrit	qd, qD	every day (once a day)
HCTZ	hydrochlorothiazide	qid	four times per day
hs	at bedtime	qod	every other day
ICP	intracranial pressure	s/sx	signs and symptoms
ID	intradermal administration	SC	subcutaneous administration
IDDM	insulin-dependent diabetes mellitus	sec	second
IM	intramuscular administration	SL	sublingual
IOP	intraocular pressure	sln	solution
IPPB	intermittent positive pressure breathing	tab's	tablets
IU	international units	TCA	tricyclic antidepressant
IV	intravenous administration	tid	three times per day
LFTs	liver function tests	TMP-SMX	trimethoprim-sulfamethoxazole
l, L	liter (= 1,000 ml)	TPN	total parenteral nutrition
MAO	monoamine oxidase	Tblsp	tablespoon (= 15 mL)
m	million	tsp	teaspoon (= 5 mL)
max	maximum	U	units
mcg	microgram	UTI	urinary infection
mEq	milliequivalents		

APPENDIX B
SCHEDULES OF CONTROLLED DRUGS

The Federal Drug Enforcement Administration (DEA) regulates the manufacture, distribution and prescribing of drugs that have a potential for abuse. Physicians are required to attach the required federal registration number to prescriptions for "controlled substances."

SCHEDULE I: No therapeutic applications. High potential for abuse. Use in research only. Requires separate DEA number.
NARCOTICS: Heroin and numerous synthetic narcotics.
HALLUCINOGENS: LSD, MDA, MDMA (ecstasy), STP, DMT, DET, mescaline, peyote, bufotenine, ibogaine, psilocybin.
DEPRESSANTS: Methaqualone, phencyclidine (PCP), all Cannabis products except THC.

SCHEDULE II: No refills, no telephoned prescriptions. Office supplies must be ordered on special federal order form. Many states add requirement of special prescription form.
NARCOTICS: Opium tincture and total alkaloids. Phenanthrene alkaloids and equivalent synthetics: Morphine, codeine except as in schedule 3, hydromorphone (Dilaudid), oxymorphone (Numorphan), oxycodone (Roxicodone) including mixtures (Percodan, Percocet), meperidine (Demerol), methadone, levorphanol (Levo-Dromoran), fentanyl, sufentanyl, alfentanil, remifentanyl (Ultiva), levomethadyl (Orlaam).
STIMULANTS: Cocaine and coca leaves, amphetamine, dextroamphetamine, methamphetamine, phenmetrazine (Preludin), methylphenidate (Ritalin).
DEPRESSANTS: Amobarbital, pentobarbital, secobarbital, mixtures of above (e.g., Tuinal), glutethimide, dronabinol (Marinol, THC).

SCHEDULE III: Prescription (phoned or written) must be reordered after six months or 5 refills.

NARCOTICS: If mixed with other active medicinal and within dose limits: codeine, hydrocodeine, 90 mg per tablet or 5 ml; hydrocodone (Hycodan), 15 mg/tablet or 5 ml Paregoric (camphorated tincture of opium). Additional restrictions in some states.

DEPRESSANTS: Schedule II barbiturates in mixtures or in suppository dose form, butabarbital (Butisol), methyprylon (Noludar).

STIMULANTS: Benzphetamine (Didrex), chlorphentermine (Pre-Sate), diethylpropion (Tenuate), mazindol (Sanorex), phendimetrazine.

ANABOLIC STEROIDS: Testosterone and analogues.

SCHEDULE IV: Differs from Schedule III only in penalties for illegal possession.

NARCOTICS: Propoxyphene, diphenoxin (Motofen).

MIXED AGONIST-ANTAGONIST: Pentazocine (Talwin).

STIMULANTS: Phentermine, fenfluramine (Pondimin).

DEPRESSANTS: Chlordiazepoxide (Librium), clonazepam (Klonopin), clorazepate (Tranxene), diazepam (Valium), estazolam (Pro Som), flurazepam (Dalmane), lorazepam (Ativan), midazolam (Versed), oxazepam (Serax), prazepam (Verstran), guazepam (Doral), temazepam (Restoril), triazolam (Halcion), zolpidem (Ambiem), chloral hydrate, ethchlorvynol (Placidyl), meprobamate, mephobarbital (Mebaral), paraldehyde, phenobarbital.

SCHEDULE V: Could be dispensed without prescription except for added state regulations.

NARCOTICS: Diphenoxylate if no more than 25 mg combined with at least 0.025 mg atropine per dose unit (generic and Lomotil). Codeine, dihydrocodeine if limited to 10 mg per 5 ml (of cough syrup). Buprenorphine (Buprenex, a partial agonists).

UNSCHEDULED:

NARCOTIC ANTAGONISTS: All

NARCOTIC: Tramdol (Ultram), Loperamide (Imodium).

MIXED AGONIST-ANTAGONIST: Butorphanol (Stadol), dezocine (Dalgan), nalbuphine (Nubain).